Working With Troubled Men

A Contemporary Practitioner's Guide

Working With Troubled Men

A Contemporary Practitioner's Guide

Morley D. Glicken
California State University, San Bernardino
and
Institute for Personal Growth, Los Angeles, CA

2005

LAWRENCE ERLBAUM ASSOCIATES, PUBLISHERS
Mahwah, New Jersey   London

MT

Lawrence Erlbaum Associates, Inc., Publishers
10 Industrial Avenue
Mahwah, New Jersey 07430
www.erlbaum.com

Cover design by Kathryn Houghtaling Lacey

Library of Congress Cataloging-in-Publication Data

Glicken, Morley D.
   Working with troubled men : a contemporary practitioner's guide /
   Morley D. Glicken.
         p. cm.
      Includes bibliographical references and index.
   ISBN 0-8058-5009-0 (cloth : alk. paper)
   ISBN 0-8058-5010-4 (pbk. : alk. paper)
   1. Men—Counseling of. 2. Men—Mental health. 3. Therapeutic alliance.
      4. Psychotherapy.   I. Title.
   RC451.M45G565   2005
   616.89'14'081—dc22   2004060657
                                                               CIP

Books published by Lawrence Erlbaum Associates are printed on acid-free
paper, and their bindings are chosen for strength and durability.

Printed in the United States of America
10 9 8 7 6 5 4 3 2 1

6/12/06

I dedicate this book to my father, *Sam Glicken*, a man who
represented so much that is truly good about traditional men.
My father never forgot his humble origins in Russia or the absolute wonder
of being an American. He was a man who had passionate beliefs about
social justice and fought hard for working men and women, believing that
being given a second chance at life by coming
to America obligated him to help others.
Like many sons, I didn't always recognize my father's
many positive qualities or honor him in the way I would today.
I do know that I miss him more each day.

Contents

About the Author   ix

Preface   xi

Acknowledgments   xv

PART I   The Serious Problems Experienced by Men

Chapter 1   The Troubled Lives of Men   3

Chapter 2   Male Development: Some Divergent Points of View   16

Chapter 3   Working With Men to Ensure Good Physical Health   33

Chapter 4   Male Bashing   52

PART II   Clinical Work with Men

Chapter 5   A Gender-Specific Approach to Diagnosing Male   67
              Clients

Chapter 6   Forming Therapeutic Relationships With Male Clients   78

Chapter 7   A Male Model of Therapy   99

Chapter 8   Storytelling, Personal Coaching, Humor, Role Plays, 127
              Men's Groups, and Other Useful Approaches for
              Treating Men

Chapter 9   Self-Help Groups With Men   146

Part III   Clinical Work With Violent Men

Chapter 10   Clinical Work With Violent Male Youths   161

Chapter 11   Clinical Work With Physically and Sexually Abusive   178
             Men

Chapter 12   Treating Male Sexual Harassment and Workplace   201
             Violence

Part IV   Clinical Work with Men of Color: Special Concerns

Chapter 13   Clinical Work With African American Men   229

Chapter 14   Clinical Work With Traditional and Newly   245
             Immigrated Latino Men (With Mina Garza)

Chapter 15   Clinical Work With Asian Men (With Steven Ino)   260

Part V   Aging and Substance Abuse

Chapter 16   Clinical Work With Male Substance Abusers   275

Chapter 17   Working With Older Adult Male Clients   296

Part VI   The Future: Improving the Lives of Men

Chapter 18   Changing the Way We Respond to Men   315

Chapter 19   Female Therapists and Academics Respond   330

References   347

Author Index   385

Subject Index   395

About the Author

Dr. Morley D. Glicken is the former Dean of the Worden School of Social Service in San Antonio; the founding director of the Master of Social Work Department at California State University, San Bernardino; the past Director of the Master of Social Work Program at the University of Alabama; and the former Executive Director of Jewish Family Service of Greater Tucson. He has also held faculty positions in social work at the University of Kansas and Arizona State University. Dr. Glicken received his BA degree in social work with a minor in psychology from the University of North Dakota and holds an MSW degree from the University of Washington and the MPA and DSW degrees from the University of Utah. He is a member of Phi Kappa Phi Honorary Fraternity.

Dr. Glicken published two books for Allyn and Bacon/Longman Publishers in 2002: *The role of the Helping Professions in the Treatment of Victims and Perpetrators of Crime* (with Dale Sechrest), and *A Simple Guide to Social Research*; and two additional books for Allyn and Bacon/Longman in 2003: *Violent Young Children*, and *Understanding and Using the Strengths Perspective*. He published *Improving the Effectiveness of Helping Professions: An Evidence-Based Approach to Practice* in 2004 for Sage Publications and is completing *Learning From Resilient People*, and *An Introduction to Social Work, Social Welfare Organizations, and Social Work*, both to be published by Sage in 2005.

Dr. Glicken has published over 50 articles in professional journals and has written extensively on personnel issues for Dow Jones, publisher of the *Wall Street Journal*. He has held clinical social work licenses in Alabama and

Kansas, and is a member of the Academy of Certified Social Workers. He is currently Professor Emeritus in Social Work at California State University, San Bernardino, and Director of the Institute for Positive Growth: A Research, Treatment and Training Institute in Los Angeles, California. The Institute's Web site may be found at: http:// www.morleyglicken.com and Dr. Glicken can be reached online at mglicken@msn.com.

Preface

By any reasonable measure, many men are doing badly these days. Almost half of America's male children grow up in single-parent homes headed by mothers where they seldom have male mentors or role models. Fewer men attend college, and when they do, increasing levels of binge drinking and date rape on American campuses paint a discouraging picture of male behavior. Male violence continues to be a serious problem with young male violence having reached epidemic proportions. Writing about male homelessness and unemployment, Marin (1991) says that 80% of the homeless in America are men. Serious health problems continue to plague men and seem to be worsening.

One would think that men and their problems would be a part of the national agenda, but that seems far from true. This disconnect between the needs of men and effective male-specific help is apparent in the helping professions where men are often the unwanted clients, seen involuntarily by clinicians, who often believe that men are unmotivated to change and resist therapy. As a result, very little has been written about men, their current problems, or what the helping professions can do to develop more effective solutions to male problems.

Working With Troubled Men: A Contemporary Practitioner's Guide is a book for helping professionals who work with men. It contains an overview of the problems men have at home, in relationships, with their children, at work, with anger, with education, with violence, with substance abuse, and, ultimately, with being fulfilled and productive human beings. The emphasis of the book is on why men are having such serious problems and how male-specific treatment approaches and social programs can assist them. The volume is intended as a sympathetic and positive effort to help professionals assist the many men who want to change their lives, and to help researchers and students better understand those men.

When a man writes a book on men, there is always a chance that a personal agenda takes over and that the book lacks objectivity. Because this is a book for helping professionals, many of whom are women, I'm including a chapter at the end of the book in which women clinicians and academics provide critical feedback.

Men are upset these days about male bashing and unfair treatment in the workplace. Necessarily, this causes a certain tone of antagonism that needs to be shared if the book is to have an impact. The male clients we see who are referred for partner and child abuse, workplace violence, substance abuse, and sexual harassment, are angry about their involuntary treatment. They believe women are able to act in abusive ways, at will, and never get punished. Whether this is true, it's important that we hear their side of the story and prepare ourselves for the reluctant, angry, and often unmotivated male clients we will increasingly see in treatment as the justice system looks to the helping professions for alternatives to expensive, nonproductive, and often harmful jail time.

I learned about male roles from the tough immigrant men I knew growing up. They were traditional men who could often be rigid, unsympathetic, and insensitive, qualities we now view with disdain. However we think about the word *traditional* now, these men often maintained commitments to their families, no matter how tough times were; stayed in loveless marriages so that children would have stable homes; served as role models for the hard work all men must be prepared to do in their lives; and taught their children strong moral values. They were not men who would use therapy or accept the need to view one's inner self. They were survivors and protectors, and if that role now seems old-fashioned or out of touch with modern views of men, their sons were often able to take the messages of their fathers and try to become better men, better fathers, and better husbands. That many of us never surpassed our fathers as good men is evidence of the strength of tradition and a reminder that traditional men are often amazing men. I dedicate this book to them.

—Morley D. Glicken

Acknowledgments

In 1991, I took my daughter Amy to a clinical social work conference in Washington, DC, to present an article I'd written on men. This was at a time when male bashing was very prevalent and there seemed to be a general lack of concern about men and our issues. Instead of presenting the academic article I'd written, however, I began to talk about my father who had passed away several years earlier and who was, in many ways, an amazing man. I realized in this eulogy for my father that I would never surpass his achievements. He was a fighter for union rights. He acknowledged the very bad behavior of many men who worked on the railroad yet always recommended some form of help as an alternative to suspension because he believed in redemption. In many ways, he was ahead of his time and modeled much that is good about male behavior. From his life, the seeds of this book began to develop.

The men I grew up with and my colleagues and friends were special men, and yet the male bashing and the attacks on men during that period made us all look like children—worse, tyrants. I wanted to write a book about men offering a more positive and helpful perspective. After many attempts to find a publisher and the dismay I felt that so many publishing houses just weren't interested in men's issues (perhaps they still aren't), Dr. Susan Milmoe at Lawrence Erlbaum Associates, Inc. accepted my book proposal and offered me a contract to write this book. So, Susan, and Lawrence Erlbaum, thank you.

I want to acknowledge two other publishers, Sage Publications and Allyn & Bacon\Longman who have published my last five books and where some of the ideas on male behavior were first researched and developed. And special thanks go to my editor at Sage, Dr. Arthur Pompino, who spent a good deal of time on the phone listening to me talk about men and who offered support and encouragement.

I am indebted to my coauthors on two chapters dealing with men of color, Mina Garza and Steven Ino. Mina and Steve are old friends and I value their insights and their help in the development of ideas about clinical work with Latino and Asian men. Thank you, Mina and Steve.

I don't think one learns about being a man until he has a daughter in his life. I've been blessed with an exceptional daughter, Amy Jennifer Glicken, who has offered a great deal of informative and sometimes eye-opening feedback about the way women view men, particularly, the way she views me. Thanks, Amy. Daughters are God's gift to men and He did a very special job when he helped create you.

I also want to thank the six female practitioners and academics who offered feedback on my book. They asked to remain anonymous and I've kept that promise. It isn't always easy to get critical feedback on an emotional subject like men, but I thank each of you for your tough and relevant responses to the material in my book. Thanks, old friends.

Finally, for the men of America who don't seem to be doing very well these days, this book is a reminder that we should never give up on people and that men will make us proud as they always have in times of need.

PART I

The Serious Problems Experienced by Men

The Troubled Lives of Men

This book about men is written for clinicians who work with male clients but often have limited research information to guide their practice. Men are not typical clients for most clinicians. If they do come for therapy, it's often because they must: courts have referred them for excessive DWIs or domestic violence, or a spouse has demanded that unwanted behaviors in the relationship must stop or the man risks losing the relationship. Men may be referred by physicians because of self-destructive behaviors that are often seen by other men as desirable, and even essential, to being a man. Employers refer men because of concerns about sexual harassment or workplace violence. The involuntary nature of a man's use of therapy is complicated by the fact that men often view therapy as feminizing and their resistance to the process can be considerable. Imagine then the clinician working with men who are often involuntary clients and who view the process of therapy as ineffective and in conflict with their roles as men, and you get a sense of the complexities of clinical work with men.

But men often respond well to therapy and make significant gains. Many men are unhappy with the self-destructive paths they've chosen. They know that continuing certain beliefs and behaviors will lead to extreme difficulty in their lives. Although they fight the idea of therapy, once it begins, they are often grateful and highly motivated to change. Real change is more likely when the help they receive is respectful, practical, intelligent, supportive, and reassuring, attributes of therapy that may be lacking in our work with many difficult clients but are frequently absent in our work with men. As I note throughout the volume in discussions of treatment attrition, length of time for change to take place, and best evidence of long-term change, our approach to treatment with men requires a uniquely different way of doing psychotherapy. Just as women have argued for a gender-sensitive approach to therapy, men require an approach that is mindful of male development and male roles. And if male therapy is still in a developmental state, hopefully this book will help bring together what we currently know about successful work with men and make our treatment with men just a bit more successful.

The following chapters explain why men are in such difficulty and provide direction from the research literature suggesting best evidence for practice. The research literature on the treatment of men is by no means extensive, but it is evolving and I have tried to use the research literature to provide guidance to clinicians working with men in today's changing clinical environment.

Many men feel discounted because they believe that the playing field in the workplace, in education, and in future life opportunities is unfair. One wants to be objective about this feeling of discontent because the gains women have made are satisfying, if still too limited. Because I want to write honestly about the way men feel, there is always the chance that a volume about men written by a man will be overly sympathetic when the purpose of the volume is rather, to share the concerns men often share with other men but are sometimes afraid to discuss publicly. There is a great deal of anxiety among men that anything they say about gender issues will reflect political incorrectness or hostility toward women. This is particularly true in the academy and in corporate America where sexual harassment and sensitivity to women are often taken very seriously and sometimes result in unfair treatment to men. To help with objectivity, a critical analysis of the volume by female clinicians and academics, offering feedback and rebuttal, is provided in the final chapter. Hopefully, you will find this a balanced way of presenting material, which can be highly emotional for both genders.

EVIDENCE OF MALE DIFFICULTIES

A considerable amount of data suggests that many men experience serious emotional, physical, and social problems throughout the life span. These data on men's lives are presented in much more detail throughout the volume but a brief summary is offered now to lay the groundwork for future chapters. Consider some of the findings reported by Courtenay (1998).

Men in the United States die seven years younger than women and have higher death rates for all fifteen leading causes of death. Men's age-adjusted death rate for heart disease is twice as high as that of women, and the death rate for cancer is much higher. Men are more likely than women to suffer severe chronic conditions and fatal diseases, and to suffer them at an earlier age. Under the age of 65, three out of four people who die from heart attacks are men. Men's cancer death rates have increased more than twenty percent over the past 35 years, while the rates for women have remained unchanged during the same period.

In additional data reported by Courtenay, among 15- to 24-year-olds nationally, more than three out of every four deaths each year are men. Among adolescents, males are more likely than females to be hospitalized for injuries. Fatal injuries account for over 80% of all deaths among 15- to 24-year-old men, and three out of four unintentional injury deaths in this age group are men. Young men in this age group are also at far greater risk than women for sexually transmitted diseases (STDs). Heart disease deaths are nearly twice as high for men as for women in this age group, and cancer deaths are also higher. Most of these deaths, diseases, and injuries are preventable

Other evidence of male problems are equally troublesome. Slater (2003) reports that 900,000 Black men are in prison as compared to 600,000 Black men attending college, junior college, or vocational training programs, or half the number of African American women attending American colleges and universities. The discrepancy between Black male and female college attendance will result in such an imbalance of college-educated men to women that it could alter the "social dynamics" of the African American community (Roach, 2001).

Epidemic increases in male juvenile crime suggest another serious problem for men. Commenting on the significance of the increase in male-dominated juvenile crime, Osofsky and Osofsky (2001) write, "the homicide rate among males 15–24 years old in the United States is 10 times higher than in Canada, 15 times higher than in Australia, and 28 times higher than in France or Germany" (p. 287). Wolfgang (1972) reports that six to seven percent of all boys in a given birth year will become chronic offenders and that these same six to seven percent will commit most of the violent crime in America throughout their life cycle. Adding to concerns about male youth violence, Svaboda (2002) writes, "Boys are in most areas and by most measures doing abysmally today" (p. 67).

In another area of serious male difficulty, men increasingly lag behind women in higher education. Women receive an average of 57% of the bachelor's degrees and 58% of all master's degrees in the United States, or, 133 women are getting bachelor's degrees for every 100 men, a number that will increase to 142 women per 100 men by 2010, according to the U.S. Department of Education (Conlin, 2003). If current trends continue, there will be 156 women per 100 men earning degrees by 2020 (Conlin, 2003). In 2002, there were 170,000 more women receiving bachelor's degrees than men (ABC Nightly News, June 16, 2003), raising the issue of an economic imbalance that could create "societal upheavals, altering family finances, social policies, and work-family practices" (Conlin, 2003, p. 77). According to Conlin (2003), men are dropping out of the work force, abandoning children, and removing themselves from community involvement. Since 1964, the rate of decline of men voting in Presidential elections is twice that of the rate of women. More women now vote than men. As the decrease in men with comparable credentials and earning power continues, increasing numbers of women will, in all probability, never marry. Currently, 30% of all African American women 40 to 44 years of age have never been married (Conlin, 2003, p. 77). As women pull further ahead of men, the lack of availability of suitable men will reduce the probability of forming families.

Citing similar problems in Canada, O'Neill (2000) says that as boys have done poorly in a number of important ways and as men are criticized in many sectors of the society, less and less is being done to help young men. O'Neill blames feminist-driven educational policies that encourage the success of girls while boys are falling further behind. Glaring discrepancies exist in Canada, according to O'Neill, in reading, writing, and math scores at grades three and six suggesting that "modern educational practices actually work against boys' best interests" (O'Neill, 2000, p. 54).

Many of the young men who reject a college education or who do poorly and drop out, complain that universities use learning styles ill-suited to the way many men learn. Complaints are raised that men must sit in classrooms and listen for long periods of time to lectures when more individualized experiential learning suits the needs of a number of otherwise qualified and motivated men. The result of fewer men on campus is increasing efforts at some universities and colleges to recruit and keep men in college, a significant change in admissions policies of the past that actively recruited female students.

To confirm the disparity between male and female performance, Allen (2003) writes, "From kindergarten to grad. school, girls now outperform boys in grades, admissions, student government, and extra-curricular activities. Women are rapidly closing the M.D. and Ph.D. gap and make up almost half of law students" (p. 34). She then provides the following aside: "Meanwhile, boys dominate in such dubious categories as remedial education, stimulant-drug prescriptions, and suicide" (p. 34).

The U.S. Census Department (1998) estimates that during a woman's lifetime, there is a 17.6% possibility of being raped (a 14.8% completion rate and a 2.8% attempt rate). However, when other aspects of violence, including physical assaults and domestic violence, are added to the rape data, American women have an appalling 55% probability of being raped or assaulted by a man sometime during their lifetime. Men have an even greater probability of some form of physical violence. Sixty-seven percent (67%) of all men face the probability of being victims of violence sometime during their lives, generally at the hands of other men (U.S. Census Department, 1998).

WHY MEN ARE IN DIFFICULTY

Lack of Child Support and Absent Fathers

There are many reasons for the deteriorating condition of men in America. Not least of all is a problem caused by men themselves. Half of the divorced fathers in America fail to pay their full amount of child support or fail to pay at all. In Los Angeles County, the District Attorney's office, which is charged with collecting child-support payments from divorced fathers who won't pay their legally mandated child support, was able to collect in only seven percent of the cases leaving 500,000 children without court-mandated support (Deadbeat Dads, 1993). The United States Office of Child Support Enforcement, a division of the U.S. Department of Health and Human Services, indicates that the amount of arrears (unpaid child support owed) that has accrued over the years is over $90 billion (U.S. Office of Child Support Enforcement, 2003). In 2002, the same office noted that over 16 million cases of unpaid child support were reported nationally. Many of these men also fail to have any consistent contact with their children, leaving boys and girls without the socializing influences of fathers.

The failure to responsibly care for children often creates social and emotional problems for single female-headed families that are prescriptions for developmental problems in children. Poverty, lack of positive male role models, abandonment by fathers, and overstressed and overworked mothers, all contribute to a deterioration in family life that frequently has a negative impact on boys. As DiIulio (1996) argues in writing about boys who become, in his words, "super predators," they all too often grow up in an atmosphere of emotional poverty

> ... without loving, capable, responsible adults who teach you right from wrong. It is the poverty of being without parents, guardians, relatives, friends, teachers, coaches, clergy and others who habituate you to feel joy at others' joy, pain at others' pain, happiness when you do right, remorse when you do wrong. It is the poverty of growing up in the virtual absence of people who teach these lessons by their own everyday example, and who insist that you follow suit and behave accordingly. (p. 3)

Freudenberger (1987) wonders where young men go who have grown up without male role models and asks the following:

> Where can these confused and vulnerable young men turn for help? At one time, men had older male role models and mentors to emulate. But that route is no longer tenable. Many older men are themselves confused and troubled by the social changes and often the only kind of man-to-man relationship that men perceive, or are comfortable with, is one of competition and rivalry in sports and elsewhere. Intimacy between men continues to be as uncertain as intimacy between men and women. (p. 47)

Levant (1997) suggests that fathers often revert to stereotypic roles in which they pledge an egalitarian marriage but revert to traditional roles of male lack of involvement with family life. This may take place because of job pressures or because they are unwilling to put the time and effort into a truly egalitarian relationship. The lack of involvement in family life fuels potential marital problems and family discord that often ends in divorce. Once a marriage has ended (Levant reports that women end marriages at twice the rate of men and that 90% of the time, children live with their mothers following a divorce), "The reality of visitation fatherhood is dismal, judging from the fact that more than half of non-custodial fathers drop out of their children's lives" (Furstenberg, Nord, Peterson, & Zill, 1983) (Levant, 1997, p. 224).

Balcom (1998) reports that abandoned sons often suffer lifelong problems of low self-worth and may develop "a sense of self as the kind of person who is abandoned and the son of a father who would abandon" (Herzog & Sudia, 1971, p. 30). Abandonment may affect the son's sense of continuity and stability in relationships and may cause the son to wonder why his father left and whether the son will do the same thing at some point in time. Abandoned sons may develop feelings of shame and stigma that affect their ability to understand and communicate their feelings (Schenk & Everingham, 1995). To mask feelings of shame and sadness, abandoned boys often turn to anger and violence because this may serve to frighten others into thinking the boy is much more emotionally competent than he really is (Krugman, 1995). Abandonment often affects men throughout their life cycle as Balcom (1998) notes:

For many abandoned sons the realization of intimacy is a mystery that eludes them. Abandoned men habitually have relationship difficulties with their parents, siblings, chosen partners, and their children. These men frequently enter treatment in response to obvious crises at family developmental transition points. (p. 286)

Abandoned sons often have two primary reactions to their father's abandonment. They proclaim that they will never be like their fathers, or they overidentify with their fathers and in Balcom's words, "The son may base his worship on the actual father he experienced, or the fantasy father that he wishes or wished for, in spite of the father's apparent lack of contact, interest, commitment, or feelings for his son" (Balcom, 1998, p. 286).

Treatment for abandonment often comes when men are in crisis over intimate relationships (Balcom, 1998). One clue that a male client is having abandonment issues is the feeling that something deeper is missing in the relationship. His partner, on the other hand, may complain of emotional and physical distance. Balcom (1998) believes that one central way to help male clients cope with abandonment issues is through grief work: "Helping an abandoned son grieve his actual and fantasy losses is perhaps the single greatest clinical challenge. The losses include the actual father, the ideal or fantasy father, aspects of childhood and adolescence, and other intimate relationships" (Balcom, 1998, p. 286).

Unemployment and Homelessness

Writing about male homelessness and unemployment, Marin (1991) reports that 80% of the homeless in America are men. Of the many interesting reasons for the number of male homeless, Marin suggests the following: "Poor families practice a form of informal triage. Young men are released into the streets more readily, while young women are kept at home even in the worst circumstances" (p. 85). Life on the streets can be very dangerous for many men and the attempt to find work, associated with traditional transient styles of life for poorer men, is often fraught with danger and violence. Marin argues that to complicate matters, transient work in the fields, on the docks, and in construction is no longer available to men and that the transient lifestyle deteriorates into homelessness and destitution. This group of men constitute the "... ghost-lovers and ghost-fathers, one step ahead of the welfare worker ready to disqualify families for having a man around" (Marin, 1997, p. 86). In their quest for work, unlike poor women with children, men have no federal or state programs to help. Although homeless men have difficulty finding work, society expects them to not only care for themselves, but to care for others. Marin (1991) believes that many men are negated as work becomes more difficult to find:

> When men work (or when they go to war—work's most brutal form) we grant them a right to exist. But when work is scarce, or when men are of little economic use, then they become in our eyes not only superfluous but dangerous. We feel compelled to exile them from our midst, banish them from our view, drive them away to shift for themselves in more or less the same way that our Puritan forebears, in their shining city on the hill, treated sinners and rebels. We are so used to thinking of ours as a male-dominated society that we tend to lose track of the ways in which some men are even more oppressed than women. [Men of color who constitute 50% of the homeless], suffer endlessly from forms of isolation and contempt that often exceed what many women experience. (p. 87)

> Finally, I must add one more thing. Whatever particular griefs men may have experienced on their way to homelessness, there is one final and crippling sorrow all of them share: a sense of betrayal at society's refusal to recognize their needs. Most of us—men and women—grow up expecting that when things go terribly wrong someone from somewhere, will step in and help us. This does not happen, and that all watch from the shore as each of us, in our isolation, struggles to swim and then begins to sink, is perhaps the most terrible discovery that anyone in society can make. When troubled men make the discovery, as all homeless men do sooner or later, then hope vanishes completely; despair rings them round, they become what thy need not have become: the homeless men we see around us everywhere. (Marin, 1991, p. 88)

Male unemployment and underemployment may lead to what Levant (1997) calls, "the loss of the good provider role" (p. 222). Levant believes that the changing emphasis on female income, where 55% of employed women provide more than half of the household income, has precipitated a role reversal for men where women not only earn more than men, they also have more stable and potentially successful employment: "The good-provider role has been such an important part of the definition of what it means to be a man that one would think that its loss would impel an immediate search for alternatives" (Levant, 1997, p. 222).

Boys Can't Be Boys

One widely held explanation for male difficulties are the limits placed on young boys as they develop. D'Antonio (1994) suggests that young men are being denied the very characteristics for which they were formally praised. "Once celebrated for their natural aggression and high spirits," he writes, "now they are branded as hyperactive, incorrigible thugs. Is society making boyishness pathological?" (p. 16). D'Antonio points out that young men have done more than a little badly of late. Boys diagnosed as emotionally disturbed outnumber girls four to one Boys have twice the number of learning disabilities as girls. Juvenile arrests, which are mostly composed of young men, increased 50% between 1987 and 1991. The murder rate for teens—most of whom are young men—has increased 104% from 20 years ago. In 1993, 7,000 boys ages 15 to 24 were killed in America.

To explain this increase in violent or dysfunctional behavior, some researchers suggest that male brain physiology creates a greater probability for difficulty than that of women. Men, as this argument goes, are more likely to be impulsive, suffer attention span disorders which interfere with learning, have more minimal organic brain damage at birth, and respond aggressively when challenged. As a result, many more boys than girls are diagnosed with attention-deficit disorder or attention-deficit hyperactivity disorder. Conlin (2003) reports that the United States uses 80% of the world's supply of Ritalin, a 500% increase over the past decade. This leads Conlin to wonder if Ritalin is the new kindergarten through twelfth-grade "management tool" and quotes Paul R. Wolpe, a psychiatry professor at the University of Pennsylvania and the senior fellow at the school's Center for Bioethics, as saying that in some school districts, 20% to 25% of the boys are taking the drug because "Ritalin is a response to an artificial social context that we've created for children" (Conlin, 2003, p. 81).

D'Antonio (1994) argues that organic problems are an irrelevant explanation for the increase in violent behavior among boys. Instead, he believes that problems with young men are a function of an increasingly hostile environment where

> ... many mothers and teachers don't understand the natural assertiveness of boys. Too often, boys are made to feel inferior or even disturbed. This notion that boys are bad is reinforced by a stream of feminist thought that argues that women are natural peacemakers while male aggression—in the form of patriarchy—is the main source of war, pollution, poverty, virtually every kind of suffering in the world. (p. 20)

This concern for the way young boys are viewed in our society is reinforced by Ellum (1994) who writes the following:

> ... it is difficult if not dangerous for boys to be raised outside the company of men. Boys are often coming of age today without a constant male model. Many women, feminists especially, are afraid that masculinity will run wild and become life threatening. If boys are in trouble, it's because too many men have abandoned their sons and adults, in general, are failing to help boys meet a social standard that requires them to be more cooperative. (p. 20)

Dubious Male Violence Data

Although no one would argue that men are without blame and that a good deal of male behavior is reprehensible and deeply harmful to women, the data used to make these arguments are often highly inflated. Consider the data reporting male perpetrators of rape and domestic violence. The 1989 Bureau of Justice National Crime Survey, which includes crimes not reported to the police as well as those that are reported, finds that about eight percent of women in America will be victimized by rape in their lifetimes (Dunn, 1994). Researchers in the 1980s, most specifically Diana Russel and Mary Koss, pegged the rate of abuse to women at 25% to 33%. Commenting on the data generated by Russell and Koss, Dunn (1994) argues that, "... their surveys are fraught with scientific flaws. Russell and Koss have included everything from consensual sex to obscene phone calls in their figures on rape and sexual abuse" (p. 26). Such practices, Dunn notes, "Inflate the statistics grotesquely" (p. 26). Reporting the work of Mark Warr, a fear researcher, whose recent work on overstressing crime is the focus of the article, Dunn reports the following:

> I asked his opinion about the numbers [of rapes]. "I am very much on the low end," he said. "Which is to say that from the National Crime Survey, we find the probability per year for a woman [of being raped] is on the order of one in a thousand. I'm certainly willing to admit that there is undercounting here. But even if the underreporting is fairly large—and I don't believe it is—we're still going to have small numbers.

> In the local rape crisis center [in Austin, Texas] they argue that one in three women is raped every year. Those people do good work. I respect it. But they are not criminologists, and they have a vested interest in inflating the numbers to convince people that they provide a necessary service. It's not like it's some innocuous academic debate. It's unnecessarily scaring people and restricting their freedom. (p. 29)

An additional argument about abuse is that because men are stronger then women, they do more physical damage when abuse is involved. In response, Steinmetz and Lucca (1988) write the following:

> ... data on homicide between spouses suggest that almost an equal number of wives kill their husbands as husbands kill their wives. Thus, it appears that men and women might have an equal potential for violent marital interaction; initiate similar acts of violence; and when differences of physical strength are equalized by weapons, commit similar amounts of spousal homicide. (p. 241)

The use of data to paint pictures of men as perpetrators is particularly galling to men who often see women misuse their power in relationships and in the workplace. Women sometimes do considerable financial and emotional harm to men in marriages and for many men, the popular notion of women as the victims of male behavior seems both inaccurate and unfair. As men see their chances for job success and promotion eroded by workplace preference for women, the political correctness of a society which sympathizes with women as underrepresented players in the workplace and as victims of discrimination seems increasingly self-serving. Contrary to the popular notion of men as avoiders of sexual harassment rules, many men fear that trivial encounters with women or an innocuous remark will be taken as sexually harassing.

The condition of men is clear in social and health data, which paint a troubled picture of men, particularly men of color. Health problems have increased, death by violence is a serious concern for men of color, and suicide rates have doubled for some male groups in only twenty years. Male bashing and a diminished view of men permeate the consciousness of men and women as they interact with one another. It is a time when men are confronted by popular descriptions of men as perpetrators and molesters. In short, it is a time of considerable difficulty for the men of America.

SUMMARY

This is a time of turmoil and change in the lives of men. Some of the change relates to an unraveling society where traditional values that keep families intact and teach boys the traditional codes and beliefs to guide male behavior have begun to breakdown. Some of the change is due to a workplace where men compete with women for jobs which once were their domain. This changing workplace offers men in poverty little opportunity for permanent or transient work. Most of all, changes in male behavior including health problems, lack of educational achievement, and violence, paint a troubling picture of men and suggest a need to take male problems seriously.

Male Socialization:
Some Divergent Points of View

No one sits down with the men of America and teaches them a male code of conduct, yet men know the code fairly early in life and try to live by it. They know, for example, that men who give in to pain are considered to be unmanly by other men and that after a certain age, you're not supposed to cry, ever. Men know that the unwillingness to compete is often seen as a sign of weakness by other men. Whatever the situation might be, there is an unspoken expectation that men will often try and outdo one another. Not to be competitive and not to try and win are considered signs of weakness. Above all, the positive judgments of other men are profoundly important.

Many of the developmental messages men learn are first given in sports where men are taught about winning and superiority. Sports have always been an acceptable way for men to show their dominance over others. Scher (1979) writes that, "Men learn early in life to compete with their fellows. Their need to win is pervasive" (p. 253). Brannon (1976) believes that there are four primary messages given to men at such an early age that, well before puberty, boys know the messages well enough to have mastered them to some extent. The primary male messages are as follows:

1. No Sissy Stuff—The need to be different from women.
2. The Big Wheel—The need to be superior to others.
3. The Sturdy Oak—The need to be self-reliant and independent.

4. Give 'em Hell—The need to be more powerful than others, through violence, if necessary.

When boys are unable to master these primary male messages, they learn to compensate through exaggerated male behavior, or what has been called "compensatory masculinity." The boy striving to become a man who also feels fearful and insecure in the process may copy male verbal patterns or the walk of men they admire. Boys see the imitation of men they admire as a way of proving to others that they are men. Boys may drink or smoke at an early age to exaggerate their need to be seen as manly. When the need to prove masculinity is overpowering, compensatory masculinity may lead young boys into violence. It is no small coincidence that violence among very young boys is often found in chaotic families or in families where fathers have abandoned their children. As Hughes (personal communication, July 7, 2003) argues in her work on gang affiliation

> Gangs are often the homes and support systems that many American boys and girls of color must substitute for actual homes and real families. In a society that creates broken and battered homes as easily as ours does, where do young boys go to get their affirmation, acceptance, and support but to gangs? And where do they learn their codes of conduct which, after all, are the same messages we have always given boys: Loyalty to your family, honesty to your friends, help and support to your mates when they need you.

> Where it gets ugly is the strong pressure on gang members to prove their masculinity through violence. All too often the cost of proving oneself is a ruined life because these vulnerable young kids are so intent on proving themselves to their peers that they will do anything required of them to be manly, even if they are still frightened, unformed, and basically very needy children.

Bereska (2003) believes that male messages are remarkably unchanged since the Victorian period. She notes that the boy's world is still

> characterized by certain types and degrees of emotional expression, naturalized aggression, male hang-out groups, hierarchies within those

groups, competition, athleticism, sound moral character, and adventure. It is heterosexual, comprised of active male bodies, and no sissies are allowed. (p. 168)

Yacovene (1990) concurs and writes the following:

The social roles of men and women, the nature of work, urbanization, industrialization, and, more generally, intellectual life, have changed dramatically since the early nineteenth century, yet the cultural perceptions of masculinity have remained remarkably static. (p. 85)

THE FOUR THEMES OF MALE DEVELOPMENT

Let's consider Brannon's (1976) four primary messages learned in childhood, when and how they are given, and their impact on male behavior.

No Sissy Stuff—The Need to Be Different from Women

Boys are taught to be different from girls almost immediately. Parents who try and encourage boys to be sensitive and to recognize their feminine side often fight an uphill battle. Boys teach one another the messages they learn from older boys, whereas the media transmits male role expectations. Men subtly influence boys to be stoic and not to give in to pain. No pain, no gain: this is a message that is given to boys by every athletic coach who has ever lived and one reinforced by every boy who plays team sports and by every fan who watches. Boys play hurt. Boys make pain a pledge of manliness. Where boys are taught to control and deny feelings, girls are often taught to express them.

As boys mature into young men, this message becomes a code of conduct: "If you can't take the heat, get out of the kitchen." The messages we pass on to young men are the messages of strength and endurance, of mastery of pain, of bravery and selflessness; male codes of conduct in which American men are so well steeped that most boys have mastered them by the time they reach adolescence, if not earlier.

A significant message that boys are given is that they are different from girls in very fundamental ways. Where girls are weak physically and emotionally, boys are tough. Where girls cry, boys never do. Where girls give up easily, boys never give up. These messages of strength versus weakness are given to boys early in life. Boys experiencing failure in school often believe that the educational superiority of girls is another example of gender differences and often come to believe that education is a feminine attribute. This may partially explain the failure of young men to seek college educations and the general superiority of women academically.

Many of the male codes of conduct may be explained by genetic differences and predisposition of men. More about that later in the chapter, but an additional thought about male codes of conduct is that they explicate certain biological differences between men and women and are really ways of justifying these differences with aphorisms that provide a way for men to conduct themselves given the considerable biological differences between male and female children. For example, male infants suffer higher rates of illness and behavioral problems than female infants. How better to protect men from their fragility than to provide messages glorifying their strength? The wise therapist should understand that attempts to give men an honest picture of their physical and intellectual limitations will be met by extreme hostility. Instead, men prefer to think that if you "Seek the positive in terms of people's coping skills, you will find it. Look beyond presenting symptoms and setbacks and encourage clients to identify their talents, dreams, insights, and fortitude" (Van Wormer, 1999, p. 54). Men work best in an atmosphere of unconditional positive regard. Negative messages or concerns about their behavior will often be met with anger, denial, and rejection of treatment because they so clearly contradict the internalized beliefs men have about their superiority and competence, even if those beliefs are patently untrue.

Returning to the notion of no sissy stuff, a ten-year-old fourth grader from California explained what happens to boys who back down from fights, even those they cannot win:

If you let the other boys get away with anything, then they think you're some kind of woman. The names they call you are always women's name. This boy I know at school, he backed down on a fight and everybody started calling him "Edna" and making kissing sounds. Or when they'd talk, they'd talk baby talk about how weak he was, or what a little baby he was, and how maybe his mommy needed to come and be with him. Pretty soon, he got into a fight just to prove he was no baby and he got beat up pretty good. But you learn fast that if you want to be one of the guys, then you got to act like you're one of the guys. (Anonymous, personal communication, June 4, 2001)

The Big Wheel—The Need to be Superior to Others at Any Cost

"Winning isn't something," said one of America's great coaches, "it's everything." "It isn't about wining or losing," said another American sage, "it's always about winning." And so it is, because boys are told in small and large ways that being first, winning, and being better than anyone else is what men strive for in sports, in work, and in love. When women ask men why they have so few real friends, the reason is that it's difficult to have friends when you're in competition with other men. Writing about the need men have to be superior to others, Cowley (2003) says, "The drive for dominance skews our perceptions, colors our friendships, shapes our moods, and affects our health" (p. 67). The put-downs and sarcasm that sometimes characterize male behavior with other men is not meant to bring men closer together but is, rather, intended to prove to others that a man is stronger, smarter, tougher, and more sexual, by far, than any other man alive. But in an almost paradoxical way, the need to be superior also serves to draw other men closer to one another. By showing that a man is better than anyone else, it also suggests that he is a leader.

We sometimes forget that historically, men have passed certain messages on to reinforce survival skills. Their lives literally depended on being superior in games, in hunting, and in war. The competitiveness that developed from having to be the very best is still with us as the following statement from a former student demonstrates:

I think women are just as concerned with winning as men are. It's just that they have more indirect ways of showing it. The women in my agency are so devious, you can't believe it. They do things behind your back. They lie, they smile and act like they're your friend, but it's always for their benefit, to get their way, to win. Men are just so much more direct. You and me, one on one, everything is out in the open. You know when you're with a man that sometime or the other, one of you will challenge the other guy. If you're out drinking, it'll be to see who can drink more or who can win at pool. It's always something. It's like the animals do when they carve out their territory by urinating around the boundaries. Men carve out their areas of expertise, their superiority every time they interact with other men. But unlike women, it's direct confrontation, no guile at all allowed. Me against you. If you lose, then I'm the king of the hill, at least for now.

The Sturdy Oak—The Need to Be Self-Reliant and Independent

When you observe very young boys at play, you will notice that their play is sometimes solitary. It will tell you how well the culture trains its boys for independence. Expecting men to be cooperative and good team players is often not a part of the social and cultural training that explains male behavior. In earlier times in our history, self-reliance and independence were necessary for survival and were considered positive male attributes. It is only lately that men have been criticized for being bad team players and too uncooperative for modern corporate or bureaucratic life. Modern life demands cooperation whereas men have often been taught to be solitary players who are independent and self-reliant. Men resent supervision. "Give me a job," they will tell you, "and let me do it." Consider this conversation among some construction workers, overheard at the author's favorite morning coffee spot.

The foreman I had on the last job, he let us alone. Do your work, he says, be on time, get it done right. You know how to do it, so *do* it. We got the project done in no time. Got bonus points for getting it done early. It was great. We all felt like he respected us. But this guy now, he can't let anything happen without poking his big nose into it. Leave us alone. We

know our job, I tell him, but he just keeps on bugging us. One of the guys
punched him out last week. They were gonna can him but the union saved
him. Been a lot better on the job now. You gotta respect a man and leave
him alone. Everybody knows that.

Although this may be an extreme example, we know that men need to
develop cooperative skills if they are to be successful in the workplace.
One way of accomplishing cooperation is what Svoboda (2002) calls
"independence with boundaries" or "sponsored independence." Independence with boundaries provides an opportunity for boys to develop
independently without losing closeness to others while gaining skills in
cooperative endeavors. Boys are given room to develop their own idiosyncratic ways of doing things. They are encouraged to share those ways
with others while accepting that the process may lead to acceptance or
rejection of their ideas, but never of them.

Give 'Em Hell—The Need to Be More Powerful Than Others Through Violence, if Necessary

Boys are often taught that if someone challenges them, they must fight
back. If they don't fight back it may be interpreted as a sign of weakness.
To show weakness is to not be a man. Fights abound in the lives of young
boys. This behavior continues on through young adulthood and sometimes, beyond. It is no doubt one of the reasons for high rates of juvenile
violence and the spread of gang violence in many American cities. The
stories men tell are all about giving the people around them hell. The author was told this story by a colleague, proving that education and rank
do not negate the need for men to give people who cross them a piece of
their mind and their bodies.

I was doing some consulting for a small school in the Midwest. I'd go
out there every few months and the dean I was to work with would tor-
pedo everything I did. I'd order something done and then when I left,
he'd countermand it. All he had was criticism for my work, but it was the
kind that was little and unimportant. Little academic put-downs.
Finally, we had a confrontation, really nasty. He actually threatened to

fight me. I couldn't believe it. This little middle-aged guy, very academic, he actually wanted to duke it out with me. I stood up when he
challenged me. I'm at least a foot taller and 50 pounds heavier, but this
guy stands up and makes a fist like he's going to hit me. Finally, I started
to laugh and walked away. They removed him, of course, but it seemed
so like our society. Even educated men, when everything else fails, resort
to violence. It made me wonder how far we've really come.

UNDERSTANDING MALE DEVELOPMENT

Male Socialization

In a review of the literature on male socialization, O'Neil (1981) suggests that men are taught a number of propositions that form their understanding of the "masculine mystique," including the notions that

> ... power, dominance, competition, and control are necessary to proving
> one's masculinity; that vulnerabilities, feelings, and emotions in men are
> signs of femininity and are to be avoided; that masculine control of self,
> others, and environment are essential for men to feel safe, secure, and
> comfortable; and that men seeking help and support from others show
> signs of weakness, vulnerability, and potential incompetence. (Robert-
> son & Fitzgerald, 1992, p. 241)

One result of the need to be independent is that men often have few support systems and a very limited number of friends. In his book, *Man
Enough*, Pitman (1993) writes

> ... sometimes there is something that a man needs to reveal, needs to talk
> over with another man, and there may be no man available to him. Some-
> times, manhood is lonely.... Loneliness is what it costs a man to be true to
> his code of masculinity. Many such men, under the sway of the masculine
> mystique, lead shockingly lonely lives. (p. 12)

Scher (1979) believes that changes in society have placed men in uncomfortable and even dissonant roles. Although men are expected to be
powerful, in control much of the time, strong, healthy, sexually robust,
and tireless, the impossibility of this creates a great deal of posing, de-

ception, and failure. As society continues to expect men to be strong, it criticizes them for all of the attributes it expects of men resulting in double bind situations that often lead to physical and emotional difficulty. Scher (1979) says that this ambiguity is difficult for most men to cope with: "Many of the attitudes that provided stability are now disintegrating and men are clinging to them in an attempt to maintain order. But their clinging creates more problems" (p. 252).

Wilson (1993) believes that our changing society creates particular problems for male socialization. Although male aggression is no longer adaptive because institutions now value conformity over physical prowess, aggressive impulses are still present in boys and young men, and weakened family and institutional controls, particularly in large urban centers, bring groups of men together with very different notions of acceptable behavior that sometimes results in violence. Wilson believes that: "From time to time we forget that young men in groups are always a potential challenge to social order, and so we are surprised when they reappear in places that we think of as tranquil and civilized" (p. 12).

Feminists have argued that sex role development is significantly influenced by socialization. Worrel (1981) writes that "the label of male or female provides a structure around which behavioral expectancies, role prescriptions, and life opportunities are organized" (p. 313). Gilligan (1982) indicates that male and female labels affect the way men and women respond to developmental challenges. Svoboda (2002) argues that from the very beginning of life, parents relate in very different ways to male and female children: "They speak differently, have different expectations, and present them with different communications and sets of signals and directions, which infants and children absorb and use as they build up mental representations of themselves" (p. 120). Kohlberg (1987) found that very young male children show more sex-typed behavior. For example, a young boy's fear of being a sissy is more intense than a girl's fear of being a tomboy. Social pressure from parents, teachers, and peers provide distinctive environments for boys and girls. Kohlberg believes that boys are socialized differently, given different messages than girls, and have internalized those values and messages into their own value system. As examples of male socialization, Kohlberg notes that boys are encouraged to play rough, to not cry, and to be strong and courageous. What would most likely be found inside most little boys' toy boxes are toy guns, plastic soldiers, racing cars, and Tonka trucks. Their idols are cartoon heroes who engage in violence against the "bad guys."

As boys enter adolescence and then young adulthood, peers become a strongly influential force in defining a young man's identity. Sexuality is heightened and the impetus to be seen as a "masculine," "heterosexual" male becomes very important. "Scoring" with maturing adolescent girls rapidly becomes a topic of discussion in locker rooms, creating feelings of inadequacy among those who have not engaged in sexual behaviors. Choosing an occupation and establishing intimate relationships are two important tasks in young adulthood (Levinson, Darrow, Klein, Levinson, & McKee, 1978). For most White men, finding a work identity seems to be much easier than establishing intimate relationships. Becoming involved with the opposite sex on a deeper level is difficult for men who have often been told to avoid nonsexual relationships with women. Yet, at this stage of life, young men are supposed to connect, communicate, and understand the dynamics of intimacy.

Because many young men have a limited understanding of emotionally intimate relationships with women, a type of "feminine mystique" sometimes develops in which men perceive women as possessing certain mysterious powers (Pleck, 1987). Pleck (1987) describes two types of power men perceive women to have over them. The first is expressive power, or the power to express emotions. Because women are given permission to express emotions, men often express their own emotions vicariously through women and may depend on women to express their emotions for them. If the woman refuses to exercise her expressive role, the man will try harder to get the woman to play this role. The second power Pleck describes is masculinity-validating power. For a man to experience himself as being masculine, the woman is encouraged to play her scripted role in behaving in ways that make him feel masculine. Once again, when a woman refuses to engage in this role, the man may feel lost and may try to force the woman back into her traditional role, sometimes through the use of coercion, manipulation, or violence.

Mahalik, Locke, Theodore, Cournoyer, and Lloyd (2001) suggest that learned restrictive definitions of male roles which are seen by others as rigid, sexist, and one-dimensional contribute to lower self-esteem, reduced capacity for intimacy, substance abuse, immature and "projective-aggressive" defense mechanisms, and rigidity in interpersonal relationships. The authors argue that adoption of rigid male sex roles are learned and as Mead (1935) reports, men can be socialized to respond to family life, work, and sexuality in a surprisingly wide variety of ways. Pleck (1995) views male behavior as a function of cultural messages that transmit socially defined roles for men. Socially defined roles may be determined by social class, education, and a society's recent history. It may suggest that rigid definitions of male roles are a function of the prevailing socializing mechanisms used by caretakers, institutions, nationalities, religious groups, the mass media, and peer groups.

Restrictive notions of male roles tend to modify themselves in middle age when men begin to integrate both male and female definitions of their roles (Levinson et al., 1978). The authors believe that with age, men shift from traditional male roles to becoming more nurturing and concerned about the quality of relationships. O'Neil and Egan (1992) report that age modifies traditional views of male gender roles and that men begin to experience less role conflict in some areas of life as they mature. Mahalik et al. (2001) believe that if traditional male role models do not modify themselves as men age, this will negatively affect feelings of intimacy and self-esteem. To adapt to changing definitions of the roles of men as they age, Wade and Brittan-Powell (2000) believes that men need a reference group to maintain changing beliefs about their roles. When a reference group is lacking, there may be negative psychosocial consequences, including feelings of isolation and confusion. Wade et al. suggest that counseling is an ideal way to help men make changes in the way they view male roles when a male reference group is either lacking or in discord with the changes a man believes he needs to make. Counseling may help men recognize that they can be less traditional in their view of male roles and still feel strongly centered in their maleness. Wade and

Brittan-Powell also believe that counseling can create affiliations between men through support networks providing confirmation that
changes men may be going through are acceptable and positive.

Warren Farrell (1992) says that many stereotypes of men exist and
that one particularly egregious stereotype is that men are unable to work
cooperatively with others. Farrell suggests that team sports teach men to
be cooperative and to work toward a unified goal. However, because
men have to deal with rejection on the job and in many parts of their
lives, Farrell believes that men are much less vindictive than women and
that male socialization often teaches men to be supportive of others. The
bad news, he points out, is that to maintain open and positive attitudes
toward others, men learn to hide their sensitivities and to deny their
feelings.

GENETIC FACTORS IN MALE DEVELOPMENT

Genetic factors may also explain differences between male and female
behavior. Parker, Keightley, Smith, and Taylor (1999) report very different levels of ability in male and female children to use emotional language from an early age. The inability to communicate emotions causes
young boys to feel uncomfortable and ill at ease, but not to really know
why, a condition many therapists find in male adult clients. Fivush
(1989) found that boys show signs of significant anger by age three, a
finding not found with three-year-old girls. A related finding is that
when boys are exposed to the distress of others, they seem far less concerned than girls. Fabes, Eisenberg, Karbon, Troyer, and Switzer (1994)
report that in a group of six-year-old boys and girls listening to a recording of a crying baby, more girls showed concern for the baby's distress,
whereas twice as many boys just turned the speakers off. Physical examinations showed the boys to be more anxious over the child's crying and
more intolerant of the crying than girls.

Other signs of gender differences are reported by Keller and West
(1995), who found that boys and girls react differently to early separation and bereavement. Boys showed little concern whereas girls were often highly preoccupied with them. The authors indicate that although

neither response is necessarily healthy, the response by the young boys is in keeping with the tendency for boys not to know how they feel emotionally and not to ask for help when it may be needed. This early behavior in boys to deny feelings and to avoid asking for help very likely carries on into adulthood. Rout (1999) reports that male British physicians (general practitioners in this study) were more anxious and depressed than female doctors, but were also more likely to avoid contact with other people when stressed, and to not seek help.

Although an argument can be made that the preceding examples of male behavior are part of the socialization process, a number of authors make strong arguments that male physiology is the primary reason for many of the differences cited. An example of the way the differences in boys and girls affects adults is provided by Kraemer (2000), who believes that early behaviors of young boys have consistent physiological patterns that continue to affect men throughout the life cycle:

> Even when ill, men may not notice signs of illness, and when they do they are less likely to seek help from doctors. This tendency will account for some of the excess suicides in males. In his despair the victim believes that no help is available, that talking is useless. If baby boys are typically harder to care for it is arguable that they will be more likely to feel lonely as adults. (p. 1611)

Kraemer also reports that male infants tend to be much more excitable than female infants and that mothers spend considerable time soothing the male infant's anxiety at some expense to normal development. Murray, Kempton, Woolgar, and Hooper (1993) found that young boys were very impacted by the moods of their mothers. In mothers suffering from postpartum depression, the impact lasted well into kindergarten and long after the mother's depression had lifted.

Kraemer (2000) believes that serious accidents among boys are largely related to poor motor skills and cognitive regulation that place boys at higher risk for accidents than girls. When compensatory masculinity and lower socioeconomic status are added to genetic predispositions, the result is a dramatic increase in violence, suicide, drug and alcohol usage, and other risky behaviors that may have a genetic base.

Hopkins and Bard (1993) have shown that girls have better literary skills than boys and are more adept at using language. This may explain why girls continue to surpass boys academically. The authors also report that "alexithymia"—the lack of an emotional vocabulary—is much more common in boys and may help to explain the difficulty men have in expressing intimate feelings. The authors note that these differences are seen very early in life and that one cannot argue that socialization alone is responsible. As Kraemer (2000) indicates in his summary of the impact of socialization and genetic causes for gender differences,

> Even from conception, before social effects come into play, males are more vulnerable than females. Social attitudes about the resilience of boys compound the biological deficit. Male mortality is greater than female mortality throughout life. The causes are a mixture of biological and social pressures: we need to be aware of both in order to promote better development and health for boys and men. (p. 1611)

Commenting on the skills of early man to access risk and use physical strength when needed, Zaslow and Hayes (1986) believe that these skills are no longer called on even if they are still part of the genetic makeup of men. In contrast, although a few men dominate top positions in government and business, modern men are now seen as lacking in characteristics usually associated with women: self-regulation of emotions and reflectiveness, characteristics which are highly valued in modern society and which suggest that women may, in time, surpass men even at the highest levels of government and business.

Male infants often require considerably more attention than female infants and are more distressed when the attention isn't given. Sackett (1972) studied this same phenomenon in male rhesus monkeys, partially or totally isolated from maternal care, and found that they are far more likely to "freeze" in test situations than are matched females, who are more active and curious.

Wilson (1993) points out that in the argument over temperament versus socialization, even in Japanese preschools where sympathy and concern for others followed by cooperation are emphasized, the same gender differences are seen in both Japanese and American preschools:

"The boys acted like warriors, the girls like healers and peacemakers. How gender differences, which seem universal, interact with culture to affect moral sentiments is a subject about which almost everything remains to be learned" (p. 27).

GENDER ROLE STRAIN

Brooks (1990) points out that an additional issue in male development, affecting the way men interact with women, is gender-role strain, or what Brooks defines as "the discomfort resulting from disharmony between early gender socialization and newer role expectations" (p. 52). When gender-role strain is minimal, as it is with men trying to understand their relationships with women and doing so in a sensitive and thoughtful way, the strain results in better male–female relationships. In more traditional men

> the challenges may be seen as precipitated by personal failures in meeting masculine role standards and the traditional man's role strain may be more intense, destructive, and devoid of compensatory benefits than the strain experienced by other men. (Brooks, 1990, p. 52)

Brooks (1998) defines traditional men as competitive, stoic, homophobic, aloof in their fathering roles, preoccupied with work and achievement, neglectful of their health needs, and distrusting women while overrelying on them on them for "nurturance, emotional expressiveness, and validation of masculinity" (p. 51). Pleck (1980) believes that men need the validation of women to feel masculine and that they are highly dependent on women for feelings of self-worth and achievement.

In suggesting that men are experiencing an increase in role strain, Pleck (1987) says that, "men as a group are experiencing more psychological distress than they did three decades ago, both absolutely and relative to women" (p. 20). Pleck believes that many aspects of traditional male–female relationships are unacceptable to women and create conflict in traditional men who see no personal benefit in having more egalitarian relationships with women. Traditional men rarely see any point in changing their perceptions of what they expect in a relationship. When change is demanded, as in the case of abusive behavior or the possibility of divorce, Scher (1990) says that traditional men see few "life-enhancing qualities in psychotherapy and come into therapy because they have no alternative" (p. 3). If therapy is chosen as the last possible alternative, Brooks (1990) says that, "Rather than acknowledging vulnerability and openly seeking help, they [men] may attempt to control therapy sessions and may provoke intellectual games or compete with the therapist for power" (p. 52). Men may also, in Scher's words, adopt "superficial changes" meant to undermine the spouse's need for empowerment in an attempt to maintain traditional forms of relationships with women that provide the man with safety and comfort.

Another area of gender-role strain is what Spielberg (1993) describes as the need for men to define themselves in heroic ways. By heroic, Spielberg means that men have traditionally seen themselves as "righteous warriors" whose behavior includes acts of bravery and good deeds. As men experience more confusion over the meaning of the word *heroic,* Spielberg believes that men have not been able to adequately respond "to the dilemma of a loss of a guiding image of manhood" (p. 173). New definitions of heroic behavior need to be found so that men can use heroic concepts of themselves in more realistic ways. But the inclusion of a heroic definition of male behavior is only part of a man's search for meaningful self-definitions, and Spielberg says the following:

> Perhaps the greatest difficulty many men face today involves the inability to construct for themselves an identity suffused with an authentic and integrated sense of life meaning. As traditional notions of masculinity fade in relevance, and as men have become more honest about their own personal histories and struggles, many have begun to question the meaning, which they previously ascribed to their life in terms of both their relationships with women and work commitments. In this regard, traditional notions of the masculine image, particularly that of the sole breadwinner, as well as that of the righteous warrior, have been under attack for the last two decades. Unfortunately, however, most men have not been able to respond to the dilemma of a loss of a guiding image of manhood. (p. 173)

Considering additional reasons for gender-role strain, in a review of a book by Pollack (1998), Sargent (1999) believes that an omission in Pollack's book is the role women play in helping boys develop notions of manhood that provide boys with traditional as well as more complex definitions of male roles in society. Sargent points to the feminization of the education system and the lack of concern for young boys, which often leaves boys without institutional support systems. Sargeant believes that mothers are frequently ambivalent about the role women have in shaping male behavior and writes, "Women, as members of society, are responsible for their part in creating and maintaining the current boy code which is so damaging to our boys and men. Women, as mothers, are responsible for their part in inflicting this code upon their sons" (p. 46). Sargent says that if society is to help boys develop a more balanced code of male conduct, then women must participate in the process.

SUMMARY

This chapter discusses a variety of explanations of the factors related to male development. Primary among those factors are the strong messages young boys get from older boys, parents, and the media that stress a male code of conduct. Genetic factors are also discussed. It seems apparent that both social learning and genetics help explain many of the complex reasons for male behavior that result in stoicism, difficulty in coping with external stress, and social isolation. Gender-role strain is an additional reason men sometimes do poorly in intimate relationships and why therapy is often a difficult but necessary process for many men.

Chapter 3

Working With Men
to Ensure Good Physical Health

In reporting data from the University of Michigan's Institute for Social Research, Gupta (2003) notes that, "men outrank women in all of the 15 leading causes of death, except one: Alzheimer's. Men's death rates are at least twice as high as women's for suicide, homicide and cirrhosis of the liver" (p. 84). The principal researcher on the study of men's health, David Williams, says that men are twice as likely to be heavy drinkers and to "engage in behaviors that put their health at risk, from abusing drugs to driving without a seat belt" (Gupta, 2003, p. 84). Gupta points out that men are more often involved in risky driving and that SUV rollovers and motorcycle accidents largely involve men. Williams blames this behavior on "deep-seated cultural beliefs—a 'macho' world view that rewards men for taking risks and tackling danger head on" (Gupta, 2003, p. 84).

Further examples of risky male behavior leading to injury and death include the fact that men are twice as likely to get hit by lightning, die in a flash flood, and are more likely to drive around barricades resulting in more deaths by train accidents and drowning in high water. As a significant difference in the way men and women approach their health, Gupta (2003) indicates that women are twice as likely as men to visit their doctors once a year and are more likely than men to explore broad-based preventive health plans with their physician. Men are less likely to schedule checkups or to follow up when symptoms arise. Men also tend to internalize their emotions and self-medicate their psychological

33

problems, notes Williams (Gupta, 2003), whereas women tend to seek professional help. Virtually all stress-related diseases—from hypertension to heart disease—are more common in men.

American men between the ages of 45 and 64 suffer an estimated 218,000 heart attacks a year, compared with 74,000 a year for women in the same age group, one of many reasons women live more than seven years longer than men (Drug Store News, 1998). Epperly and Moore (2000) report that men are at much greater risk of alcohol abuse than women with the highest rates of alcoholism occurring in men between 25 and 39 years of age. However, age is not a deterrent for risk factors in men and fourteen percent of men over 65 are alcohol dependent as compared to 1.5 percent of women in the same age group. Male suicides in men over 65 are six times the rate of the general population, according to Reuben, Yoshikawa, and Besdine (1996).

These findings of greater health problems among men are not explained by biological differences related to gender. Harrison, Chin, and Ficarrotto (1988) indicate that:

Research suggests that it is not so much biological gender that is potentially hazardous to men's health but rather specific behaviors that are traditionally associated with male sex roles which can be (but in the case of women are not) taken on by either gender. (p. 275)

Saunders (2000) reports that a poll by Louis Harris and associates in May and November 1998 indicated that 28% of the men as compared to 8% of the women had not visited a physician in the prior year. Although 19% of the women didn't have a regular physician, 33% of the men didn't have one either. More than half of the men surveyed had not been tested for cholesterol or had a physical examination in the prior year. Waiting as long as possible to receive needed medical care was a strategy used by a fourth of the men studied and only 18% of the men surveyed sought medical care immediately when a medical problem arose.

Additional health data paint an equally troubling picture of male health. Drug Store News (1998) reported the following information for American pharmacists: (a) Women still outlive men by an average of six to seven years, despite advances in medical technology; (b) the death

rate from prostate cancer has increased by 23% since 1973; (c) oral cancer, related to smoking, occurs more than twice as often in men; (d)
three times as many men suffer heart attacks than women before age 65.
Nearly three in four coronary artery bypasses in 1995 were performed
on men; (e) bladder cancer occurs five times more often in men than
women; (f) nearly 95% of all D.W.I. (drinking while intoxicated) cases
involve men; and (g) in 1970, the suicide rate for White men was 9.4 per
100,000 as compared to 2.9 for White women. By 1986, the rate for
White men had risen to 18.2 as compared to 4.1 for women, and by 1991,
the rate for White male suicide was 19.3 per 100,000, as compared to a
slight increase to 4.3 for women (National Center for Chronic Disease
Prevention and Health, 2001, 2003). In 1991, suicide rates for Black and
Latino men were 11.5 per 100,000 or almost six times the rate of suicide
for Black and Latino women. Suicide is the third leading cause of death
among Black men. By 2001, suicide rates for all men had increased,
whereas suicide rates for men over 60 were from 10 to 12 times higher
than suicide rates for older women, with men over 85 having an astonishing suicide rate of 54 per 100,000, as compared to women in the same
age group, of 5 per 100,000 (CDC, 2004).

One of the primary health concerns for men is prostate cancer. The
National Center for Chronic Disease Prevention and Health Promotion
(CDC, 2003) reports that prostate cancer is the second leading form of
cancer among men after lung cancer. The CDC (2003) reports an American Cancer Society estimate for 2003 of 220,900 new cases of prostate
cancer and that 28,900 men will die of the disease. Most diagnosed prostate cancers (about 70%) are found in men 65 years or older. Because of
earlier diagnosis and better treatment, the survival rate for prostate cancer has increased from 67% to 97% over the past twenty years. The prostate cancer death rate is higher for Black men than for any other racial or
ethnic group, whereas Asian and Pacific Islander groups have relatively
low rates of prostate cancer incidence and mortality. Among all racial
and ethnic groups, prostate cancer death rates were lower in 1999 than
they were in 1990. Decreases in prostate cancer death rates between 1990
and 1999 were almost twice as great for Whites and Asian and Pacific Is-
landers as they were for Blacks, American Indian and Alaska Natives,
and Hispanics, suggesting a difference in the use of doctors for early di-

agnosis, the quality of medical care received, dietary or genetic influences, or taking no action once the cancer is diagnosed.

The decision to treat prostate cancer is made more complicated by the fact that the two most commonly used tests to detect prostate cancer, the digital rectal examination (DRE), and the prostate-specific antigen (PSA) test, sometimes give false-positive readings or fail to detect cancer when it is present. It is not unusual for men to have negative findings on both tests only to discover a rapidly growing cancer a year later. Men with prostate cancer are often symptom-free, making detection even more difficult. The National Center for Chronic Disease Prevention and Health (CDC) is ambivalent about what to do if results for prostate cancer are positive and indicates that

> Although there is good evidence that PSA screening can detect early-stage prostate cancer, evidence is mixed and inconclusive about whether early detection improves health outcomes. In addition, prostate cancer screening is associated with important harms. These include the anxiety and follow-up testing occasioned by frequent false-positive results, as well as the complications that can result from treating prostate cancers that, left untreated, might not affect the patient's health. (National Center for Chronic Disease Prevention and Control, 2003, p. 3)

The CDC recommends the following for men with diagnosed prostate cancer:

- CDC promotes informed decision making, which occurs when a man understands the seriousness of prostate cancer; understands the risks, benefits, and alternatives to screening; participates in decision making to the level he wishes; and makes a decision about screening that is consistent with his preferences.
- CDC supports a man's right to discuss the pros and cons of prostate cancer screening with his physician and to make his own decision about screening.
- CDC does not recommend routine screening for prostate cancer because there is no scientific consensus on whether screening and

treatment of early stage prostate cancer reduces mortality. (National Center for Chronic Disease Prevention and Health, 2003, p. 3)

Regarding male vulnerability to other diseases, Kraemer (2000) reports that men are physically more vulnerable than women. Although there are more male than female embryos, the male embryo is much more at risk of being terminated before conception than the female embryo. After conception, the male fetus is at greater risk of death or damage, and

> perinatal brain damage, cerebral palsy, congenital deformities of the genitalia and limbs, premature birth, and stillbirth are commoner in boys. By the time a boy is born, a newborn girl is the physiological equivalent of a 4 to 6 week old boy. (p. 1611)

Kraemer (2000) indicates that after the male child is born, a pattern sets in and male children are more prone to developmental disorders. Hyperactivity, autism, stammering, and Tourette's Syndromes are three times more prevalent in boys than girls and conduct disorders are twice as prevalent among boys. Kraemer (2000) believes that to cope with the variety of problems faced by boys, "Males are attempting something special all through life" (p. 1609).

Despite the problems identified with male health, Courtenay (2000) believes that "policymakers and health professionals alike have paid very little attention to men's health risks, or to their greater risk of premature death" (p. 84). Courtenay goes on to say that: "The consistent, underlying presumption in medical literature is that what it means to be a man in America has no bearing on how men work, drink, drive, fight, or take risks" (p. 84). She notes that few articles have been written regarding the health of men in general and men in the 15 to 24 age range, in particular, although younger men have serious problems with sexually transmitted diseases (STDs), testicular cancer, and mental health. "Despite this dearth of literature, men's health was recently ranked by American College Health Association members as their fifth top priority for continuing education" (Courtenay, 2000, p. 84).

AVOIDABLE REASONS FOR MALE HEALTH PROBLEMS

In covering sessions on men's health at the 2000 American Psychological Association's annual convention, Kogan (2000) reports that panelists all agreed that the pressures men feel to maintain a strong image of masculinity is literally making them sick. She notes that many men don't get regular checkups because the feelings of vulnerability and passivity in the role of patient are incompatible with their view of male behavior. Men shy away from psychotherapy because talking about their feelings is often felt to be feminizing and inconsistent with male roles. Because men let their health slide, they place themselves at particular risk for preventable diseases and illnesses. Men live shorter lives than women and have higher risks for all fifteen leading causes of death, according to Kogan.

Kraemer (2000) indicates that men are more vulnerable to health problems from the beginning of life, but that caregivers assume that a boy should be tougher than a girl. Cultural expectations about the way boys should react to social and emotional stressors shape the experience of boys as they grow up. Kraemer believes that the boys most at risk of developing serious health-related problems are "the boys who don't talk. They become ashamed of being ashamed, and try to stop feeling anything. This makes them seem invulnerable, even to themselves. This is not a safe strategy" (p. 1610). Kraemer suggests that male patterns of mismanagement of risk lead to dangerous behaviors including drug and alcohol abuse and violence and reports increasing rates of male suicide, death by violence, and death by avoidable accidents, which he attributes to "poor motor and cognitive regulation in developing males" (p. 1610).

Harrison, Chin, and Ficarrotto (1988) indicate that as much as three fourths of the seven-year difference in life expectancy between men and women is attributable to socialization. Although parents often believe that boys are tougher than girls, boys are far more vulnerable to illness and disease than girls. Male children are more likely to develop a variety of behavioral difficulties such as hyperactivity, stuttering, dyslexia, and learning disorders. There seems to be little evidence that these behavioral health problems experienced by boys are genetically determined.

In explaining the difference in health data between men and women, Harrison et al. write the following:

Male socialization into aggressive behavioral patterns seems clearly related to the higher death rate from external causes. Male anxiety about
the achievement of masculine status seems to result in a variety of behaviors that can be understood as compensatory. (p. 306)

In explaining some of the reasons for poor health care by men, Harrison et al. (1988) believe that health choices made by men are associated
with strongly defined masculine roles and write the following:

... men's basic needs are the same as women's: all persons need to be
known and to know, to be depended upon and to be dependent, to be
loved and to love, and to find purpose and meaning in life. The socially
prescribed male role, however, requires men to be non-communicative,
competitive and nonloving, and inexpressive, and to evaluate life success in terms of external achievement rather than personal and interpersonal fulfillment. All men are caught in this double bind. If a man fulfills
the prescribed role requirements, his basic needs go unmet; if these
needs are met, he may consider himself, or be considered by others, as
unmanly. (p. 297)

One way children cope with anxiety derived from sex-role expectations is
the development of *compensatory masculinity* (Tiller, 1967). *Compensatory masculinity* behaviors range from the innocent to the insidious. Boys
naturally imitate the male models available to them and can be observed
overemphasizing male gait and male verbal patterns. But if the motive is
the need to prove the right to male status, more destructive behavioral
patterns may result, and persist into adulthood. Boys are often compelled
to take risks that result in accidents; older youth often begin smoking and
drinking as a symbol of adult male status (Farrell, 1974); automobiles are
often utilized as an extension of male power; and some men find confirmation of themselves in violence toward those whom they do not consider confirming their male roles (Churchill, 1967). (p. 298)

In reporting the health consequences of compensatory masculinity,
Karlberg, Unden, Elofsson, and Krakau (1998) studied Type A behavior
and its relation to automobile accidents. Type A behavior has been stud-

ied extensively for its impact on coronary heart disease and includes several components the authors found to be risk factors for automobile accidents: Impatience, easily aroused irritability, hostility, and being in a hurry even when hurrying wasn't necessary. The authors found that men with Type A behavior had higher rates of automobile accidents when in a hurry than women with similar personality traits. Aaron et al. (1985) found a strong relation between Type A behavior and alcohol ingestion in a study of 12,886 men aged 35 to 57 years. The authors concluded that Type A men have a high need for relaxation which makes them more inclined to drink alcohol.

Moore (1995) reports an interesting paradoxical finding on Type A personality and coronary heart disease. In a 1974 study, over 3,000 men ages 35 to 59 were interviewed and classified with either type A or type B personalities. Of those who had heart attacks over the next nine years, 69% had been classified as Type As. However, if a Type A man survived an initial first attack, he lived longer than Type Bs who had also had heart attacks. Moore believes the reason for this is that Type A men are more responsive to the need to change their health patterns. As men who are achievement-oriented and highly motivated to succeed, they relish a challenge, change their lifestyles, and enjoy the results of better health and knowing that they are doing well.

In describing the many differences in health-related behaviors between men and women, Courtenay (2000) believes that

> men's behavior is a major—if not the primary—determinant of their excess mortality and premature deaths. Furthermore, this review reveals that the leading causes of disease and death among men are clearly linked to over 30 behaviors and lifestyle habits that are controllable and can be modified. (p. 110)

Courtenay (2000) identified the following behaviors that negatively affect health: (a) combining alcohol with drugs and smoking, which increases the risk of cancer by 15 times; (b) unbelted driving, which increases the risk of brain injuries and other disabilities; (c) violent behavior and fighting; (d) the lack of regular health checkups; (e) a continuation of unhealthy lifestyles including obesity; (f) the lack of exercise; (g) The tendency to self-medicate with alcohol and illicit drugs; (h) the lack of use of vitamins; (i) less sleep or less quality sleep than women which increases the risk of accidents and health problems; (j) lack of helmet use when driving motorcycles; (k) risky sexual behavior leading to STDs (sexually transmitted diseases) and AIDS; (l) an unwillingness to use sun protection to prevent skin cancer; (m) the underuse of dietary fiber and the overuse of fat, which often leads to cardiovascular problems in men; (n) the use of anabolic steroids in sports and weight training, which increases the risk of cardiovascular disease and cancer; (o) dangerous jobs that require unsafe risk-taking (although men constitute only a little over half of the workforce, they account for 94% of the fatal injuries on the job (National Institute of Occupational Safety and Health, 1993); (p) unsafe driving, driving while under the influence of alcohol or drugs, and driving without proper use of safety equipment; (q) involvement in risky sports and recreation; (r) criminal activity (men are involved in 85% of the crimes in America); and (s) unemployment, underemployment, and job discrimination against men, men of color, and older men.

Courtenay (2000) believes that these risk factors for poor health and lessened longevity are avoidable. However, he also thinks that there have been few attempts to find out why men choose behaviors that negatively affect their health and asks the following:

> ... why do men behave more self-destructively than women, and why do they do less to promote their health? The failure to identify and examine men's risk taking as problematic perpetuates the false, yet widespread, cultural assumption that these behaviors are "natural" or inherent. Indeed, the failure to question men's risk-taking behavior and violence reflects an underlying social assumption that it is normal, that men just are violent or are risk takers. (Courtenay, 2000, p. 111)

In answering these questions, Courtenay (2000) suggests that risk-taking behavior helps men define themselves as masculine and manly. He urges us to learn more about this process, particularly, when it happens, who influences the behavior, and what we can do to change it. He also wonders why we have so little research on ways of influencing men to improve their health-related behavior. Although there has been a great deal of emphasis on the use of psychological interventions with men, seldom do these interventions help reduce health risks or provide services to specific portions of the male population by race or ethnicity and sexual orientation, or for incarcerated men or men in poverty. And as significant as the prior concerns are, Courtenay reports that when men do see doctors, they receive less advice and information about changing their health-related behavior than do women. Misener and Fuller (1995) indicate that only 29% of the physicians surveyed routinely provide instruction on performing testicular self-examination as compared to 86% of the physicians surveyed who provide instruction to women on performing breast self-examination.

To help reduce the risk of poor health and early death among men, Courtenay (1996) suggests the use of a health-risk assessment which includes physical and emotional indicators of "at risk" behavior, and that medical and psychological personnel use this type of assessment to help men deal with risky but avoidable behaviors which needlessly affect their health. Among the assessment items with relevance for health is information pertaining to the following: (a) satisfaction with work, personal life, and relationships; (b) work-related problems including frequent job changes, fighting, or sexual harassment charges; (c) the date of the last health checkup and if any problems were noted; (d) how often a man sees a physician and under what circumstances; (e) weight, amount of exercise, and caloric or fat intake; (f) existence of serious health problems in a man's biological family; (g) involvement in risky sports or recreation; (h) the number of times a man has been married or divorced; (i) financial problems; (j) the average amount of alcohol or illicit drugs consumed per week; (k) all current prescription and over-the-counter drugs taken; (l) indications of metabolic syndrome (high blood sugars, high blood pressure readings, waist size greater than 36 in., and high cholesterol, all of which are related to cardiovascular problems in men); (m) sexual history including STDs, unprotected sex, number of sexual partners, recent sexual activity, erectile problems, or other sexual problems; (n) last prostate checkup; (o) smoking history; (p) level of danger at work or the existence of dangerous chemicals in the workplace; (q) the length of a work commute; (r) the average number of hours of sleep per night; (s) any history of violent behavior including fights and domestic violence; (t) evidence of problems with temper or irritability; (u) problems with depression or anxiety and any prior experiences and the reasons; (v) early life health or emotional problems including fighting, abuse, gang membership, fire setting, animal cruelty, and other problems that might suggest early life traumas and subsequent acting-out behavior, or internalized emotional problems; (w) any history of accidents or brain injuries; (x) any history of abusing children; (y) prior surgeries or medical problems; (z) the number of close friends and how often the client sees them; (aa) attendance at church or synagogue; (bb) quality of the relationship with parents and how long parents lived or their current age, if alive; and (cc) educational level and achievement (grades).

One final reason for health problems in men is explained by a series of studies in which the level of self-involvement in health care correlated strongly with good health and longevity. The studies (Seligman, 2004) show a very high correlation between self-involvement in one's own health care and the level of education. One study Seligman (2004) refers to is a 2001 study conducted by the CDC which found that college graduates were "three times as likely to live healthy lives as those who never went beyond high school" (p. 114). With men increasingly opting not to pursue higher education, the study predicts a high correlation between male health problems and the lack of self-involvement in their own health care. It further predicts that uninvolved patients will misuse what medical care they do get. According to Seligman, half of the 1.8 billion prescriptions issued annually are incorrectly taken and over 40% of the patients with diabetes (a large number of whom are men) don't understand blood sugar values or what to do if those values are high. Seligman goes on to say,

> Intelligent people tend to be the most knowledgeable about health related issues. Health literacy, matters more than it used to. In the past, big gains in health and longevity were associated with improvements in public sanitation, immunization and other initiatives not requiring decisions by ordinary citizens. But today, the major threats to health are chronic diseases—which, inescapably, require patients to participate in the treatment, which means in turn that they need to understand what's going on. (Seligman, 2004, p. 114)

DEPRESSION AND SUICIDE

Cochran and Rabinowitz (2003) write that, "Psychologists increasingly recognize depression as a serious, albeit often undiagnosed, condition in men. In fact, undiagnosed and untreated depression in men may be one reason why many more men than women commit suicide" (p. 132). Anderson, Kochanek, and Murphy (1997) indicate that suicide rates for men are estimated to range from 20 to 25 per 100,000 for men in their late teens to mid-30s and as high as 30 to 70 per 100,000 for men over age 65. Heifner (1997) reports that for men of all ages and races, suicide is a significant mortality risk factor, far exceeding rates for women in all age categories. The author believes that male suicide is an effort to "take control" of a life that may be tragically out of control with no apparent alternatives in sight. Cochran and Rabinowitz (2003) write the following about male depression:

> Although men are often perceived to be immune to depressive disorders, there is mounting evidence that many men do in fact suffer from various manifestations of depression. These manifestations, which may include typical depressive episodes, are often associated with alcohol and drug abuse, interpersonal conflict, and externalizing or acting-out behavior patterns. Effective diagnosis and treatment of men who suffer from the many manifestations of depression remain a challenge for psychologists, educators, and scientists. (p. 13)

THE MID-LIFE CRISIS

MacDoniels (1997) describes the mid-life crisis as a period in mid-life lasting about four years, when men are in transition and where their future direction is in doubt. The transition is often caused by physical changes in men and the realization that life goals may not be met. MacDoniels writes the following:

> This period of time is one in which adults take on new responsibilities at the workplace and therefore often feel a need to "reappraise previous life structures with an eye to making revisions 'while there is still time'" (Huyck, 1997). The term of "mid-life crisis" was originally coined by Jaques (1965) who claimed that people encounter a crisis as they realize

their own mortality and a change in time frame from "time since birth" to "time left to live" (Shek, 1996). Specifically, the mid-life crisis is often thought to include: worries about the future, inability to enjoy leisure time, a feeling that health is deteriorating, a negative evaluation of the marital relationship, a negative evaluation of work life, and stress arising from taking care of the elderly. (Shek, 1996, p. 1)

Daniel Levinson (1979) writes that men hope life starts at 40 but begin to anxiously believe that it actually ends there. Fearing that the latter is true, many men frantically try and make changes in their lives that permit early stages of youth to continue. Levinson believes that the mid-life crisis is the middle stage between youth and adulthood and that it creates a crisis in up to 80% of the men studied. The remaining men are actually in crisis but are in a state of denial. Levinson describes a number of developmental stages in adult life and delineates an early adult era from the mid-20s to the late 30s. He also discusses a middle adult era from the mid-40s to the early 60s. What is in-between is what he calls the years of mid-life transition. He sees these years as a bridge between young adulthood and senior membership in one's occupational world, a period dominated by self-examination, difficult life choices, and questions about life meaning that often result in cataclysmic social and emotional changes in men and certainly qualify as a legitimate crisis.

In seeking an alternative reason for the concept of a mid-life crisis, Kruger (1994) believes it can be identified as an adjustment disorder related to specific stressors experienced by men, such as getting married, having children, job stress, and so forth. Krueger believes that the mid-life crisis may have its origins in the leisure time we have in our society which often leads to self-absorption and acting-out, providing many men with a belief that it's acceptable and even necessary for emotional health, to leave wives and children, find new relationships, and develop new families to offset a sense of failure. In America, the crisis of mid-life usually occurs between ages 35 and 50. In many other countries, social events take place at much earlier times. In those societies and among men from different countries who are still coping with the traditions of their country of origin, the mid-life crisis may occur in men in their 20s and 30s or as late as their 60s and 70s.

For our purposes, the mid-life crisis is a period of severe discontent in men and a belief that if major changes aren't made and made soon, life will spiral downward and bad marriages, unhappy children, boring work, and lack of challenge will plague a man for the rest of his life. For this reason, Kruger's (1994) idea of an adjustment disorder provides therapists with an opportunity to help men with meaning-of-life issues and in practical ways, to help them cope with defining social and emotional challenges which may affect their lives throughout the remainder of the life cycle. As an example, a client described his treatment for a mid-life crisis:

> I was going through a hell of a mid-life crisis. I was unhappy, irritable, and mad at my wife for getting older and heavier and feeling that my life was over and there was nothing I could do about it. I was 38. I went to a male therapist and he listened and nodded a lot and let me talk until I was blue in the face. When I was done bitching about my life, he looked at me very closely and asked me what I would do about my life if I could ... if I wasn't constrained by anything. Why, I stammered, I'd be a writer. I'd be with a cool woman who appreciated my writing. I'd quit my job and make a living writing, and I'd smoke dope and drink good liquor, and have a ball. I'd go live in Mexico where it's cheap and I could live on $100 a month.
>
> He asked me what was stopping me now from doing exactly what I wanted to do. Well, I said, you can't just pick up and leave. Why not, he asked? He was persistent. Well, because I have responsibilities, obligations, mouths to feed, payments to make. Why not give your wife an allowance and do what you really want to do? Well, shit, I thought, because I really love my wife, and kids, and my house, and my job, and what the hell is going on with me anyway? That's what I asked him. What the hell is happening to me?
>
> He explained about mid-life crises and Levinson's work on middle adulthood and his findings that a lot of men have trouble getting through mid-life. He said it sometimes precipitated a crisis, which many men handled badly and who often made terrible decisions that ruined other people's lives, and how he didn't want that to happen to me. He gave me a number of things to read and the next time I came to see him, he asked me if I was ready to work and I said, yes, I was, and that was that. We worked

on my feelings of discontent, what was causing them, and we concluded that the death of my parents had precipitated a secondary crisis in my life and that perhaps what I was feeling was a sort of hopelessness and a freezing of my emotions. Maybe I thought some upheaval in my life would make me feel better, but that was wishful thinking. We worked a lot on my feelings about my father and I was struck by how ambivalent they were. The same with my mother.

I have a wonderful wife. She was very generous and supportive. Maybe it took a year and I was in a better place than when we started. And you know, the Mister Smith before my dad died was my dad. Now I'm the Mr. Smith and it feels darn good to know that when people are talking about Mr. Smith, it's me they're talking about and not my dad. And simply put, I didn't want to be Mr. Smith, and now I do.

SEXUAL PROBLEMS

One of the leading reasons men seek help from physicians is for the treatment of sexual problems. Because of the way dating is done in America with its pressure for early sexual encounters, it's not unusual for many men to experience situational impotence and premature ejaculation. Both problems are usually related to performance anxiety and can be dealt with by working with the man's partner if he has a stable relationship. Men often obsess that having failed once in a sexual encounter, suggests the man has a serious problem. Reassurance, letting men read about performance anxiety, and suggesting more stable relationships all help to remove issues of anxiety about sexual performance. There are also techniques to help men stop premature ejaculations, such as helping men focus on things other than sex, or having the partner squeeze the shaft of the man's penis if he feels he is about to have a premature ejaculation. Most men in time develop their own techniques, but sometimes, premature ejaculation occurs anyway, and it's true that men often feel anxious when this happens and think that their partner is going to discount their sexual prowess.

It's also true that some men (about 10%) have physical reasons for impotence related to spinal injuries, diabetes, and strokes. Many medications also cause impotence, and reduced libido, including blood pressure medications. One easy way to find out if a man has a physical reason for impotence is to have his partner check to for erections while he sleeps. Spontaneous erections occur during the sleep cycle every 90 minutes in normal men.

American men often think they should perform well while using alcohol and drugs, but both may inhibit having an erection. Helping men cycle off the use of drugs and alcohol before sex is always a much better approach than suggesting they use Viagra or any of the other medications available for erectile problems that are situational or intermittent in nature. Viagra causes severe headaches and upset stomachs. It also places a severe amount of pressure on the heart which may be bad for men with heart problems or older men developing heart problems who may not know it. Although the newer drugs have a longer staying power than Viagra (30 min until it works and four hours for maximum effectiveness), men still have to be sexually stimulated for the medication to work. Far too many men become dependent on drugs like Viagra and don't think they can have a complete erection without it. Ads for the drug showing fairly young men using Viagra are indications of the misuse of the medication. And contrary to popular belief, Viagra is not an aphrodisiac. It doesn't increase sexual drive but only helps men have harder and longer erections. Some men have difficulty having orgasms with Viagra while others claim it leads to more premature ejaculations. As one of my clients told me,

> I was using Viagra regularly. I'm still only in my 40's and I hated the way it made me feel. My nose would plug up and I'd get these awful headaches. So I stopped using it and you know, I was fine. I realized I was using Viagra as a crutch and I was dependent on it. It's pretty hard to enjoy sex when you have a headache and your nose is plugged, and I just figured that women aren't always as wet as they'd like to be, but it's OK and it doesn't interfere with sex. So what if I'm not as hard as I'd like to be? We still have sex and it's great without the side effects. I'm worried that a whole generation of men are going to dependent on drugs to do what they can do without drugs.

SUMMARIZING REASONS FOR MALE HEALTH PROBLEMS

In summary, the primary reasons for the health problems of men are as follows:

1. Men are more vulnerable to a range of health and mental health problems from birth. This vulnerability to health and behavioral problems continues throughout the life span. There is evidence that male vulnerability is both genetic and related to male socialization.

2. To maintain traditional notions of masculinity and because of reduced cognitive skills, poor judgment, and peer pressure, boys and young men are likely to engage in dangerous activities that lead to physical disabilities and shortened lives. This need to maintain traditional notions of masculinity may continue throughout the life span in some men. Men are far more prone to accidents and homicide than women. The need for men to prove themselves is often called *compensatory masculinity*.

3. Men are less likely than women to seek help for physical and emotional problems. When they do seek help, it is usually at a more advanced stage in an illness or emotional problem. Many researchers believe that the unwillingness to seek help for physical and emotional problems is explained by an unwillingness to feel vulnerable, passive, and out of control. If men feel vulnerable and passive when they receive medical care, perhaps part of the problem is explained by the way care is given and men are treated.

4. Men tend to internalize stress and convert it into physical problems, substance abuse, or emotional difficulty. To complicate this problem, men sometimes live solitary lives with no one to talk to, or they may find it difficult to communicate their feelings to others.

5. Men often believe that being careful about health is a sign of weakness and that going to doctors may cause bad luck. This belief often causes them to take health risks.

6. Heavy drinking is sometimes encouraged among men as a sign of masculinity. Popular sayings such as "drinking someone under the table" or "he can sure handle his liquor" are often positive reinforcers

for men to drink too much or to binge drink. Although drinking too much may not be a sign of addiction, it is a dangerous behavior and may lead to sexual aggression, assaults, and accidents. Drinking as a sign of manliness is often reinforced by the popular culture, which romanticizes drinking and portrays it as an acceptable way for men to resolve personal problems.

CLINICAL WORK WITH MEN WHO HAVE HEALTH PROBLEMS

Getting men to initiate contact with their physicians, following through on medical advice, and maintaining healthy lives are often primary tasks in clinical work. The following suggestions might help clinicians in their work with men:

1. Don't separate physical health from emotional health. If you're seeing a man for a mental health problem, you need to be equally concerned about his physical health. Many therapists encourage and even require men in therapy to receive a complete physical examination as part of their treatment. Not only does this help rule out medical reasons for the client's emotional difficulties, but it also establishes a baseline for health. Effective therapy should not only result in better social functioning but it should also facilitate better health.

2. In the psychosocial assessment, it's important to get a full health history. If there are any problems that have significance for health (erectile problems, more than two drinks a day, obesity, shortness of breath, heart palpitations, smoking, heavy use of caffeine), the client should be told that health issues dictate that he see a physician for a complete evaluation. A health history will also confirm prior family illnesses which might suggest that men are at risk for certain types of health problems (for example, high blood pressure, heart problems, diabetes, stroke, and cancer). We also need to know every medication the client uses, even over-the-counter medications. Men often self-medicate and certain medications are sometimes used by men for emotional rather than health problems. For example, the use of Motrin to help men sleep or control anxiety is not unusual. The

health history should also determine if drug addictions are present. Often men are addicted to legal drugs they were placed on for a short period of time but have continued using. This might include painkillers such as Vicadin and Percadan, and tranquilizers such as Valium, Ativan, and Xanax. Interestingly, a number of men the author has spoken to who are members of H.M.O.s (health maintenance organizations) indicate that addicting drugs are often very easy to obtain well past the time of their original use.

3. Keep a list of physicians who are sympathetic to men and easily establish rapport with men because male clients will often see a physician who is kind and considerate. If the referral comes from you, it may help the client seek help when he might otherwise be reluctant to contact a doctor on his own. Suggest that finding a good doctor often requires shopping around and it may take a bit of time to find the right person.

4. A number of health clubs will work with men to help them get in better shape. When the author was executive director of a family service agency, he was able to get health clubs to provide reduced costs and specialized help for many of his staff and their clients. Men receiving individualized help can often make significant changes.

SUMMARY

This chapter reports the serious health problems of men and the reasons men often fail to take care of themselves physically and emotionally. Suggestions are provided for ways of helping men see doctors more often, cope with early signs of physical and emotional health problems, and follow through on treatment.

Male Bashing

Let's take a moment and read the average man's mind: Sex, sex, sex, red meat, sex, sex, sex, beer, sex, sex, sex, Cheetos, sex, sex, sex, baseball, football, sex, sex, sex ...

—*Alkon* (2003, pp. 17–23)

Male bashing is one of those serious problems in America we tend not to take very seriously. But just as women and ethnic and racial minority groups have been bashed in the past and often continue to feel the sting of pejorative jokes and name calling, bashing is a harmful and insensitive way of responding to any group since the essence of bashing is hostility and a feeling of superiority. This chapter discusses the bashing of men and what we can do to stop it.

Cary (1998) says that examples of male-bashing can be found all around us

in books and movies that denigrate men as ridiculously immature and entirely ruled by their little heads, in sitcoms that make husbands the butt of every family joke, in TV commercials that disparage male pride or portray them as unable to care for themselves. (p. 15)

Wetzstein (2000) wonders if greeting cards have become another indication of public male bashing and writes the following: "If a man belittles a woman, it could become a lawsuit; but if women belittle men, it's 'a Hallmark card' as noted by the 'increasing number of greeting cards that carry a message of misandry, or man-hating' " (p. 1).

Why the upsurge in male bashing? According to Farrell (1999), part of the reason is that some women are obviously angry at men. Farrell believes that many women have had to fend for themselves as men abandon families leaving women as primary breadwinners and responsible for child care. Cary (1998) writes the following: "... many women have found themselves divorced, often facing the double burden of child care and financial responsibilities that used to be divided among couples" (p. 16). Cary further suggests that it may be easier for women to say that they don't need men and that they're useless when the needs women have are often not met by men. Cary quotes Stephen Johnson, founder and director of The Men's Center of Los Angeles as saying, "I have a hunch that at the heart of it, women are lonely and longing for good relationships with men, but they're afraid such relationships are few and far between" (p. 16). Johnson speculates that in addition to their anger at men, women often say: "If I can't have the kind of man that I want, I'm going to throw stones at the image" (Cary, 1998, p. 16).

In a review of Warren Farrell's 1999 book, *Women Can't Hear What Men Don't*, Young (2000) writes that the gender debate has been primarily about women's problems and men's faults. As a result, "Male bashing flourishes not only in the feminist movement but in popular culture, from sitcoms to greeting cards" (p. 53). Young indicates that arguments made by Farrell are persuasive when he writes that male disadvantages in education, health care, and criminal sentencing have received little attention in the academy, in government, or in the media. Citing Farrell, Young (2000) points out that initiatives to empower girls ignore the fact that boys are the ones who are falling behind in education and that institutions have closed their minds to nonfeminist perspectives because feminism, or what many call the lace curtain, is a concept of gender politics with only one point of view.

Kaufman (1999) says that unlike Lamb, Frodi, Hwang, and Frodi (1982), who found fathers to be as competent as mothers in the care of children and the time spent in activities related to the home, men are portrayed in American commercials, particularly daytime commercials, as uninvolved, passive, incompetent, and dependent on their wives. Very few commercials portray men as involved in the lives of their families. Because many children get important messages from television, this inaccurate portrayal of men in the home has a particularly negative impact on young men and women trying to understand their models of adult male and female behavior. To further confirm the way men and women are portrayed in commercials, I watched television commercials for a week across a number of different channels and noted that many commercials show women and children without a man present. Conversely, similar ads showing men almost always had women and children present. Many of the commercials without men present were for home repair and paint supplies, giving rise to a sense that women will be alone with their children without a man in the home or without a man to help them. This is an interesting finding because divorce in America has been gradually declining in the past ten years.

Abernathy (2003) gives an example of the type of ad that denigrates men. In a digital camera ad, "a young husband walks through a grocery store, trying to match photos in his hand with items on the shelves. Cut to his wife in the kitchen, snapping digital pictures of all the items in the pantry so that hubby won't screw up the shopping" (p. 2).

Two Verizon ads I watched in November 2004 stand out for special mention. In the first ad, a father is trying to help his daughter as she works on the computer. He clearly doesn't know what he's doing and the daughter has an annoyed look on her face. The mother comes into the room and literally shouts at the husband to do what he was supposed to do, which is to take out the garbage and leave *her* daughter alone. That ad resulted in numerous complaints from men's groups. A second Verizon ad shows a father giving his daughters phones so they can call home from school. The daughters have a dismayed look that suggests that calling home is the last thing on their mind and particularly calling their father. At the same time, the mother comes into the room and tells the daughters that they can always use the phone to call their friends. The daughters and their mother embrace and leave the father in the room looking sheepish. He tries to touch one of the daughters as she leaves with the mother but she eludes his touch. Another imbecilic man, the ad says to us.

A Mexicana Airline ad, however, shows that in the Latino culture, men are portrayed in a very different way. In that ad, which I watched in

November 2004, a little girl wakes up in the middle of the night, goes to the window and looks at the moon. She walks to her parents' bedroom and stands by the bed until her father wakes up with a smile, happy to see her even though he'd been fast asleep. The daughter asks her father if they can go to Mexico to see relatives. He smiles and the little girl is embraced by her mother and father and snuggles in bed with both parents. The scene changes and the little girl, holding hands with her parents, walks to the airplane. Both parents are smiling and obviously proud of the little girl as the commercial fades to a scene of Cancún.

I've never seen a male bashing ad on Spanish-speaking television because I suspect they would offend people, but I see them almost daily on English-speaking television. These ads are insulting and play to the most base emotions of people. I doubt very much if they're effective.

Abernathy says that the bashing of men continues in other ways on television and writes,

> It has also been studied by academicians Dr. Katherine Young and Paul Nathanson (2001) in their book *Spreading Misandry: The Teaching of Contempt for Men in Popular Culture.* Young and Nathanson argue that in addition to being portrayed as generally unintelligent, men are ridiculed, rejected, and physically abused in the media. Such behavior, they suggest, "would never be acceptable if directed at women." Evidence of this pattern is found in a 2001 survey of 1,000 adults conducted by the Advertising Standards Association in Great Britain, which found that 2/3 of respondents thought that women featured in advertisements were "intelligent, assertive, and caring," while the men were "pathetic and silly." The number of respondents who thought men were depicted as "intelligent" was a paltry 14%. (While these figures apply to the United Kingdom, comparable advertisements air in the U.S.) (p. 2)

Obviously, ads that portray men in highly negative ways often reinforce harmful stereotypes of men. As Abernathy (2003) argues, "Young men learn that they are expected to screw up, that women will have the brains to their brawn, and that childcare is over their heads" (p. 2).

Morrow (1994) argues that a common theme in feminist literature is that all men are rapists at heart. Quoting Marilyn French, Morrow writes,

"All men are rapists. They rape us with their eyes, their laws, and their codes" (Morrow, 1994, p. 57). In response, the author writes,

> Fine. But the charge that "all men are rapists" is a slander and an outrage. It is also not true—all men are not even potential rapists. All-men-are-rapists is a moral stupidity as well, since it annuls the distinction between a decent man, who does not rape, and a barbarian, who does. If there is no difference between the two men, then there is no meaning to civilization. (Morrow, p. 57)

The author goes on to ask why men are so angry at male bashing:

> Why do men get angry? Are they angry because something in their con-ditioned or instinctive social roles as men revs them up in order to ex-pose them to the worst dangers, like dying in war, like being killed in the line of duty as policemen and fire fighters, or otherwise doing the dirty, dangerous work; 93% of people killed on the job are men. The more dangerous the job, the greater the percentage of men who are doing it. Federal, state and local governments spend hundreds of millions of dol-lars protecting women workers from sexual harassment, while millions of men are still left substantially unprotected from premature death by industrial hazard. Actually, the real reason men get angry is not the dan-ger or premature death. It is mostly because they feel unappreciated. (Morrow, 1994, p. 56)

Kelly and Hall (1994) suggest that another form of male bashing is to unfairly blame men for problems that are not their fault or are inaccu-rately reported. As an example, they point out that The Association for Advanced Training (AAT) publishes study guides for professionals pre-paring for licensing examinations. The following quote regarding spousal violence is taken verbatim from that study guide: "Because adult violence in the home most often involves the male as the aggressor, the research on spouse abuse has traditionally focused on the battering hus-band and the battered wife, and the following review of literature re-flects this emphasis" (AAT, 1991, p. 55). Kelly and Hall (1992a) indicate that the AAT material is inaccurate and that they have provided evi-dence that "men and women are equally violent perpetrators of domestic abuse ... there remains an urgent need to dispute mistaken beliefs and assumptions regarding men" (p. 480).

Leo (1994) furthers the discussion when he writes:

The current emphasis on men as beasts and women as needing special protection makes it all the harder to forge partnerships between women and men. The most important need is to break the hold of victim feminism and an agenda wholly centered on women. (p. 24)

Leo (1994) believes that anti-male attitudes are filtering into counseling and psychotherapy. One therapist told him that at a Wisconsin conference for therapists, "The air was thick with anti-male gibes. Later, when a man complained about these comments, one of the women running the conference muttered, 'What that man deserved was a "f---you" ' " (p. 24). Many of these remarks, according to therapists Leo interviewed, came from people involved in counseling couples.

In what has become standard fare for discussing men, Allen (2003) asks if men are obsolete and answers that they are, except in the area of violence:

There remains, to be sure, one large sector in which men retain unquestioned domination: crime. In 2001, the FBI reports, men arrested for violent crime outnumbered women by roughly 5 to 1. (For murder the ratio was 7 to 1.) Even in nonviolent categories males prevailed (11 to 1 in illegal weapons possession; 5 to 1 in drunken driving). Indeed, aside from prostitution, only in the categories of fraud and embezzlement have women begun to close the gender gap. And even in these office bound areas—witness the latest round of corporate scandals—when it comes to big-time booty, the boys are still way out in front. (p. 33)

STEREOTYPES OF MEN

Men often feel (a) confused about their role in society, (b) blamed for the misdeeds of some men, and (c) unrecognized for their good work as fathers and husbands. Because television portrays men as passive, weak, and incompetent, Kaufman (1999) argues that television commercials are socializing agents for men. Because men often look to television for their messages about male roles, particularly the roles of fathers, they often get distorted, incorrect, and even harmful messages that support a distant and passive role for men as fathers.

Morrison (1994) wonders if a tax on men to cover the costs to women and children of rape, physical and sexual abuse, abandonment, harassment, and emotional abuse might not be a good idea. Grant-Bowman (1994) proposes laws to fine and jail men who make leering and offensive remarks about women on the streets of our country. In defending her position, she discusses

> ... the revelation of the secret history of sexual aggression: domestic violence; rape by friends and husbands as well as by strangers; sexual harassment in the workplace, as well as in the academy, church and street; and similar abuse of relationships of unequal power and trust, such as those between clergy and parishioner, divorce lawyer and client, teacher and student. (p. 15A)

Lehrman (1994) believes that highly pejorative statements about men such as the ones by Grant-Bowman (1994) and Morrison (1994), although hurtful and offensive to men and often having a small following, "are being voraciously employed by university administrations and corporate offices that fear being called 'sexist' " (Lehrman, 1994, p. 15A). These policies often place men in difficult and sometimes indefensible positions in terms of common behaviors for both men and women that may, however, be seen organizationally as sexually harassing or indicative of workplace violence. Morrow (1994) believes that men often feel they are "fair game, a payback for the years, the centuries of male domination and oppression ... A man who objects to male bashing must be anti-woman" (p. 56). Morrow believes that male bashing, although insulting to men and suggestive of hostility to men by women, is often discounted by women who continue to male bash in a belief that men can take it and that it may have a positive socializing effect on men. Stillman (1994) says that although sexual harassment is a problem we should all take seriously

I feel that in the unfettered pursuit of gender politics, women have made a grave mistake in not examining broader issues, such as that of office harassment in general. What men have had to put up with over the years to rise through the corporate and bureaucratic marketplace, frankly, is as odious to me as sexual harassment. But men have never lobbied against such wage-slave requirements as mandatory lying to cover up company crimes, mandatory company retreats, mandatory obsequiousness toward higher-ups, mandatory cocktails with the bosses brother-in-law, and so on. Maybe they should. However, in their fight against sexual harassment, women have failed to take into account that power always resists challenge, and change is always met with resistance. If women could stop taking the general unfairness of the workplace so personally, they would find allies rather than enemies among their fellow worker-bees. (p. 32)

In a further negative response to male bashing, Heckard (1998) writes that humor often helps reduce exasperation in relationships but admits that jokes about husbands and other men in a woman's life often "… deviate from tasteful wit into male bashing when they capitalize on failures and exploit weaknesses, pitting the genders against each other" (p. 46). Heckard (1998) goes on to say that

Male bashing threatens our relationships with men. Because it's essentially gossip, male bashing undermines trust—the foundation of relationships—and makes it difficult for men to be vulnerable. Jeff, a church friend, once admitted to me that he avoided committees on which a particular woman served because she often used her husband's weaknesses as amusing anecdotes. "If she talks like that about him," he confided, "what might she say about me?"

Male bashing hurts our children. Initially, I was amused to hear my five-year-old son tell a baby sitter we have four children in our family: himself, his brother, his sister, and his father. But I was embarrassed when I later learned he'd merely repeated my own words. As my son and I talked, he asked me, "Mommy, what do you say about me?" I realized when my children hear me belittle their father, they question their own security. After all, if someone as powerful as Daddy is vulnerable to such disregard, aren't they also? (p. 46)

MALE BASHING THEMES

To better understand male bashing, the author collected Internet jokes sent to him by women friends who say that their e-mail folders are clogged with male bashing jokes. In trying to understand male bashing themes, the following categories are noted: male insensitivity and stupidity, women are better without men, and male sexual inadequacy.

Theme 1—Male Insensitivity and Stupidity

1. Question: What do you call an intelligent, good looking, sensitive man? Answer: A rumor.
2. Male Prayer: I pray for a deaf-mute nymphomaniac with huge boobs who owns a liquor store. Amen.
3. Question: Why do little boys whine? Answer: Because they're practicing to be men.
4. Question: Why do female black widow spiders kill their males after mating? Answer: To stop the snoring before it starts.
5. Question: Why do men whistle when they're sitting on the toilet? Answer: Because it helps them remember which end they need to wipe.

Theme 2—Women Are Better Without Men:

1. Question: What should you do if you see your ex-husband rolling around in pain on the ground? Answer: Shoot him again.
2. A couple are lying in bed. The man says, "I am going to make you the happiest woman in the world," and the woman says, "I'll miss you."
3. Question: How can you tell when a man is well hung? Answer: When you can just barely slip your finger in between his neck and the noose.

4. Question: What does it mean when a man is in your bed gasping for breath and calling your name? Answer: You didn't hold the pillow down long enough.

5. A Woman's Perfect Breakfast: She's sitting at the table with a tall, vanilla latte. Her son is on the cover of the Wheaties box. Her daughter is on the cover of Business Week. Her boyfriend is on the cover of Playgirl. Her husband is on the back of the milk carton.

Theme 3—Male Sexual Inadequacy

1. He said: Since I first laid eyes on you, I've wanted to make love to you really badly. She said: Well, you succeeded.

2. He said: Shall we try swapping positions tonight? She said: That's a good idea ... you stand by the ironing board while I sit on the sofa.

3. My husband came home with a tube of KY jelly and said, "This will make you happy tonight." He was right. When he went out of the bedroom, I squirted it all over the doorknobs. He couldn't get back in.

4. Why don't women blink during foreplay? Answer: They don't have time.

5. "It's just too hot to wear clothes today," Jack says as he stepped out of the shower. "Honey, what do you think the neighbors would think if I mowed the lawn like this?" "Probably that I married you for your money," she replied.

RESPONDING TO MALE BASHING

As professionals, we should not allow male bashing in our practice. When female clients make sweeping statements about men that imply something generically negative, we have a responsibility to call them on it just as we would with a client who made racist or hostile religious statements. This also applies to people in our personal life. When others send me jokes with a racial or gender theme, I tell them to stop because I find the jokes offensive. You can do the same and you can urge your clients to stop accepting male bashing jokes. Trading information and insights about male bashing can also help. We should all start educating our friends not to bash anyone and that male bashing is intolerable.

What if you hear male bashing from friends, family members, even clients? How should you handle it? In my opinion, male bashing is every bit as hurtful and suggestive of bigotry as racial bashing and homophobia. It's not funny and it's decidedly hurtful. If you secretly agree with female clients and friends who bash men and either passively accept or encourage male bashing as a form of catharsis, you aren't helping your female clients at all and you need to consider the reasons for your behavior and to do something serious about changing it. Male bashing has no place at all in therapy. It's a sign of bias and it needs to be dealt with gently but firmly.

When a woman tells me a male bashing joke, I let her know it isn't funny and remind her that she's talking to a man who believes that men should be treated with respect and dignity. I never retaliate by telling female bashing jokes because I believe they are hurtful and have no place in the interaction between people, even among friends. When I hear female bashing jokes from male clients and students, I immediately let them know I don't find these jokes funny and I assume that telling me jokes about women means that they want to talk about problems they are having with women. Being Jewish, I've heard every anti-Semitic joke under the sun and I can tell you they hurt as much now as they did when I first heard the term *Jewing them down* when I was five years old.

I've heard more male bashing in the academy than in any other environment in which I have worked. The lack of civility between men and women and the gender wars I see in the academy where male bashing and anti-male sentiment are at their strongest are signs of a deteriorating workplace. I suspect those of you who work with academics in therapy have heard the bitterness that exists between men and women on issues of tenure, promotion, and leadership roles. Out of male bashing comes behavior that creates a miserable work experience for many men and women. It just has no place in education, in civil society, or, particularly, in therapy.

SUMMARY

This chapter discusses the prevalence of male bashing, the impact it has on men, central themes and reasons for male bashing, and strategies to deal with clients, friends and family members who bash men.

PART II

Clinical Work With Men

A Gender-Specific Approach to Diagnosing Male Clients

This chapter discusses the difficult issue of diagnosis with men and the stigmatizing nature of labels which tend to present male behavior in ways that men believe are unfair, inaccurate, and stereotypic. A case presenting a misdiagnosis of a male client is used to show how gender bias and incompetence when working with men can have disastrous results.

CONCERNS ABOUT DIAGNOSIS WITH MALE CLIENTS

Diagnosing male problems seems particularly fraught with ambiguity, worker bias, and politically correct notions of men as dysfunctional without question. The major diagnostic tool used with all clients in America, the *Diagnostic and Statistical Manual of Mental Disorders* (DSM–IV; 4th ed.) has been criticized for a number of these reasons. Cloud (2003) has fundamental concerns about the accuracy of the DSM–IV:

> ... can even a thousand PhDs gathered at a dozen conferences ever really know the significance of such vague symptoms as "fatigue," "low self-esteem" and "feelings of hopelessness"? (You need only two of those, along with a couple of friends telling the doctor you seem depressed, to be a good candidate for something called dysthymic disorder.) Though it's

fashionable these days to think of psychiatry as just another arm of medicine, there is no biological test for any of these disorders. (p. 105)

Other concerns about the DSM–IV include the criticism that diagnostic categories were determined by ad hoc committee decisions that were often contentious and were only resolved by pleas for agreement and consensus, and that the DSM–IV is just a checklist of symptoms used to justify a worker's preconceived notions about the client (Cloud, 2003). To improve the DSM–IV or diagnostic manuals like it, Cloud (2003) suggests the use of four categories of disorders:

> Those arising from brain disease, those arising from problems controlling one's drive, those arising from problematic personal dispositions, and those arising from life circumstances. While such groupings are imperfect they at least get clinicians focused, not only on the symptoms of an illness, but on its possible causes as well. (p. 106)

The DSM also has been criticized because it fails to provide an individual framework from which to fully understand many of the environmental and historical factors affecting clients, and, as a result, is thought to be overly focused on pathology (Saleebey, 1996). The client's uniqueness is seldom represented by a DSM diagnosis, and neither are the positive behaviors clients bring with them to treatment that often determine whether the client will improve. In his appraisal of the DSM–IV, Saleebey (1996) writes the following:

> The DSM–IV (American Psychiatric Association, 1994), although only seven years removed from its predecessor, has twice the volume of text on disorders. Victimhood has become big business as many adults, prodded by a variety of therapists, gurus, and ministers, go on the hunt for wounded inner children and the poisonous ecology of their family background. These phenomena are not unlike a social movement or evangelism. (p. 296)

Whaley (2001) believes that White clinicians often see Black male clients as having paranoid symptoms that are more fundamentally a cultural distrust of Whites because of historical experiences with racism. He believes that the diagnostic process with Black male clients tends to discount the negative impact of racism and leads to diagnostic judgments about clients, suggesting that they are more dysfunctional than they really are. This tendency to misdiagnose Black men, or to diagnose a more serious condition than may be warranted, is what Whaley calls "pseudo-transference" and believes that cultural stereotyping by clinicians who fail to understand the impact of racism leads to "more severe diagnoses and restrictive interventions" (p. 558) with Black male clients. Whaley's work suggests that clinicians may incorrectly use diagnostic labels with male clients they either feel uncomfortable with or whose cultural differences create some degree of hostility. This casts doubt on the accuracy of diagnostic labels with an entire range of male clients.

DeGrandpre (1999) provides an egregious example of gender misdiagnosis when he reports that a diagnosis of Attention Deficit Hyperactivity Disorder (ADHD) made solely from observation of children in a physician's office routinely resulted in misdiagnosis. Sharp, Walter, and Marsh (1999) found that boys were diagnosed with ADHD at rates three and four times higher than girls although ratios as low as two to one have been found in community studies. Wilke (1994) argues that men are diagnosed with alcoholism because of stereotypes of drinking that apply to some men but not all men. As a clear misdiagnoses in the mental health field

Morey and Ochoa (1989) asked 291 psychiatrists and psychologists to complete a checklist of symptoms for a male client whom they had diagnosed with a personality disorder. When the checklists were later correlated with the DSM criteria, nearly three of four clinicians had made mistakes in applying the diagnostic criteria. (McLaughlin, 2002, p. 259)

In a sample of 42 psychologists and 17 psychiatrists, Davis, Blashfield, and McElroy (1993) had the sample read and diagnose case reports containing different symptoms of Narcissistic Personality Disorder (NPS). Ninety-four percent of the sample made mistakes applying the diagnostic criteria, whereas 25% diagnosed NPS when less than half the DSM criteria were met.

In another example of incorrect diagnosis based on first impressions, Robertson and Fitzgerald (1990) randomly assigned 47 counselors to watch videos of a depressed male portrayed by an actor. The only changes made in the videos were the client's type of employment (professional vs. blue collar) and the client's family of origin (traditional or nontraditional). The researcher found that counselors made more negative diagnostic judgments when the actor portrayed a blue-collar worker and came from a nontraditional family. The signs and symptoms of any specific emotional disorders were secondary to the worker's bias.

In an example of another type of bias, self-confirmatory bias, or diagnosis based only on the information collected by the clinician that confirms his or her original diagnosis, Haverkamp (1993) had counseling and counseling psychology students watch a video of an initial counseling session and then write down the questions they wanted to ask in a follow-up session with the client. The majority of students (64%) wanted to ask questions that confirmed their original diagnostic impression of the client. A follow up study by Pfeiffer, Whelan, and Martin (2000) came to a similar conclusion.

In a related type of error, the error of using treatment approaches that confirm one's original diagnosis, Rosenhan (1973) had research associates admitted to a psychiatric hospital after complaining of auditory hallucinations. Although the researchers stopped complaining of the symptoms, the treatment staff continued using a diagnosis indicating a serious mental illness when none was present.

REDUCING ERRORS IN DIAGNOSIS

McLaughlin (2002) suggests the following ways of reducing errors in diagnosing, which are very applicable to male clients: (a) Don't make too much or too little of the evidence at hand; (b) try and note the biasing effect of your workplace which may routinely diagnose everyone in the same way; (c) use falsification to try and disprove a diagnosis; (d) consistently use all of the DSM diagnostic criteria and keep current about revisions; (e) be aware of other disorders or a dual diagnosis, and delay making a diagnosis until you have more data; (f) use symptom checklists to make certain your diagnosis adheres to DSM categories and follow a logical protocol to collect and evaluate data about the client before finalizing a diagnosis; (g) if you use psychological instruments to diagnose, make certain they're valid and reliable with the type of client you're diagnosing (by age, ethnicity, race, etc.); (h) make absolutely certain your expectations of clients don't reflect racial, ethnic, gender, or religious biases, or self-fulfilling prophecies about certain categories of diagnosis; (i) remember the importance of social factors in diagnosis and that the DSM may have a built-in bias against certain groups; (j) consider other diagnostic possibilities and understand that the more time you take getting to know the client, the more likely you are to arrive at a correct diagnosis; (k) consider the pros and cons of a diagnosis before formally using it with a client; (l) use multiple diagnostic instruments to determine a diagnosis and accept a diagnosis only if those instruments are in agreement with one another; (m) focus on what may be atypical about a client and follow those leads to help determine a correct diagnosis; (n) follow ethical standards; and (o) use training to improve your diagnostic work, particularly with men from diverse ethnic and cultural groups.

THE AVERSIVE IMPACT OF LABELING MEN

Men find psychological labels very demeaning. Labels are often an accumulation of words used in pejorative ways to describe men that are almost never used with women. Words such as troublemaker, uncooperative, out of control, irresponsible, and lazy are words often used to describe men to their faces. Other words that make men angry are dishonest, lush, crazy, failure, and impotent. I could go on but the point is that even sophisticated diagnostic labels are stigmatizing because they contain a collection of negative attributes. The term *personality disorder,* for example, implies a flaw in character. Markowitz (1998) believes the term *mental illness* suggests a lifelong illness whose label compounds feelings of low self-worth and depression in clients. Franklin (1992) argues that Black men react badly to labeling and suggests that Black men want to be recognized for their many positive attributes, not just their negative ones. Because of the subtle and overt use of labels as a function of racism, they dislike labeling and want to see themselves as partners in treatment. And Black men are particularly sensitive to male bashing and stereotypes of men, which they find demeaning and insulting.

USING BEST EVIDENCE IN DIAGNOSING MEN

The reader can find out more about best evidence and evidence-based practice (EBP) in a volume I wrote on the subject (Glicken, 2005). EBP is a paradigm with a great deal of potential for correctly diagnosing and helping male clients. In EBP, diagnosis is based on concrete evidence from the research literature. Although clinical experience is still important in diagnostic work, the Evidence-Based Medicine Working Group (1992) of the American Medical Association describes EBP as follows:

> The new paradigm [EBP] puts a much lower value on authority. The underlying belief is that [practitioners] can gain the skills to make independent assessments of evidence, and thus evaluate the credibility of opinions being offered by experts. The decreased emphasis on authority does not imply a rejection of what one can learn from colleagues and teachers whose years of experience have provided them with insight into methods of history-taking and diagnostic strategies that can never be gained from formal scientific investigation. (p. 2422)

In a statement with significance for men, the Evidence-Based Medicine Working Group (1992) suggests caution in making more of clinical observation than may be warranted and write that, "In the absence of systematic observation, one must be cautious in the interpretation of information derived from clinical experience and intuition, for it may at times be misleading" (p. 2422). The Evidence-Based Medicine Working Group (1992) goes on to note that a strong factor in making a correct diagnosis is the recognition of the client's discomfort and emotional distress. The group believes that clinicians must be compassionate in their approach to clients and that the diagnostic process must directly involve the client. As Gambrill (2000) writes, "EBP begins and ends with clients" (p. 1).

One example of how an incorrect diagnosis can have long lasting negative consequences for men is in our work with highly aggressive male children and adolescents where strong, life long consequences are predicted. As examples, Moffit (1994) believes that children who develop early aggressive tendencies are much more likely to move on to more seriously violent behaviors than children who show no violent tendencies before adolescence. He calls these two cohorts early and late starters. Late starters show signs of violent behavior in late middle school and even high school. Early starters often show signs of disobedience, bullying, intimidation, and fighting when they begin kindergarten and elementary school. According to Sprague and Walker (2000), "Early starters are likely to experience antisocial behavior and its toxic effects throughout their lives. Late starters have a far more positive long-term outcome" (p. 370). Walker and Severson (1990) suggest that diagnostic signs of "early starters" include disobedience, property damage, conduct problems, theft, the need for a great deal of attention, threats and intimidation, and fighting. Although it's wise to remember that diagnostic labels can be misleading and incorrect when applied to children, labels that have been used with boys that sometimes correlate with violent behavior include the following: (a) inattention and impulsivity (Lynam, 1996), (b) antisocial personality disorder, (c) conduct disorder, (d) oppositional defiant disorder, and (e) serious emotional disturbance (American Psychiatric Association, 1994).

In considering the literature on early onset violence in very young children, Sprague and Walker (2000) write:

> Well-developed antisocial behavior patterns and high levels of aggression evidenced early in a child's life are among the best predictors of delinquent and violent behavior years later. Over the developmental age span, these behavior patterns become more destructive, more aversive, and have much greater social impact as they become elaborated. (p. 369)

Dwyer, Osher, and Warger (1998) believe that we can diagnose potential violence as early as age five, but that few at-risk youth will commit serious violent acts throughout their life span. Many at-risk youth with early diagnoses of aggression and violent behaviors, however, will display such major life problems as drug and alcohol abuse, domestic and child abuse, divorce or multiple relationships, employment problems, mental health problems, dependence on social services, and involvement in less serious crimes (Obiakor, Merhing, & Schwenn, 1997).

Although signs of early aggression in male children may lead to future aggression, I (Glicken, 2004b) believe that we are, after all, discussing children whose behavior is not completely formed. Many factors contribute to the continuation or end of violent behavior in young children. One of the strongest reasons for the discontinuance of violent behavior is early intervention. Further, although profiling children for early signs of violence may lead to needed treatment, we should be cautious about using indications of violent behavior to project into the future. Many changes occur in a child's life and the benefits of positive influences, including helping professionals, teachers, mentors, religious affiliations, parents, siblings, and extended family members, should not be discounted. Children with early signs of violent behavior should not be labeled but an evaluation should be made to find out why the violent behavior is beginning to show itself so early in life. There are many reasons for early violent behavior. Violent behavior is often a reflection of early childhood physical and sexual abuse and neglect. Early violence may be associated with parental drug and alcohol abuse, learning difficulties, poor peer relationships, and a host of treatable conditions. If we do not show caution and humanity in our work with children who act out, we run the risk of so categorizing these children that they may live with a stigma that only exacerbates their anger.

People often change, even those we diagnose with serious problems. In longitudinal studies begun in 1955 by Werner and Smith (1992), the researchers found that one out of every three children who were evaluated by several measures of early life functioning to be at significant risk for adolescent problems, actually developed into well functioning young adults by age 18. In their follow-up study, the authors report that two out of three of the remaining two-thirds of children at risk had turned into caring and healthy adults by age 32. One of their primary theories was that people have "self-righting" capabilities and that an important reason children do well is because of a consistent and caring relationship with at least one adult or peer. These relationships provide the child with the self-protection to help initiate and develop the child's self-righting capacities. Werner and Smith believe that it is never too late to move from poor functioning to achievement and fulfillment.

This finding is supported by similar findings of serious anti-social behavior in children. In summarizing the research on youth violence, The Surgeon General (Satcher, 2001) reports that, "most highly aggressive children or children with behavioral disorders do not become violent offenders" (p. 9). The Surgeon General also notes that most youth violence begins in adolescence and ends with the transition to adulthood. If people didn't change, these early life behaviors would suggest that all violence in youth would certainly continue into adulthood. The report further suggests that the reasons for change in violent children relate to treatment programs, maturation, and biosocial factors (self-righting tendencies, or what has more recently been termed, *resilience*) that influence the lives of even the most violent youthful offenders. This and other research suggests that people do change, often on their own, and that learning from prior experience appears to be an important reason for change.

Consequently, it should be understood that a diagnosis, although supported by best evidence from the research literature, is not written in stone. Like so many activities related to helping professionals, a diagnosis is our best attempt to accurately define what is happening to the client at a particular moment in time. A diagnosis is not for life. It is subject to change, can be influenced by many psychosocial factors, and is always to be done in the least stigmatizing and most socially appropriate and positive way possible. The strengths perspective (Glicken, 2004a), which focuses on positive behaviors, is one way to remove stigma from a male diagnosis.

CASE EXAMPLE: A MISDIAGNOSIS

Jake Wright is a 32-year-old blue collar worker whose behavior has become erratic of late. Suspecting alcohol or drug abuse, his supervisor required Jake to attend counseling or lose his job. Jake has missed a great deal of work in the past two months. When he does come to work, he is absent at inappropriate times, seems to be losing weight rapidly, often has problems paying attention to his work, and is inappropriate with his coworkers, displaying signs of poor judgment, grandiosity, and feelings of invincibility. He openly talks about his sex life which seems to be very dangerous and violent. He has come to work with bruises on his face and body which he proudly shows everyone.

Jake was referred to a female therapist by his family doctor for substance abuse counseling. The diagnosis of substance abuse was confirmed by his doctor through the use of the CAGE questionnaire which asks the following:

> 1) **Cut**: Have you ever felt you should cut down on you drinking? 2) **Annoyed**: Have people annoyed you by criticizing your drinking? 3) **Guilty**: Have you ever felt guilty about your drinking? 4) **Eye-Opener**: Have you ever had a drink first thing in the morning (eye-opener) to steady your nerves or get rid of a hangover? (Bisson, Nadeau, & Demers, 1999, p. 717)

Stewart and Richards (2000) write the following: "A patient who answers yes to two or more of these questions probably abuses alcohol; a patient who answers yes to one question should be screened further" (p. 56).

After an initial interview, the drug and alcohol counselor concluded that Jake had a serious substance abuse problem and initiated individual and group treatment. Although Jake's use of substances began to modify itself after a few months, much of the behavior that got him into trouble on the job continued and he was fired. In fact, a careful interview with substantial medical and historical information would have confirmed a diagnosis of bipolar disorder with a secondary diagnosis of substance abuse to self-medicate the symptoms of bipolar disorder.

When asked how she could have ignored the symptoms of bipolar disorder, the therapist explained that she was a substance abuse counselor and expected the clients she saw to have substance abuse problems. It never occurred to her that he might have had a dual diagnosis. When asked if she saw changes in his behavior after therapy, she said that many men she'd worked with were what she called "dry drunks" and that the underlying personality disorder she found in many male alcoholics remained the same once the drinking and drug use stopped. When the guidelines for personality disorder and bipolar disorder were brought to her attention, she admitted she hadn't used the DSM–IV and was only vaguely familiar with the symptoms of bipolar disorder. "Men who drink and use drugs," she said, "behave the same way that Jake does."

The results of her misdiagnosis were that Jake was fired from his job and, in one of his very depressed states, tried to commit suicide. A psychologist who interviewed Jake in the emergency room of a community hospital after his suicide attempt immediately diagnosed bipolar disorder, ordered a psychiatric consult, and Jake was placed on medication that worked well enough for him to return to work. In trying to explain the misdiagnosis, the psychologist said

> It's understandable that the substance abuse was identified immediately and treated. What I find incongruent with this episode is why the counselor didn't recognize bipolar disorder. I suspect that she was so focused on the substance abuse that she just ignored the other behavioral signs and, although I don't want to admit it, many people in the substance abuse field have a fair amount of hostility toward substance abusers, particularly if they're male. We tend to use terms like "dry drunk" with men because the bias is that the drinking or drug use may stop but the dependent and immature personalities of male substance abusers will remain. I've never heard the term "dry drunk" used with women and I suspect we're much more compassionate with female substance abusers because their behavior is less noticeable and often somewhat more private. They hide their drinking and drug use better than men and, consequently, we have more compassion for them. I think what happened to Jake not only suggests incompetence, but it points out gender bias that I frankly think is all too common with men. Jake is suing the

78

therapist, and while I hate to see this happen to any of us, in this case it's well deserved.

SUMMARY

This chapter discusses concerns related to accurate diagnosis of men, including the negative influence of stereotyping. The chapter provides a number of suggestions to improve diagnosis and encourages the use of cooperative relationships in pinpointing male problems and their severity.

Forming Therapeutic Relationships With Male Clients

The therapeutic relationship is obviously a very significant aspect of effective work with men. In discussing the importance of the relationship, Warren (2001) writes the following:

> The relationship between the quality of the patient–therapist relationship and the outcome of treatment has been one of the most consistently cited findings in the empirical search for the basis of psychotherapeutic efficacy. (p. 357)

Saleebey (2000) suggests that: "If healers are seen as non-judgmental, trustworthy, caring and expert, they have some influential tools at hand, whether they are addressing depression or the disappointments and pains of unemployment" (p. 131). In a review of evidence-based practice for psychotherapy, Kopta, Lueger, Saunders, and Howard (1999) say the relationship is of key importance in the helping process.

In an assessment of a study done using *Consumer Reports* data on the effectiveness of psychotherapy, Seligman (1995) notes that clients have the wisdom to "shop around" for therapists who meet their own particular needs, and that the type of therapy they receive is far less important than the intangible aspects of whether they like the therapist and think that he or she will be able to help.

> Patients in psychotherapy in the field often get there by active shopping, entering a kind of treatment they actively sought with a therapist they

screened and chose. This is especially true of patients who work with independent practitioners .... (p. 970)

DEFINING THE THERAPEUTIC RELATIONSHIP

Brent and Kolko (1998) define psychotherapy as a

> modality of treatment in which the therapist and patient(s) work together to ameliorate psychopathological conditions and functional impairment through focus on (1) the therapeutic relationship; (2) the patient's attitudes, thoughts, affect, and behavior; and (3) social context and development. (p. 1)

Entwistle, Sheldon, Sowden, and Watt (1998) say that clients are actively involved in decisions regarding their treatment in three ways: (a) the care a patient will or will not receive, (b) the research information indicating the effectiveness of certain interventions that include risks and benefits of an approach with the alternatives of using one of the recommended approaches showing good research validity or doing nothing, and (c) being involved in all decisions regarding treatment. The Evidence-Based Practice Medicine Working Group (1992) of the American Medical Association writes that an important skill required of practitioners "is sensitivity to patients' emotional needs. Understanding patients' suffering and how that suffering can be ameliorated by the caring and compassionate practitioner are fundamental requirements for practice" (Evidence-Based Practice Medicine Working Group, 1992, p. 2422).

Orlinsky, Grawe, and Parks (1994) indicate five variables that have consistently been demonstrated to positively affect the quality of both the therapeutic alliance and treatment effectiveness: (a) the overall quality of the therapeutic relationship, (b) the skill of the therapist, (c) patient cooperation versus resistance, (d) patient openness versus defensiveness, and (e) the duration of treatment. Alan Keith-Lucas (1972) defines the relationship as "the medium which is offered to people in trouble and through which they are given an opportunity to make choices, both about taking help and the use they will make of it" (p. 47). Keith-Lucas says that the key elements of the helping relationship are "mutuality, reality, feeling, knowledge, concern for the other person, purpose, the fact that it takes place in the here and now, its ability to offer something new and, its nonjudgmental nature" (p. 48). In describing the key elements of the relationship, Bisman (1994) says that therapeutic relationships are a form of "belief bonding" between the worker and the client and that both parties need to believe that "the worker has something applicable for the client, the worker is competent, and that the client is worthwhile and has the capacities to change" (p. 77).

Weiss, Sampson, and O'Connor (1995) suggest that clients are unusually motivated to resolve their problems and that they work actively throughout treatment to obtain experiences and knowledge that will help them do this by coaching their therapist about what needs to been done and the best way to do it. The effective therapist recognizes the significance of the client's coaching and rather than seeing it as controlling or divisive, accepts it as an important part of the client's need to be highly involved in the process. Writing about the importance of the relationship, your author says the following:

> The relationship is a bond between two strangers. It is formed by an essential trust in the process and a belief that it will lead to change. The worker's expertise is to facilitate communications, enter into a dialogue with the client about its meaning, and help the client decide the best ways of using the information. (Glicken, 2004a, p. 111)

In a statement with significance for work with men, Saleebey (1996) writes,

> We [helping professionals] must engage individuals as equals. We must be willing to meet them eye-to-eye and to engage in dialogue and a mutual sharing of knowledge, tools, concerns, aspirations, and respect. The process of coming to know is a mutual and collaborative one. (p. 303)

EVIDENCE OF THE IMPORTANCE OF THE THERAPEUTIC
RELATIONSHIP WITH MALE CLIENTS

In a review of evidence-based practice for psychotherapy, Kopta, Lueger, Saunders, and Howard (1999) found that the relationship is of key importance in the helping process. Horvath and Greenberg (1994) report research evidence of the central role of the relationship in successful therapies. Major advances, according to Horvath and Greenberg (1994), have been made in (a) understanding the important role of relationships in the helping process; (b) how to operationalize the relationship for effectiveness for research purposes; (c) a better understanding of the variables that suggest potential for a successful therapeutic relationship; (d) and the ways in which the relationship may change as treatment progresses, including "ruptures" in the relationship. Krupnick et al. (1996) evaluated data from the large-scale National Institute of Mental Health Treatment of Depression Collaborative Research Program that compared treatments for depression. The authors found that the therapeutic relationship was predictive of treatment success for all conditions.

In a large study of diverse forms of therapy for alcoholism with male clients, the therapeutic relationship was also significantly predictive of success (Connors, Carroll, DiClemente, Longabaugh, & Donovan, 1997). Horvath and Symonds (1991) note that a positive relationship between scores on the quality of the initial (early) relationship and positive outcomes have been repeatedly found regardless of how the relationship is described by the practitioner. Kopta et al. (1999) write that, "Bordin (1994) argued that—regardless of the modality—the alliance always involves agreement on tasks and goals as well as a sense of compatibility or bonding" (p. 8). Brent and Kolko (1998) report that, "The contribution of therapeutic empathy and a good working alliance to positive clinical outcome has been demonstrated in several clinical trials of adult patients (Burns & Nolen-Hoeksema, 1992; Cooley & Lajoy, 1980; Luborsky, McLellan, Woody, O'Brien, & Auerbach, 1985; Murphy, Simons, Wetzel, & Lustman, 1984)" (p. 2). Brent goes on to say that, "From the patients' points of view, provision of support, understanding, and advice have been reported as most critical to good outcome (Cooley & Lajoy, 1980; Murphy et al., 1984)" (p. 2).

In further comments about the correlation between the relationship and effective therapeutic outcomes, Brent and Kolko (1998) write:

> The adult psychotherapy literature strongly supports the central role of the therapeutic relationship and therapeutic empathy in mediating the efficacy of treatment across many treatment models and psychopathological conditions. (p. 8)

Finally, Brent and Kolko (1998) summarize the research on the importance of the relationship as follows:

> According to Henry, Schacht, and Strupp (1986), in "good outcome" therapy, the therapist is described as "helping and protecting, affirming and understanding," whereas the patient is seen as "disclosing and expressing." In "poor outcome" psychotherapy, the therapist tends to be "blaming and belittling," whereas the patient is depicted as "walling off and avoiding. (p. 2)

GENDER AND THE THERAPEUTIC RELATIONSHIPS

Clinical wisdom usually suggests that gender is a neutral variable in clinical outcomes and that the quality of the help is more significant than issues related to the genders of the worker and the client. However, studies by Gehart-Brooks and Lyle (1999), and Sells, Smith, Coe, Yoshioka, and Robbins (1994), indicate that a therapist's gender is an important factor affecting a client's therapy experience. Although clients specifically state that gender is important, parallel interviews with therapists suggest that it isn't important. Gehart and Lyle (2001) believe that this "potential oversight has significant implications for the practice of ethical, gender-sensitive therapy and training" (p. 444). Gehart and Lyle go on to note that:

> Jones and Zoppel (1982) found that clients, regardless of gender, agreed that female therapists formed more effective therapeutic alliances than male therapists; however, both male and female clients of male therapists also reported significant improvements as a result of therapy. (Gehart & Lyle, 2001, p. 444)

Gehart and Lyle (2001) reports that further inquiry into the relationship between gender and therapeutic outcomes indicates that, "male and female therapists interrupted females three times more often than male clients" (Werner-Wilson, Price, Zimmerman, & Murphy, 1997) (p. 444). Shields and McDaniel (1992) indicate that families made more directive statements to male therapists but more openly disagreed with each other in front of women. Shields and McDaniel (1992) also found that male therapists explained issues more fully than female therapists and that male therapists provided more advice and direction than female therapists. Werner-Wilson, Zimmerman, and Price (1999) report that men were more successful at suggesting issues for discussion in family treatment whereas women did better in marital therapy. Gehart and Lyle (2001) believe that these "studies provide further evidence that gender may significantly affect the therapeutic process in ways in which therapists are currently unaware" (p. 444).

Gehart and Lyle (2001) describe three types of gender-related connections made by clients: (a) The connection is stronger with a therapist of the same gender because it offers a common language and knowledge base; (b) the connection is stronger with a therapist of the opposite gender. Gender differences may provide motivation to work harder in treatment; and (c) the client develops a good relationship with a therapist of the same gender but often reports that therapists of the opposite gender are also effective (p. 451). In summarizing their work on gender, Gehart and Lyle write,

> ... clients described women as more feeling-focused, but only half found this helpful. Conversely, almost all clients described male therapists as more direct and problem-focused, yet only half found this approach helpful. What is consistent is that clients reported that they experienced a distinct and consistent difference between male and female therapists. (p. 452)

Your author (Glicken, 1995) argues that the therapeutic relationship with men is of primary significance and that men will not enter into a productive relationship without the following elements: (a) A cooperative working relationship which values the male client's observations, insights, and goals for treatment; (b) a supportive and respectful working environment; (c) an understanding and appreciation of male socialization; (d) a recognition of the male client's positive accomplishments; (e) a willingness to listen to the client and not give negative feedback even when the client is dishonest about his behavior; (f) an understanding of the stressors in a man's life and the pressures on men to succeed at all costs; (g) a willingness to never openly use labels or psychological terms with negative connotations; (h) an understanding that men may take longer to develop trust than female clients; (i) a recognition that although men may not want to talk directly about their problems, they are listening and learning while they talk about disconnected issues; (j) a kind, respectful, and supportive worker will generally have more impact on the relationship, and ultimately, on treatment success than a critical and unsupportive worker.

Scher (1979) believes that although men often hide their need for a warm and nurturing relationship, in reality, they crave the attention, support, and advice of others. Instead of focusing on the cognitive aspects of a problem in treatment, Scher suggests the need to, "impress on the client that his emotions, not his thoughts and cognitions, are causing him difficulty, because thoughts can always be ordered and forced to assume a logical sequence" (p. 254). To help men better understand their emotional lives, the part of a man's world Scher describes as deeply suppressed and almost "banished" from awareness, the therapist must, "gain trust, be honest, patient and indulgent of the client's wishes. If the therapist is genuine and accepting," (p. 254), the client will relax. Although testing and competing with the therapist are common ways of coping with discomfort, the male client will ultimately begin the process of trusting the worker, which will lead to a real breakthrough and changes in behavior. Scher concludes,

> Men are not easy clients to deal with at the outset. Once the therapeutic contract is established, men generally become hard-working and productive clients. The counselor who works successfully with men will exercise restraint, candor, and affection. (p. 254)

In a discussion of therapy with traditional men, Lanzillo (1999) writes,

> The traditional man is committed to representing himself as strong, independent, rational, competent, and fearless. This man does not want to put himself in a situation (like a therapist's office) that may challenge his perception of being in control and powerful. (p. 119)

Lanzillo (1999) believes that therapists must have ways of feeling empathy for their traditional clients which promote the relationship and create a safe haven for clients to share highly personal and sometimes embarrassing information with the worker.

TWELVE ELEMENTS OF THE HELPING RELATIONSHIP IN WORK WITH MEN

Some of these elements of the helping relationship with men were first written about in Glicken (2004a).

Cooperative Relationships

When working with men, there should be no power differential between the client and the worker. Beginning the relationship with the assumption that we know less than the client about their problem is humbling and accurate. Only the client knows what's really happening in his life or how he feels about it. We need information from the client that only he can provide if we are to be helpful.

What the Client Wants From Us

It is important to know what male clients want from us and, if possible, to honor that request. It is not OK with men for workers to believe that they know what's best for their clients or that they always act in the client's best interest. This need to know what the client wants should be spelled out immediately in the very first client contact, even if the client is an involuntary client and sees us in an adversarial role. The purpose of the work we are to do together should be specified by developing a contract between the client and the worker that identifies the issues to be resolved and the therapeutic processes required. As one male client told me,

> It's frustrating. You go to see someone for a personal problem and it's hard to get up the energy and courage to see him or her in the first place. You come full of what you want to say and how you think the therapist can help, but before you know it, the therapist is asking questions and leading you in a different direction. The story you wanted to tell doesn't get told and you leave with this sad feeling that the therapist hasn't heard a word you've said. It makes you feel that the therapist isn't interested in your point of view, and isn't going to take much of what you say, or want, into consideration. It's very frustrating.

Work on Developing Rapport

It is important to establish an early rapport with men. Rapport has been defined in many ways but it is simply the level of comfort the client feels with the worker. There is no particular trick to establishing rapport, but it is often thought to be a process by which the worker helps the client feel relaxed, valued, and confident. Some workers use part of the initial session to help men overcome the "stage fright" they initially experience. As Bisman (1994) suggests, the initial contact with the client establishes whether the worker and the client will be able to work together. The developing relationship, based on the comfort level between the helper and client, defines whether the degree of "belief bonding" will be adequate to help resolve the client's problem.

Rapport is established, or not established, almost immediately. The contributing factors in establishing rapport are: the helper's level of warmth, the helper's comfort level in just chatting, the closeness the contact has to the client's usual social interactions, and the warmth and comfort of the physical setting. The client takes all of these factors in immediately and a judgment is made about whether the worker can be trusted and how much of a commitment the client will make to treatment. As one male client told me,

> I went for therapy over the loss of my job and I was feeling very distrustful of people at the moment. The therapist I went to had come very highly

recommended. She had a very nice voice. In the first minute or two, as I was sizing her up and trying to get my thoughts together, I couldn't help notice that she was wearing suede shoes and that a little piece of suede was missing. Maybe other people would have seen it differently, but to me it was endearing. I thought to myself, this is a regular human being who has flaws and she'll be easy on me and I can trust her. And the fact was that she was excellent and she did help. I came to that conclusion in the first minute or two I was in her office.

Active and Attentive Listening

A core ingredient of work with men is the ability of the worker to help the client clearly communicate the nature of the problem and the impact the problem is having on his life. For this to happen, the worker needs to allow male clients to tell their stories unfettered by questions or observations until it is clear to both the client and the worker what the problem is and what the client would like the worker to help him do about it. This process of active and attentive listening requires patience, time, and a willingness to let clients tell their story in ways that feels right to them. At some point in time, if we listen closely, if we are nonjudgmental and keep interpretations of the material from influencing us, we will accurately know the client's version of the problem.

Evidence-Based Practice

To assist in the process of communication, the worker must be able to access and share information from the research literature that might lead to change. This means that the worker must know the sources of empirical information, must be able to explain those sources to the client, and must help the client consult those sources by encouraging independent reading, thinking, and evaluation of the information. The client needs to know what the worker knows and if the client is confused about the information, he should be guided by the worker, or by others, to better understand the material. The purpose of therapy with men is empowerment. One way to achieve empowerment is to help men know that they have the internal and external resources available to them to resolve a problem. Gambrill (1999) explains information-guided practice as follows:

> Honoring our own code of ethics to inform clients and to draw on practice-related research will help us to have the courage and integrity to challenge puffery, avoid propagandistic appeals, and value truth over winning arguments. Embracing a justification approach to knowledge in which we seek support for our views rather than rigorously try to falsify them, encourages authority-based decision making. One option is to prepare books for clients critically reviewing the literature in relation to key areas of concern in social work (e.g., child welfare) that describe what has been tested to what effect and what has not been tested. (see for example Enkin et al., 1995) (p. 358)

Encouraging Independent Client Solutions

Male clients are encouraged to gain knowledge by reading available literature and by reaching their own conclusions about its meaning, even if it differs from that of the worker. The same process is encouraged when the client explores his past life experiences, cultural and social roots, family origins, and significant conflicts, failures, and successes. As one client told me,

> The therapist suggested that I keep a journal of my past history and jot down the things that happened to me that might be related to a depression I was going through. As I was driving to work one day, I remembered having this terrible argument with my father about a girl friend. He told me that my girl friend was an indication of how poorly I thought of myself, and that if I was a healthy person, I'd be involved with healthier women. And I mean he used to say the same thing about every one of my friends. Here I am in my forties and I'm alone and very lonely. I have no friends at all and if someone reaches out to me, I have the same troubled feeling that they're all inferior and that I'm an unhealthy person. It's not true, any of it, but I really got in touch with what I've been feeling lately just by being encouraged to think about my past history and by reading about loneliness and isolation. And what was so good about it is that the therapist started the sessions by

asking me about any insights I'd gained through my journal writing. She was interested and encouraged me to talk about my thoughts and feelings. It was really empowering.

Sharing Opinions

The worker can certainly share his or her opinions, but these opinions need to be explained in a way that utilize the male client's ability to comprehend and process them and to disagree when they seem incorrect. Change comes from knowledge, and the function of treatment is to help the client critically evaluate information. This approach recognizes that clients have inner resources, critical thinking competencies, and the ability to rationally determine what is best for them. The worker's opinion is just that. It isn't truth and it's not written in stone.

Focusing on the Positives

The worker should help men realize that they have used successful approaches to problem-solving in other areas of their lives that may be transferable to their current life difficulties. It is the worker's role to help the client reflect back on his prior successes because the same process that led to success can be applied to the current task of resolving personal problems.

Humility As a Key to Helping

In the real world, people expect the helper to do just that—to help them. They want the person to be nice about it, but, more to the point, they expect honesty and humility from the worker. It is a privilege to help someone. The privilege is from the client opening up his heart, barring his internal conflicts and pain, and trusting the worker with private and often distressing information. That process should promote a sense of humility and deeply felt respect for the brave and often painfully troubled men we work with who place their pain and the expectation that their suffering will end, in our hands.

The Client Needs to Understand Our Work

The client has the right to know what we're doing. Our work is not mysterious. It's a process between two people that constantly needs to be explained, discussed, and evaluated. If the client doesn't know what we are doing and why, it only serves to confuse him and to negatively affect the relationship. The worker who asks the client to do a role-play very soon into treatment, but doesn't explain its purpose, is going to have a client who feels confused and discounted. The insights from the role play will be diminished and the exercise will end with the client feeling that the worker is playing games. Some male clients hate role-plays and some of the other techniques of the profession. It is the worker's obligation to search for the techniques of treatment that promote the most comfort in the client and come closest to the client's usual way of problem-solving. This is a very important rule to remember, particularly for the man who is new to treatment and is anxious to please the worker (as most men are), but may be confused about what the worker is doing. An informed male client who is in a cooperative relationship with the worker will have a sense of strength knowing that he can ask questions, disagree with the worker, and provide feedback to achieve a successful outcome in treatment.

Working With Transference

Freud believed that clients tended to see workers as substitutes for the loved ones they never had in their life. The loved one they want the worker to represent can be a parent, a sibling, a friend, or someone to fill a void in their life left by the absence of a suitable parental or adult love relationship. Freud believed that it was inevitable that clients experienced a transference relationship with workers because the worker, particularly if he or she was kind, empathic, and concerned, would represent something so unusual in the client's life that the worker could easily be placed in a role of intimacy that might help or hinder treatment.

In my opinion, transference occurs when the worker subtly encourages the client to place the worker in a role of importance he or she should not hold. If a client is beginning to develop strong, emotionally charged feelings for the worker that could create problems in treatment, it should be discussed in a positive and gentle way. It should be done as early as possible to avoid the dependency problems associated with transference.

A client I know told me about his experience with a female therapist and how the worker dealt with it:

> I was seeing a therapist regarding a problem I was having with my love relationship. My therapist wasn't particularly attractive but she was very warm and kind, two qualities lacking in my love relationship at the time. I started writing short stories and showing them to her. I'd dress extra well for our sessions. I'd notice what she was wearing and comment to her about it. She was very professional and she accepted each gesture objectively. It was driving me crazy. It wasn't that I wanted to see her outside of the office or to be involved with her physically; I just wanted her to love me beyond any love she'd ever felt. I even wrote her a short story comparing her to my love relationship and describing all of the things I loved about her but didn't love about my lady friend. It was a bit more complicated than that but she remained objective, said very little to encourage these feelings, although a few times I got irrationally angry at her for discounting me but, in time, I felt how safe I was working through the feelings I had for her with someone who was, at all times, very professional. I still like her a lot, appreciate the help she gave me, and am thankful, in a curious sort of way, that she didn't fall for my baloney since it was the same stuff I was using in my love relationship and it was ruining any chance I had for the relationship to work.

The client gave me permission to reprint the story he wrote. It can be found at the end of this section.

Writing Summaries of the Work After Each Session

One of the techniques that some workers describe as effective with men is having them write summaries after each session so that issues to explore during the next session might be identified. Giving men something active to do is always a good idea. A colleague of mine who had

just begun therapy with a therapist he liked very much used this technique. After nine sessions and just as they were beginning to progress
in treatment, my colleague accepted a new job in a small community
thousands of miles away. Because of the absence of therapists in the
new community, the original therapist and my colleague decided to
continue treatment by telephone. The day after the first telephone session, my colleague sent the therapist an e-mail outlining what he'd
learned during the telephone session, what he intended to do about it,
and the issues(s) he wanted to discuss during the next session. He said
that in many ways, the work they did together on the phone was much
more powerful and relevant than the work he'd done with the therapist
in person. The client said the following about his experience:

> First of all, it *is* possible to do therapy on the phone. I had to be very fo-
> cused, but since I was in a room with no distractions, that was easy.
> Then, we had to have a sense of where we wanted each session to go or
> we would misuse the time. Therapy seemed to last longer on the
> phone, because, I suppose, there were no distractions. In my prior ses-
> sions, we must have spent a lot of time warming up because I'd leave
> feeling sort of half-done. On the phone, I felt as if we'd covered the ma-
> terial in a more concise and usable way. The day after the first tele-
> phone session, I began to sit down and write about what I'd gotten
> from the session, what I was doing about it, and what I wanted to talk
> about during the next session. Then I'd e-mail it to my therapist. It
> started a process I found extraordinarily helpful. Of course, the thera-
> pist was terrific and after a session or two, I think we both knew that
> something pretty special was taking place. The other thing our phone
> calls did was for me to take a more proactive role in my treatment. I be-
> gan to read everything I could about mid-life depression and loneli-
> ness. What I found was a very strong literature that was really helpful. I
> discussed medication with my therapist and then went to see my physi-
> cian about it. In the end, they didn't recommend medication because
> of the side effects, but my goodness, I felt as if I was being consulted
> and cared for in an extraordinary way even though my therapist was
> thousands of miles away.

> I should add that one of my sessions was held the day of the World Trade
> Center bombings, 9–11. We were both in such a troubled state of mind
> because of the horrible loss of life that the session was electric. I still

can't quite believe how powerful it was or how touched I was that my therapist was in her office waiting for my call when she had family members in New York who may have been harmed by the bombings.

A CLIENT'S STORY ABOUT TRANSFERENCE

This story is used with permission of the author, a colleague and a friend. It does, I think, a superb job of describing the way some men respond to treatment, their reaction to their therapists, and the meaning of love in their lives.

CASE EXAMPLE

I'm sitting in my therapist's office and my guts are on the floor. We're talking about the woman I've been seeing, the therapist and me, and I'd rather spend some time just having a cup of coffee with her, shooting the breeze, having some Joe together. Talking about Rachel is costing me $110 an hour. From my point of view, that's a lot of money to be talking about someone who seems to enjoy tearing my heart out, raising it above her head, and letting everyone see that it's still beating before I keel over and die.

My therapist wants to know why I'm staying in the relationship. Well, for one thing ... I can't find the words for the one thing. I'm stuck. I can't think of a reason. Maybe because a guy like me deserves a woman like Rachel, that's why. I'm waiting for my therapist to say something profound to get me out of my state of eternal stuckness, but she looks sympathetically at me, and smiles. She has a nice smile, warm and tender. Why can't I find a woman like my therapist? Well, of course. If I even recognized a woman like my therapist and let her seriously enter my heart, I wouldn't be in therapy, would I?

Rachel. I love the name. I imagine that anyone with a name like Rachel has to be somehow biblical. And it's true that her father was a minister and she has the plain, middle aged looks of a minister's daughter; short hair, severe features, small breasts, large hips, and yet we have an incredible amount of primal sex. She isn't very good in bed and feels heavy and awkward, but there's something about her ... the shyness, the lack of knowledge, the heat I feel radiating from her body that makes me want to do everything to her I know about sex.

I don't want to tell the therapist about my lust for Rachel. I want my therapist to love me, to have fantasies about me, to think about me in bed when she lies awake longing for someone to love her in the same way I long for someone to love me. Rachel isn't able to love anyone. I know it and maybe she does too. I feel a kinship with her in this loveless relationship we have together. Two lonely people with nothing more than our primal lust to keep us together.

The therapist suddenly has little tears in her eyes. I can't imagine why. Maybe I've said something to hurt her. Maybe in my descriptions of Rachel, she sees something of herself. I look carefully at the therapist to make sure she's OK. I want to walk over and hold her and tell her that whatever is hurting her, whatever sits heavy on her heart, it will go away. I wonder what her lover is like. Does she have someone? Is she married? Does she have children? Is she happy? I want to know and yet I don't want to know. If I knew, it might change these little moments of intimacy we have together. I want to think that my therapist loves me even if Rachel doesn't.

Rachel says hurtful things to me just as we're about to make love. In the midst of beginning to make love, she wonders what we'll need at the store, or she'll remember that she forgot to get some cosmetic and asks me to remind her about it the next morning. This intrusion into our intimate moments makes me want her all the more, but when we're done making love, an anger passes over me and I want to say cruel and hurtful things to her. I want to tell her how plain she looks and, for Christ sake, why does she wear her hair so short? And Jesus, why can't she wear some nice clothes instead of the sterile, shapeless, middle-aged ladies clothes she buys at the end of the year sales? But

I don't. I listen to her fall asleep, the softness of her breathing almost imperceptible in the quiet room where we make love so often. Like the stillness of her breathing, maybe she feels so invisible that no one sees her but me.

It's what my therapist says about me. That I make myself invisible. It's true, of course, and Rachel is my mirror image. The two of us ... loveless, invisible, plain, deep in each others arms, aloof from love, and substituting our mutual dislike for nights in bed.

My therapist has long blond hair and a kind face. I keep looking at her shoes. Today she has on scuffed clogs. I like them better than the plain sensible shoes she often wears. Maybe my success in therapy will be related to the shoes my therapist is wearing. I don't know. Why am I even here? It feels as if I'm doing penance for something awful when something awful has just been done to me. I've been fired from my job. It feels like my insides are about to spill out all over the floor. I laugh and joke and tell everyone I'm fine, but I'm not fine at all. I'm as unfine as I can be. I drink too much, I'm depressed most of the time, life feels hopeless and, of course, I've chosen Rachel as my mate.

I like Rachel's dog Andy who has soulful eyes and a wonderful smile when you tickle her. Andy is funny and spirited, unlike her owner. Rachel has a kind of simpatico with her dog that I wish she had with me. With me she sits and stares at the floor most of the time or does crossword puzzles. It's no wonder we're in bed so much. We have nothing much to say to one another. My therapist knows all of this and looks hurt when I talk about how bad it is between Rachel and me. Maybe the person inside somehow takes over and what I say to her reminds her of moments in her own life. I don't know. It's very odd telling someone you don't know intimate things about yourself.

I like my therapist's voice. It sounds genuine and full of caring. I like talking to her on the phone. Sometimes I wish she'd just call me up at home and shoot the breeze. I wish I'd known her when I was getting into trouble at work. Maybe it wouldn't have happened. Maybe she would have listened and told me that the job was impossible and to leave as soon and as gracefully as I could.

My therapist has a way of sneaking the important questions in before I leave. This time she looks at me and wonders if I trust her. I don't trust anyone, of course, but the question goes right to my heart and so touches me that I fight back tears. Why couldn't Rachel say something so smart and caring? Why do I need to pay someone to ask me something so important?

When we're done with my session, I'll go home and drink myself into a stupor and then, numbness settling over me, I'll sleep, wake up, feel a panic coming over me and wonder, before I go to work, before the sun comes up and the next day starts, whether I'll make it through the day. A few times on the way home from seeing my therapist, I start to cry and have to pull over and watch the people with angry looks on their faces drive past me, oblivious to a middle-aged man sitting in his car, hunched over the steering wheel, and sobbing.

Our 50 minutes are up. We say goodbye and it feels as if we've just made love. I hate to leave therapy and I have to throttle an impulse to ask for more time. Please, I want to say, can't I just sit on the couch and talk for a while? I don't want to go to my empty house and sit and stare at the walls and drink myself into a stupor again. I just want to sit here where I feel loved for 50 minutes and shoot the breeze, maybe tell a bad joke, tell lies about all the women I've been with, act like a kid, and laugh for a change. But, of course, I say nothing of the kind and dutifully pay my bill and walk to my car.

Before I leave the therapist's office, I sit in my car for a while and listen to Bach on the car stereo. Sometimes I watch the other therapists coming out of the building where my therapist has her office and wonder what they're like. The other clients shuffle in and out with the same hang-dog look on their faces that I've begun to notice on mine. And then a sadness settles over me and I know, in my actual visceral heart, how it will end with Rachel ... the lovers arguments, the stillness of no one speaking, the feigned touching at night and being rejected, the click and the clack of dishes in the evening of sorrow and the wine, and the crying, and the hurt that slowly washes everything away. The look of betrayal, the sleeping next to someone turned to ice, the fear of loss, the love-making that's really hate-making, the loss of passion, the requiem for a thousand nights of solace and the emptiness of a room, a house, a life. Who will repair me if I fail again? Who will warm my heart at night, the lonely night, the flowers withered where she placed them fresh and her smells gone and forgotten but lingering in the corners of every empty room? The empty bed, the loveless substitutes, the dates without a future, the silly people who fill the void, the empty shopping cart, the buying for one person, the movies watched alone, the books read to myself, the yin and the yang and the endless reprises of what could have been, what might have happened, who was to blame, what would be lost and will she call me, sometime, and tell me she misses me and, God in heaven, can I be with her again?

Please let me love somebody and let them love me back. It isn't asking so much, is it? Just someone nice. Just let me love someone for an hour and let them love me back, and the empty house, the click and the clack of dishes, the rain and the wind, the sorrow, and the crying, and the despair will wither like smells of perfume in the corner of an empty room, and the days, and the nights, and the trips, and the dinners, and the growing of flowers, and the planting of love seeds, and the wanting to get home as fast as possible to be with my love; maybe God will be kind this time and let it happen. It isn't asking so much, is it?

SUMMARY

This chapter discusses the important issue of the therapeutic relationship and its significant impact on treatment effectiveness. The significance of client–worker gender and race and ethnicity were raised with many authors believing that both issues have an impact on treatment efficacy and that much more time must be spent in training new workers for effective work with diverse client populations, particularly men.

A Male Model of Therapy

Because male socialization values independent solutions to problems, men often find it difficult to seek help. Even when men do seek help, they may not be able to clearly state a relation between why they feel discomfort and what may be causing it. And because men often grow up believing that others are unable or unwilling to help, or that the process of seeking help may be a waste of time, they often deal with extreme emotions by themselves.

   In discussing male socialization and the assumptions of counseling and psychotherapy, Robertson and Fitzgerald (1992) argue that traditional notions of psychotherapy are often ill-suited for men for the following reasons: (a) Although psychotherapy and counseling require self-awareness, men are encouraged to hide their feelings; (b) counseling and psychotherapy often require clients to admit that they have a problem, but men have been taught to deny that they have problems; (c) therapists often encourage clients to share their vulnerabilities, but men have been taught to hide their vulnerabilities so they can maintain a competitive edge; and (d) counseling and psychotherapy ask clients to openly explore their problems with another person, but men have often been socialized to distrust others, to maintain rational control over their lives, and that "self-exploration should be done independently and on an intellectual level" (Robertson & Fitzgerald, 1992, p. 241). In further explaining male resistance to therapy, the authors write:

Comparing the goals and processes of traditional counseling and psy-chotherapy with those emphasized by traditional masculine socializa-tion processes leads to a series of paradoxes, if not contradictions. For example, many approaches to personal counseling require that clients bring a sense of self-awareness to the counseling room (client-centered, humanistic, gestalt, existential, and others); yet men appear to be so-cialized away from self-awareness and encouraged to control (or hide) their feelings. In addition, personal counseling is designed for people who admit they have problems, but men are generally taught to com-pete on their own and not admit that they need help. Many counselors further invite clients to disclose their vulnerabilities; men, however, are taught to hide their vulnerabilities to maintain a competitive edge. Finally, counseling asks clients to explore their lives openly with an-other person, whereas men are socialized to be in rational control of their lives, implying that any self-exploration should be done independ-ently and on an intellectual level.

Given these considerations, it seems reasonable that men avoid a process that requires them to consider failure instead of success, cooperation in-stead of competition, and vulnerability instead of power. Although these comparisons certainly do not suggest that men bring "wrong" attitudes to therapy or that traditional counseling assumptions are "right", they do highlight the differences between masculine socialization and the expec-tations of many traditionally trained counselors. (p. 241)

Robertson and Fitzgerald (1990) considered another reason men do poorly in therapy: mistreatment by therapists. In their research, the authors found that men who deviated from predetermined roles such as work and caregiving were viewed more negatively by therapists than men who maintained those predetermined roles. The authors also found that many therapists view a man's desire to work out a problem by himself as resistance to treatment or a lack of motivation. Many of the elements of O'Neil's (1982) masculine mystique were, in fact, seen as negatives by therapists in the study. Robertson and Fitzgerald (1990) conclude, "… psychotherapy may be as unprepared to deal ef-fectively with such men (men who do not conform to traditional role expectations) as it was with nontraditional women a generation ago" (p. 243).

Scher (1990) believes that therapy is almost always about women and that, "... what it means to be a man in our culture and what impact that has on men as clients in psychotherapy has frequently not been addressed" (p. 322). Scher (1979) also believes that men are reluctant clients because therapy intrudes on their need to be independent. Glicken (1995) notes that therapy is primarily a process used with women and it may, in its present form, so discount or ignore male socialization as to render it ineffective with men. Not only does it often not work in its present form, but men don't use it in anywhere near the numbers that women do. Men have been taught to be logical in the way they problem-solve and to use themselves to resolve problems. Before a man will consider the possibility of using someone else in a helping role, there are trust issues that need to be resolved. Just as many intimate relationships deteriorate because of lack of trust, men go into therapy with a very limited sense that it will help because the therapist will let them down. Consequently, they often fail to disclose important material, or they may enter therapy half-heartedly in the belief that it won't help them and that, perhaps, it might even hurt them.

Cochran and Rabinowitz (2003) argue that men have been culturally programmed to repress the emotional aspects of loss. This pertains to all aspects of loss including loss in the workplace, in relationships, with children, with parents and siblings, and with intimate relationships. The authors believe that "gender-sensitive therapists" should help male clients identify repressed experiences of loss across the life span:

> Some common experiences of loss include early maternal disconnection, boyhood experiences of rejection by peers on the playground, experiences of rejection and loss in relationships, failure in occupational achievement, and loss of physical health due to the aging process. (Cochran & Rabinowitz, 2003, p. 135)

The authors suggest that if experiences with loss are left unresolved, one consequence is the development of depression. The key to men's work is an empathic response to their loss and to their feelings of depression. Cochran and Rabinowitz (2003) indicate that: "Psychotherapeutic interventions provided from an empathic, gender-

sensitive perspective provide a means by which to counter the mixed
and often conflicting messages many men have internalized about
their feelings of depression" (p. 135).

In another example of the unwillingness of traditional men to seek
help for emotional problems, Robertson and Fitzgerald (1992) studied
the relation between levels of traditional maleness and the willingness to
seek psychological help. Two primary findings are significant:

> First, traditional masculine attitudes *do* seem to be negatively related to
> the willingness of men to seek professional psychological help. Second,
> men who express highly masculine attitudes react more positively to de-
> scriptions of interventions that are consistent with masculine socializa-
> tion processes. (Robertson & Fitzgerald, 1992, p. 245)

In discussing the willingness of men to seek help if it is framed in a way
that stresses male socialization, the authors report a relation between
the willingness to seek help and two types of traditional men: Technical
and realistic types of men who, although highly traditional in their outlook on life, are also changeable when the need arises, and men who feel
independent, competitive, self-confident, and decisive. Robertson and
Fitzgerald (1992) conclude that their

> study implies that to reach new groups of men, counseling psychologists
> need to offer programs that emphasize self-help and problem-solving
> approaches, rather than offering solely counseling for deeper insight into
> self-development and personal emotions. (p. 245)

WHEN MEN USE TREATMENT

Men often respond positively to help when it is offered in a collaborative
way. Gambrill (1999) believes that effective work with clients "requires
an atmosphere in which critical appraisal of practice-related claims
flourishes, and clients are involved as informed participants" (p. 345).
Men respond well to therapy when the therapist understands and appreciates male socialization. Rather than being critical of their beliefs and
attitudes, men want therapists to understand how well they've done in

their lives and how close to being "real men" they've been, even if the results are problematic.

This need to understand and even admire many aspects of male socialization and male behavior is what defines successful therapy with men. Many therapists enter the relationship determined to show men how dysfunctional their socialization has been when a much more effective approach is to admire men for their achievements and to work collaboratively with them. The tendency to criticize men discounts a great deal of very positive and socially important behavior and often ends in unnecessary treatment attrition or complete rejection of treatment.

Male attrition rates have been found to be as high as 50% (DeMaris, 1989). Although some researchers have looked at demographic reasons for attrition (DeMaris, 1989), others have focused on the degree of masculinization of participants, believing that the more highly internalized the masculine role, the less likely participants are to stay in treatment. In work with abusive men, DeMaris (1989) found that sociodemographic issues correlating with attrition and noncompliance with treatment were as follows: employment status, use of substances, arrest record, age, income, desire to reduce violent behavior, age of partner, and the timing or reason for the abuse. The author, however, found that demographic explanations explained attrition at a level only twelve percent above chance. In other words, it's difficult to find precise reasons for male attrition rates in treatment. Other theories suffer from similar problems in that a man's reasons for staying in treatment may be less therapeutic than legal. In diversion projects, for example, one stays in treatment or goes to jail. It may be very useful to study the reasons men actually stay in treatment rather than why they drop out.

In a study of how men view therapy, Robertson and Fitzgerald (1992) devised two brochures: one described counseling in a traditional way while the other described therapy using terms such as *classes, workshops,* and *seminars.* Both brochures discussed reasons for coming for counseling (depression, academic failure, relationship problems, etc.) and described staff competence, waiting periods, and cost. Both brochures looked alike. The study found that men with traditional attitudes toward masculinity were reluctant to come for counseling. Interestingly, these same men reacted more positively to descriptions of counseling that were consistent with male socialization processes. The authors concluded that men are more likely to stay in treatment when the service offered is supportive, reinforcing, instructional (advice giving), and nonconfrontational, and write,

> ... counseling psychologists need to offer programs that emphasize self-help and problem-solving approaches, rather than offering solely counseling for deeper insight into self-development and personal emotions. Our findings are consistent with the tradition in counseling psychology that encourages the use of culturally sensitive formats for providing services to clients representing ethnic minorities and those designated as "special populations." Although it is not usual to think of men in this fashion, it is also true that the masculine mystique generates a unique assumptive world that appears to function as a barrier to men in many areas (e.g., emotional, psychological). (Robertson & Fitzgerald, 1992, p. 245)

In a review of a book by Brooks (1998), Lanzillo (1999) reports that Brooks warns against trying to force male clients into the "alien" world of psychotherapy. The culture of therapy, as Brooks calls it, "is a culture of asking for help, being open with our feelings, and admitting that we may not be able to fix the problem by ourselves" (Lanzillo, 1999, p. 120). This definition of therapy creates a struggle within men that may prevent them from entering therapy because, "Traditional men see psychotherapy as a direct threat to their identity as men" (Lanzillo, 1999, p. 120). Lanzillo also notes that, "According to Brooks, the traditional man is committed to representing himself as strong, independent, rational, competent, and fearless" (Lanzillo, 1999, p. 120), a self-perception that bodes poorly for psychotherapy as it is now practiced. Instead, Brooks suggests that:

> Therapists must have some way to feel empathy for their traditional male clients. Although many traditional men engage in some unattractive behavior, they must be understood as persons who can be valued and deemed worthy of a therapist's most dedicated efforts. (p. 79)

Brooks goes on to say the following:

We need to have a strong sense of the traditional men's culture if we are to effectively communicate and collaborate with these men in a therapeutic environment. As health-care professionals, it is important to stop demanding that our male clients simply adapt to the rules of psychotherapy and that we begin to become familiar with our clients' culture when we reach out and engage men. It is through this "culturally sensitive therapy" that we adjust our interventions to meet the values and needs of the traditional man. (p. 79)

In a study of the willingness of men to talk about feelings and to discuss their emotional life, Robertson, Lin, Woodford, Danos, and Hurst (2001) report that, although men may be unable to answer questions posed to them about their emotional life, they readily answer questions that involve problem-solving, task-completion, and structured activities. The authors suggest, as alternatives to spoken responses to questions about feelings, that men do better when given written assessments and structured expressive assignments. However, men with lower levels of gender stress are perfectly able to effectively discuss emotions. The authors found that stress is one of the most common problems men want to discuss in treatment and that 80% of the men in their study readily participated in a discussion of the best ways to relieve stress. The authors suggest that focusing on physical and emotional awareness of stress may lead to changes in behavior and attitude.

One of the common problems with many forms of therapy is a failure to recognize that when men enter therapy, they are experiencing forms of physical discomfort (anger, anxiety, depression, stress, and confusion). As the therapy is focused on the reduction of these physical discomforts, the client feels relief and there are probably biochemical changes that result. The client who feels better will continue on in treatment because there appears to be a direct link between therapy and the relief of symptoms. This seems obvious but many therapists practicing forms of process-oriented therapy seem not to realize that the longer men are in discomfort, the less likely they are to think that therapy works. Therefore, the initial focus of work with men should be on symptom removal. I can't stress this enough. When men go to doctors, if they don't feel better after seeing a doctor, they either see someone else or they see no one and try and handle the problem on their own. Telling a man that he might feel better months later is the same as inviting him to leave the office.

THE PRIMARY ISSUES OF THERAPY WITH MEN

Robert Bly (1986) believes that there are four primary issues men must resolve to become healthy adults and calls these issues the "initiation rites" of men into the mature acceptance of their maleness. They are, in short, the agenda for therapy with men. Bly's four primary issues are:

1. Resolving ambivalence toward the role their mothers played in their development and learning to accept the inevitability of life without her support.
2. Learning to resolve incongruent messages from aloof or absent fathers.
3. Learning to trust and respect the wisdom of others.
4. Learning to choose mates whose positive attributes transcend physical appeal.

Resolving Issues Related to the Influence of Mothers

The first therapy issue considers the mother's role in the family, her alliances, her conflicts with the father, and her willingness or ability to prepare her son for autonomy and independence. The exploration of a man's view of his mother helps explain many of the client's notions about the role of men. It may also help explain the origin of problems in relationships with women including codependence, abuse, and problems with intimacy. A discussion of the relationship between mother and father can also help in understanding the way men view commitment to their spouses and families. Problems in separation from the mother may further suggest difficulty in accepting adult responsibilities. As one client said during a discussion about his mother,

I always thought she was very seductive. I don't mean sexually, but she used our relationship to distance my father from her and it made me feel very special growing up. I felt like a prince. No woman was good enough for me. I'd been loved by the most important woman in my world. Who could ever compare to that? No one, of course. It created terrible conflicts with my father who, I always felt, hated me, and it made me go through a series of relationships with women so dysfunctional, I can only wonder what was going on at the time. But, you see, when you're loved in a truly dysfunctional way by your mother, you come to believe that the role of every women in your life is to love you with the same intensity. And when it doesn't happen, you feel hurt and confused. In therapy, I've begun to see the many troubled messages my mother gave me about myself and about relationships. She could never talk about love without complaining about my father and comparing me to him by saying that I was the sort of man she should have married, not that loser of a father of mine. She always used that word to describe him, "loser."

When your mother loves you more than her husband, the little crazy things that go on in your head tell you that you're really the husband and that the guy in her bed is just a temporary visitor. When she died, I went into a two-year depression. I'd lost my only lover and I didn't think anyone would ever replace her. I was wrong, of course, and with some very hard work that helped me define the type of woman I want to be with, I've been able to make much more satisfying choices. But it took me until I was 50 to do it. I think all men have confused relationships with their mothers, and if I could say anything to other men, it would be to work out your feelings about your mother. If you don't, you'll have a very rough time with relationships and with becoming a mature and healthy man.

Defining Absent and Aloof Fathers

Messages regarding love, commitment, male conduct, and responsibility are frequently given to sons by fathers. When sons discuss fathers, there is considerable denial. The father's hard work and his dedication to the family may be forgotten by the son to be replaced by memories of abandonment, aloofness, weakness, or abuse. Confusion may also exist regarding the father's intentions, his actual behavior, and his impact on family life. Sometimes a mother's view of the father forms the basis of the son's memories and considerable work may be necessary to separate reality from memory. Fathers are powerful figures in the lives of men. Their behavior, their beliefs and values, their worldviews, take on added importance in the man's life and should be explored thoroughly. This exploration can help men resolve long-held patterns of behavior influenced by their fathers which distress and confuse men as adults.

In a men's group, a participant who was also a therapist had a very confused memory of his father which he shared with the group members:

> My father was an FBI agent. Very macho, you know. The strong one. In fourth grade he took to driving me out into the country and telling me how useless his life was. At these times he would take his gun out and put it in his mouth. "If I had the guts," he'd tell me, "I'd pull the trigger." He never did, you know, until I was in tenth grade. By then, he'd lost his job because of his drinking. We never did know what the trouble was, it was so deep inside. By the time he killed himself, I wasn't surprised, I was relieved. I vowed that I'd never be the wimp *he* was and here I am at 38 with the same preoccupation with death and the same pain inside I can't explain.

The men in the group tried to help the client understand the source of his pain. In time, it became clear that at an early age, the client was required to rescue his father from his suicidal inclinations. Failing at that, the client always believed that he was responsible for his father's progression into alcoholism and depression and that he was also a failure as a therapist. This sense of failure defined him as a therapist and resulted in a profound fear that he was harming his clients. The client later told the group that as much as he had tried to understand his behavior, it was not until the group allowed him to discuss his experiences with his father that he was really able to make changes in his life. The group also helped the client remember more positive attributes of his father and to focus on his father's strengths. He told the group that he didn't think a man could have a healthy view of himself if he felt emotionally betrayed and abandoned by his father. Many of the group members felt the same way and had gone through a process of finding out more about their fathers by talking to others who knew them. One client with very negative feelings about his father told the group of an insight he had about his father and how it had changed him:

> I was trained to be successful by my father. Survival and winning, that's what I was taught. Don't depend on anyone else, be above it all, and don't trust anyone. Now I've reached a point in my life where everything is falling apart. I'm *not* strong or confident. I'm weak and confused and I can't find a friend who will help because I was taught by my father not to have friends. And I can't go to my family because they have the same problems I do. Before he died, I asked my father what to do about the confusion I felt and he reminded me that he walked across Russia and worked for three years as a kid in Europe to get the money to come to America. Once he got here, he learned a new language, and even though he talked with an accent, he made it and so would I. He said that this was just a bad time that I was going through. I discounted everything he said and then he passed away suddenly and I had a very long period of grief that I'm not fully over.
>
> I started thinking about what he said and asked some of my relatives about his life. They thought my father was the most generous and giving man they'd ever known. I was dumbfounded. My dad was a union man and when I went off to graduate school after he died, at every train stop along the way, men would meet me on the platform and give me cookies, or homemade bread, or a sandwich. They'd get teary eyed when they'd talk about my dad. He'd helped them keep jobs when they were deteriorating as men and he believed in them.
>
> I began reconciling the view I had of my father with the view everyone else had, and I came to realize that he gave me messages that helped him survive. They were loving messages because the intent was to help me survive even if they were messages that sometimes make me aloof and isolated. After my father passed away, I began having conversations with him in my mind. These conversations are the ones I never had with him when he was alive. They are funny, and sexy, and they fill me with joy. I wish I'd had them when he was still alive but, thankfully, he's allowed me to have this connection with him and it's amazing to me how wise and tender and supportive he seems to me now. Maybe I'm fooling myself into believing that he was always that way, but I don't think so.
>
> I think he was tough on the outside but tender on the inside. When I was away at undergraduate school and he was still alive, he used to write me 30

page long letters about the way snow sounded when he walked on it, or the way the smoke hung over our town when it was really cold. Long, beautiful, poetic letters without punctuation marks or a numbering system that made following the letter almost impossible. I used to think they were silly letters, but then I went back and I read them, and they made me cry. They were beautiful, caring letters, full of his happiness that I was bettering myself, and praise for my achievements. I don't think men move on in their lives until they really know their fathers, even if it comes after they've passed away. It's never too late to know your father, and you may be surprised that your memory and the reality don't match at all.

Accepting Advice From People of Wisdom

The third issue to explore with adult men is their choice of people for advice and guidance. This exploration of who represents truth and wisdom in a man's life can help identify a man's value system and his larger worldview. It may also explain whether the current choice of people of wisdom has a positive or a negative impact on the client because not everyone chosen by the client to provide advice and guidance demonstrates positive or healthy behavior. Sometimes a man's choice of a person of wisdom may be someone who reinforces abusive or self-destructive behaviors. He or she may represent the same dysfunctional attitudes of the client toward the role of men. Highly dysfunctional men (those who abuse and terrorize wives and children) almost always choose close friends who support their own abusive views. In explaining this, one client told me the following story:

> My best friend is a guy I work with named John. He doesn't take crap from anybody. I've seen him beat up his wife for disagreeing with him. I admire that, you know. I wish I could be more like John. Nobody hassles him, that's for sure. Maybe if I was more like him, my wife would treat me better. My dad was a lot like John. He'd slap you around if you even looked at him wrong. Everybody respected him, too. I guess I'm too soft. That's what John says, anyway.

In trying to understand the choice of John as his man of wisdom, clearly the client hoped to find someone who would prod him into being more like his own abusive father. The choice of an abusive friend explained an important decision the client had made—to incorporate the abusive patterns of his own father as a way of dealing with the complexities and unhappiness in his life. That path would lead to the same destruction of his family and the march toward alcoholism experienced by his father. Nonetheless, his man of wisdom represented authority, power, and certainty, attributes lacking in the client's confused understanding of how to deal with family issues he was increasingly unable to handle. After some months of mandatory therapy for spousal abuse, the client came to recognize that accepting advice from John led to serious problems in his own life:

> John is really a mean bastard. I'm starting to see things a lot different since I've been coming to the group. When I told him what I was learning, he just made fun of me. He said that this sissy stuff I was learning would make me more "pussy whipped" than I was before. His wife was sitting there when he said that and she had bruises on her face and a couple of front teeth were missing. She used to be a nice looking woman, but now she looks old and worn out. Anyway, I told John that I didn't agree with him. I told him since I'd been coming to the group, I was doing better at home. There were still rough times, but not like before. I said it took a real man to face up to what you were doing to your wife and kids and to change that before you really hurt people. Then he said something my dad would have said. He said, "Men don't treat kids and wives good. That's not our job. Sometimes you got to hurt them a little to help them see the way." Well, it reminded me of how much my pa hurt me. So I thanked him and left. I've been chumming around with this guy who isn't like John at all. He used to be a boozer and a wife-beater but he got religion and he changed. We meet for coffee before work and I can really talk to him. He gives me good advice and it usually works. I'm meeting other men like him and they're good men who have happy families and good lives. I'm happy about it. Friends are as important as family, and I've got some good ones now.

The Ideal Mate (The Czarina of the Heart)

The final issue men need to resolve is the hidden or eternal woman who represents a man's adult fantasy of his ideal mate. The difference between the fantasized ideal woman and the woman a man may choose as his mate helps to explain the degree of contentment or unhappiness he will experience in the relationship. The perfect woman is a combination of the nurturing and loving qualities of the idealized "Good Mother," as well as someone who, unlike a current wife or girlfriend, is completely safe emotionally and will be continually nurturing and giving regardless of the man's behavior. Trying to help men understand that an idealized view of women often results in unhappy relationships, demystifies women and helps men enter into intimate relationships based on a realistic understanding and appreciation of women rather than on fantasy. As one client said,

> I had this thing about women being beautiful, gentle, tender, loving, kind, endlessly considerate and supportive, never challenging or unhappy and, positively in love with me even when I was acting like a jerk. I never found that woman and I never will. Just as I'm no perfect man, neither are women perfect. I think you have to make a list of the qualities you want in a relationship, narrow the list down to something attainable and realistic, test the waters out to see if your list is right, and then make the adjustments necessary for a compatible relationship. Maybe all men are obsessed with beauty, but as I started this journey, I found that inner beauty almost always outweighs outer beauty. Women who were unkind, but beautiful, suddenly stopped being beautiful to me. Gentle women had an attraction that was overpowering. I discovered I found them much more beautiful than the really gorgeous women I'd been dating. I respect intelligence and accomplishment in women but I'd date needy and dependent women because it made me feel superior.

> The women I see now listen, they relate, they offer suggestions, they provide companionship I never really had before, and they allow disagreements to be worked out without a change in my feelings for them. It amazes me, really. What was I thinking all these years? I think I was thinking what a lot of men think: The better looking the woman, the more that says about you as a sexual and attractive man. It's really baloney, you know. The power women have isn't in their beauty, it's in the way you feel as a man when you're with someone compatible, someone who loves you for who you are. You get old, you change physically, you lose your job, you get ill, and they still love you and you love them. If a man can achieve that sort of a relationship, he's made it as a man in my book.

GUIDELINES FOR WORK WITH MEN CONSISTENT WITH MALE SOCIALIZATION

The Developmental Model

Kelly and Hall (1992a, 1992b, 1994) suggest the use of what they call the "developmental model" for work with men. In the developmental model, male behavior isn't viewed as pathological. Instead, the model views men in the context of lacking an opportunity to learn necessary skills to function well in certain situations. Those skills can be learned if men are given a chance. To work effectively with men, helping professionals need to acknowledge the client's strengths and respect him for his history of positive behavior. Development of social skills, in this model, can be learned through education if the behavior is seen within a social context. Although men often don't respond well to therapy in its present form, the following guidelines show how the developmental model can be used effectively with men and how the model serves to define a different type of therapy.

GUIDELINES FOR WORK WITH MEN

Treatment Must Be Collaborative

Men often accept help when it is given collaboratively and with an appreciation for their input. Men are doers, so giving them assignments to gather and read material that may help them better deal with an issue may be one way of responding to their attempts to change behavior. It's always wise to listen carefully as men discuss what they have found out about themselves through readings and attempts to problem-solve, and to be supportive, even if their interpretation of the material they've found and its relation to their problems isn't quite right. It's not effective to downplay their efforts by focusing on what they did wrong. Men resent people who think they know it all or insist that their way is the only way, and they resent therapists who seem aloof or unwilling to share information. Saleebey (2000) correctly describes the collaborative experience when he writes,

Healing, transformation, regeneration, and resilience almost always occur within the confines of a personal, friendly, and dialogical relationship ... the more the power of a caring relationship is actualized with those served, the better the individual's future .... (p. 128)

The need for collaboration in treatment is discussed in the following description of therapy:

I went to see a therapist about my marriage. He was this very aloof guy and he said that before I could resolve the problems in my marriage, that I'd have to explore my early life experiences. The past always explained the present, he said. I mean I had some very good ideas about why the marriage was going bad and I wanted to talk about them, but he said we needed to explore the past first. He was very insistent. So we explored the past and the more we did it, the more I started hating the guy. He wasn't listening to me at all. I just got sick of it and found a new person, a young woman who made it clear that she valued my ideas and perceptions and wondered what I thought was happening in the marriage and how it might be fixed. Well, we had this incredible discussion and it was like a breath of fresh air after the other guy. She was really interested in what I had to say and she listened very attentively. In no time, we were testing things out we thought might work, and they did. I mean it was great. She actually thought my insights into the relationship were very profound and she kept telling me how easy it was to work with me and how motivated I was. We almost never talked about the past but focused on why things were going badly with my wife and what I could do to make them better.

I'm happy in my marriage now. I think my therapist is a very wise person and I get a little emotional when I think about how good the help was she gave me. She asked my opinion and she made me feel competent at a time when I was feeling like a failure. Praising my ideas just made me feel like a million bucks.

Treatment Should Define Male Socialization in a Positive Way

Men don't often change when the process that defines their belief systems is considered dysfunctional. They improve when their belief systems are viewed with pride, understanding, and appreciation. The tendency to ridicule men for what they believe is hurtful to men and will usually end in termination of therapy or staying in therapy halfheartedly. There are many positive aspects of male socialization that lead to admirable behavior. Men should be praised for their hard work and their efforts to provide for their families. They should be recognized for their toughness, endurance, and for their efforts to resolve problems. As Kelly and Hall (1994) state, "As long as we hold men solely responsible for all negative events in their lives, in their families, and in the world, we have no hope of helping men" (p. 482).

As an example of treatment that failed to value male socialization, a male client going through a severe adjustment to retirement shared the following experience with me about how difficult it was for him to seek help from the counseling service in his HMO, and, when he sought it, how unsuccessful it was:

I retired because I was really burned out on my job. All I could think about was quitting. I'd written resignation letters on the computer for many years. They were categorized by how angry I was and some of them were doozies. I finally quit without a retirement plan and after 4 months of feeling great, I started missing work, or at least something to occupy my time. I don't have hobbies and I've never been good at filling spare time. So I looked for some work and got turned down by every place I applied. It was really hurtful after all the years I'd spent working so hard. The more I got turned down, the more anxious and depressed I became. I don't like the idea of medication for down moods and I talked to my primary care doctor who suggested therapy. I reluctantly went, but I didn't feel very optimistic because I don't think most therapists know the first thing about men.

The therapist I saw made a joke out of what I was going through and said she knew lots of men who would be "tickled pink" to be in my shoes. She suggested a group called "Getting off your Rockers." Most of the people were easily 10 to 15 years older than me and did activities I really dislike, like square dancing. I saw her twice and decided she was making me more upset than I was before I first came in. I mean, a side of me knows there are better therapists, but it just makes me mad that I did something that was so hard for me to do and the results were worst than doing nothing. I don't think I have the energy to go back and try someone else. Most of the therapists in my HMO are women and, from what I can see in the waiting room, almost all of the clients are women. I don't think the therapists know what to do with older men at my place in life, and I doubt if they see retirement the same way that most successful men do. I've used work to put off dealing with my non-existent personal life. I would think that would be evident to any therapist in 5 minutes. For me, retirement is about getting old. Being turned down for other jobs just reinforces that feeling. Not to be taken seriously is just plain hurtful. I don't know who I'm more angry at: Therapists for being incompetent, or me for getting myself in this situation and going for help when I knew it wouldn't work in the first place.

Treatment Should Not Be a Power Struggle

If you get into a power struggle with a man, you may win but you won't help him. Brooks (1999) points out that, although men may be antagonistic toward therapy in ways that often make therapists defensive, we shouldn't assume that they are unwilling to participate or to change. He suggests that there are aspects of personal involvement in a problem where men may deny culpability to avoid change. The therapist should be aware of the arguments men make to avoid personal responsibility for their problems with their families and with intimate relationships, but they should neither collude with men to ignore problems nor should they unnecessarily confront them. Being neutral and focusing on positive behavior will ultimately lead to discussions of troubled behavior.

One of the common mistakes therapists make with men is using stereotypes of male behavior without first checking them out with the client. Some common stereotypes of men are as follows: (a) Men believe that success and stress at work are justifications for a lack of involvement with families; (b) men do almost nothing to help run homes and leave everything, including raising children, to spouses; (c) men are rational at work but irrational when it comes to issues of intimacy and relationships; (d) men always act strong even when they don't feel strong; (e) men resist new approaches to fatherhood, marriage, and other close relationships because they are threatened by change; (f) men resist hearing about the destructive impact of stoicism; (g) men need sexual gratification and have few needs for emotional intimacy; (h) men think that people who praise them are manipulative; (i) pain strengthens feelings of masculinity and symptom relief only discourages men from making needed changes; (j) although men may change with age and become more focused on relationship and intimacy needs, real change doesn't take place until age 50 or later, if at all; (k) men go through a mid-life crisis during which time they have affairs with younger women as a way of proving their masculinity; (l) a corollary is that men are more interested in the conquest of women than in love or intimacy; (m) and a further corollary is that men will say anything to have sex with a woman, even the dreaded "I love you"; (n) men usually look for women who will be like their mothers, whereas they almost always act like their fathers, repeating the family pathology; (o) fathers are usually competitive with sons; (p) as men age, they lose their interest in sex; (q) men aren't interested in the finer things in life and asking them to read or see films will usually result in noncompliance; (r) alcohol abuse is so prevalent among men because the culture of drinking is a form of male bonding; (s) men will usually try and seduce a female therapist, which helps explain the stereotypes of men having affairs with their therapists (or is it women having affairs with their therapists?); (t) the word *traditional,* when used with men, almost always suggests potential for spousal abuse and the need to dominate; and (u) although the list is endless, men don't work as hard as women and get by because of the old boy network. If it weren't for the old boy network, women would have many more high positions in government and business because women are more conciliatory and understand cooperative relationships in a way that most men don't.

Labels Should Not Be Used with Men

Men resent labels. They really have no purpose in treatment. Instead of using terms such as *anxiety* or *depression,* suggest problems men might be experiencing including problems at work, problems in relationships, problems with substances, and so forth. Don't use pejorative terms such as *alcoholic,* when drinking a bit too much is a gentler and less pejorative way of saying the same thing. Never use diagnostic terms like *personality disorder* or *bipolar disorder* unless there is a clear reason, as in management of a problem through medication. A brochure I developed to promote services to male clients in a family service agency used the following terminology.:

A Description of Therapy for Men.   Short term consultation is offered to men having concerns about work, their relationships, or in other areas of their lives that cause stress. Consultations are with an older trained licensed male social worker with many years of experience in helping men with practical life problems. Usually, one or two meetings are sufficient, but if you'd like to spend more time talking to your consultant, that's perfectly O.K. Some examples of the reasons men come for consultations might be an unappreciative employer or work setting; children and spouses who aren't as caring as you'd like them to be; not knowing when you'd like to stop working or when a good time might be to change jobs or careers; work that isn't satisfying; feelings that seem different from how you usually feel, and other common experiences men have that respond well to brief consultations. All information provided to our male worker is confidential. Evening and weekend hours are available to accommodate your schedule. Grants permit us to offer the first two consultations at no cost. Further meetings are based on what you think a reasonable fee would be.

Frame Treatment As a Form of Short-Term Problem Solving

Don't describe therapy as something that may fundamentally change a man. Instead, describe it as a way of reducing stress through problem-solving or seeing a problem in a different way. Focus on specific problems and how they affect a man's physical and emotional health. Descriptions of therapy as a way of changing people often meet with resistance from men. Describe the process as something similar to consulting a specialist in a field the client understands. Focus on the fact that much can be accomplished in very few sessions and that many of the same skills men use at work or other successful areas of life can be used to reduce unwanted emotional states. Stress the fact that men will feel better as a result of therapy.

Describing Therapy As Problem-Solving.   In another section of the brochure I developed for a family service agency, I described services offered to men as follows:

> Many times it's hard to think through the best way to handle a tough life problem. Our trained worker is very skilled at helping men problem-solve in a quick and logical way. Help with problem-solving is often what many men find very useful to feel better. You will find our problem-solving suggestions very easy to understand and useful in many other areas of your life. When you finish meeting with your worker, you should feel more optimistic, less stressed, and a lot clearer about the way you intend to handle a life concern. There isn't anything magical about the services we offer because we think that men are able to solve problems with just a little practical assistance.

What Men Are and What They Think They Should Be

Many of the problems men experience result from the lack of congruence between how they think they should be as men and how they actually are. The messages men get in childhood and adolescence about expected male behaviors are often confusing and anxiety-provoking, primarily because they may seem so absolute and impossible to achieve. An adolescent client explained his feelings about male expectations this way:

> I get picked on all the time by the kids at school. Boys and girls both, and ever since I can remember. They put me down because I'm fat and I'm not very coordinated. I'm interested in science, and I wear clothes that aren't very cool, and I love computers. Kids call me "freak," "Doctor Weirdo," "Pussy Face," "Nerd" and other names that really hurt my feelings. I've never been interested in sports, so that makes me different, and I'm not very good socially. Being picked on just makes me feel like crying sometimes. So I'm not like the other kids, so big deal. Who says you have to be? I know I'm going to be successful in my life and I have a great family who

see all the potential I have, but these years in school, I can hardly wait until they're over. It's like there's a screenplay and if you don't follow the script then there's something wrong with you. I'm a guy and I'm happy about it, but the way some of the guys act, and some of the girls, you'd think they were the most insecure people around. If you don't follow the script, it makes them—I don't know—it makes them feel like something is wrong with them.

My dad was in Desert Storm and he was brave and won medals. He's a warm person and he tells me he loves me, and all, but when he tells me about school, it was the same way for him, being bullied and all. I think the things we're supposed to be as men are great. It's when men go overboard that it gets bad, and picking on other people, like I'm being picked on, it's the worst thing I see in the other kids. They need someone to feel superior to or they begin to feel rotten about themselves. My mom says that when I'm older and dating, that more mature girls will like me for my intelligence and my niceness, but that right now, girls like guys who are jerks, pretty much. She said she went out with her share before she met my dad. When she met him she said there was something so good hearted about him that she fell in love with him right away, and my mom is a babe and my dad isn't very handsome, so I guess there's still a chance for me. I wish it wasn't so bad at school, though, I really do.

What Works With Women May Not Work With Men

A new model of treatment is needed if psychotherapy is to be used successfully with men. The new model of therapy will view men in a positive way. It will be collaborate in helping men to find solutions and it will use a supportive and positive orientation to men and their achievements. Applying models of therapy to men that are useful for women may be just the reason many men are reluctant to use therapy. Just as women called for a new understanding of their emerging roles in a changing society, men are asking for the same thing. Consider a client discussing his past experiences with therapy:

> I went for therapy because my life was falling apart. So far, it's falling apart even faster now that I'm in therapy. I leave therapy sessions feeling like a failure. I don't think I ever get the therapist to hear my side of the

story. She already thinks she knows what's going on with me better than I do. I asked her for advice and feedback when I first came in and what I got was all this fishy insight. It's because of my father, or my mother, or my dog dying when I was at a vulnerable age. That's not what I want. I want someone to recognize that I've been successful in many ways. I want someone who can praise my good stuff and give me ideas about what to do about the bad stuff. I'm smart, I can take a hint. But what I get in therapy are these endless fishing expeditions instead of what I really want which is straight talk, done nicely, with a plan: If I do this, this, and this, that, that, and that will happen. If it doesn't, we'll try something else. What's so hard about that? What's so hard about knowing that if you listen to a man, you'll hear everything you need to know in order to help him?

I don't think men have much guile. I think we're pretty straightforward. I don't know, it's like what women have been saying to men: "You don't hear me and you don't understand what I'm saying." OK, I get it. Then why can't a man say the same thing? Why can't people get it that if they had some skill in doing therapy, men would be falling over each other trying to get help? Have you ever gone to a bar? Well, men can't talk enough about their problems, but at least people listen. In therapy, we get this bad rap that we discount therapy because we don't use it. Well, for sure. Men aren't dumb. They don't use therapy because it doesn't help them. What *would* help is to try and find out what men expect in therapy, test out some approaches that men and therapists agree on, and see if it works. My God, this isn't the middle ages. Why would that be so hard?

Trust Develops Slowly

Men don't bond easily and are generally suspicious of attempts to form relationships before they're emotionally ready. Don't assume that an intimate therapeutic relationship exists with a male client even when the client suggests that it does exist. Men are often very fearful of getting hurt by those they believe they should trust the most. Allow the relationship to dictate when self-disclosure is most appropriate. If trust hasn't developed, you may find men self-disclosing and then not returning for treatment because the self-disclosure has prompted feelings of vulnerability and self-loathing which men mistakenly believe therapists share. Scher (1979) says that, "competition trains men to be suspicious. The best way to gain trust is to be honest, patient, and indulgent of the client's wishes" (p. 254). Be certain that you are supportive, reassuring, and positive about the client and his self-disclosures. Men often have few outlets to discuss emotional difficulties. When they freely self-disclose, it often brings with it feelings of weakness. Pollack (1990) says that therapists must learn to reach out to male clients, mindful of the man's need to "save face" in the process of self-disclosure and intimacy.

In developing the relationship with a male client, assure him that you will value him as a person regardless of the problem he discusses. Make certain that you're being honest about it. As an example of what can happen when therapists are insincere about how much a man can trust them, a client said that a therapist he went to

> Yawned her way through therapy. The more troubled I was, the more she yawned. Of course I called her on it but she made up every reason in the book for her yawning, like having just eaten. She was very defensive about it, too. I began to suspect that she didn't know what to say to me about the painful things I was telling her and that she yawned because she was anxious. At a time when I really needed to tell someone what was honestly happening to me, I began to censure what I told her. The more superficial I was, the less she yawned. I was living in a small town and everyone I called for help was too busy to see me, so I had little choice but to continue with her. Finally, I just stopped going. I didn't trust her a bit, not at all. This was further validated when she double billed two insurance companies for the same sessions and received double payments. I was long gone from the community by the time I found this out, but it certainly said what I thought all along: She wasn't trustworthy. And I guess I'm using the word trust more as a way of describing her personal integrity with me. Rather than being up front, she hid behind her lack of ability to help me. If you can't trust someone to help you, what's the point? I'm very troubled about the whole thing because my life was going to hell at the time and someone I could have worked with might have made a big difference.

> As a manager in a large company, I've worked indirectly with a number of therapists. They just don't seem like very caring people. They joke about their clients and they share information that seems very close to breaching confidentiality. I think the issue of trust is at the back of every man's

mind when he goes for therapy, and I think the inability to trust a lot of therapists comes from the messages they give men that they could care less about us, and that they don't think we're worth working with. And I'm not saying this about women therapists alone because male therapists do the same.

If you're going to be effective with men, you need to realize that therapy is a big step for most men. Therapy implies that men can't handle their lives using their own devices and that they're going to have to share dirty little truths that embarrass them and make them feel weak. If you want to help men, you have to like us, you have to consider us worthy people, you have to realize that we take our lives seriously and that you can't stereotype us or think of us like the men portrayed in bad male bashing jokes. And you have to do what's necessary for us to develop trust. You have to give us the absolute feeling that what we say will be held in confidence, that it will be taken with all humility and seriousness, and that you'll work as hard as you possibly can to help us. Most men believe that professionals don't take us seriously. Maybe that goes for the way women feel, too, and maybe it says something about the doctors and therapists we meet in our lives. If that's the case, there ought to be a lot higher level of training than there is now and it should help therapists learn the importance of building trust and developing meaningful and helpful relationships with male clients.

Structure Therapy

Men generally need order in their lives. It's a good idea to structure therapy carefully so that it has a logical set of steps to achieve an end result with a predictable point in time when it will end. Share your plan with the client and involve him in a discussion of whether the plan is appropriate for his needs. Therapy that seems to meander along with no focus will ultimately go nowhere with male clients. Perhaps it's an old canard to suggest that women are more comfortable with a lack of focus in treatment than men, but for certain, men need structure. To reinforce the need for structure, a client shared the following experience:

I went for therapy with someone who was highly regarded in the community. She was one of a couple of people I heard unequivocally good things about, although all my feedback came from women. I was in a lot of turmoil at work. I thought I needed some very focused help since I was depressed and drinking a lot. The therapist was quite gentle and her observations were often brilliant, but after a few sessions I started complaining that we weren't going anywhere. She seemed to be reacting to whatever I said with no specific goal in mind. I, of course, was worried I'd get fired and that I'd end up destitute. I felt an urgency for practical help that would allow me to put my energies into my problems at work. Instead, we'd just amble along with nothing specific happening. When I'd leave the sessions, I'd go home, drink too much, and end up bawling. I was feeling very suicidal and shared that with her. The more I asked for focus, the less we seemed to have any. I switched therapists and she was very hurt about it. When I told her I was going to someone else, she had tears in her eyes, so I think I mattered and that she was concerned about me. The new therapist was very focused and very practical. She was also very positive and kept on getting me to look at my past achievements in life, insisting that someone with my skills would overcome this setback, and I did. I adored the first therapist. I didn't feel very much at all about the second one, but she helped me most since I could see where we were going and I thought she knew exactly what needed to be done.

I didn't get fired but I took a new job. When I moved, the first therapist called me in the new community I'd moved to. Ostensibly, the call was about my bill but it was really to have closure. Her closure. She said that I'd misunderstood the way she worked and had I given it more time, I would have done a lot better. I tried to get her to see that I was falling apart and very close to doing something that was self-destructive, but she said that you have a hurt a lot before you get better. I couldn't believe my ears. How much more could I hurt than what I felt about possibly being fired? We ended on a very bad note and to this day, I'm confused about it all. I felt that her lack of direction was going to be my undoing.

Focus on Strengths

Keep the discussion focused on strengths since men are often reluctant to discuss negative issues unless they are operating from a positive emotional position. One approach that may work for men is the strengths perspective which I (Glicken, 2004) define as a way of viewing the positive behaviors of clients by helping them see that problem areas are secondary to areas of strength. Out of what they do well can come helping solutions that have their origins in the successful strategies they use daily in their lives to cope with a variety of important issues, problems, and concerns. (p. 3)

One client complained that everything he believed was good about himself was being attacked by a therapist he had gone to see for help with a work-related problem:

I went to a therapist, an older woman in my HMO. It was clear she didn't especially feel comfortable working with men because she kept on saying how most of her clients were women. When I told her about the problems I was having at work, she went into this little lecture about how what men believe always gets them into trouble. I'm working almost two people's jobs and I'm starting to get very irritable about it. Some woman complained and my boss accused me of potential for workplace violence. Instead of seeing my irritability as coming from working so hard, they actually threatened to fire me if I didn't go for counseling. So I went, and here's this lady lecturing me on male pride and the idea that I can do superhuman things, and my stoic attitudes, and all this stuff that I actually think are positives. She wanted me to use more female approaches to the job, like being more sensitive, and working better with others, and talking to others about the things that upset me. OK, so not bad ideas, but why not be positive about the fact that I'm working two people's job and that, for the most part, I'm doing very well? Why not assume the woman who complained was in the wrong, or that the organization I was working for was treating me badly? I really don't get it. You go for help and you're told to be more like a woman, but all this stuff I read about the women's movement is about women being more like men. If we're so bad, why are we the model for women to do better in their lives?

SUMMARY

Therapy offers men an important way of changing troubled behavior when done cooperatively and with respect and support. A treatment approach using social learning as its model is discussed along with the primary issues of treatment which Bly (1986) calls the initiation rites to healthy adult male behavior. A number of short feedback pieces suggest problems men have had in therapy and their ideas about what went wrong and what might have been done to make their treatment much more effective. A call was made for a new type of therapy for men which parallels the call for a new type of therapy made by women in the 1960s and 1970s. In this new therapy, male socialization would be supported and symptom removal would be a primary treatment concern. Several model descriptions of services to men are offered as a way of explaining that treatment isn't something men should fear and that significant change might result in a short amount of time using very concrete, problem-solving approaches.

Storytelling, Personal Coaching, Humor, Role Plays, Men's Groups, and Other Useful Approaches for Treating Men

This chapter discusses several treatment approaches that have relevance for men, including the use of stories, humor with metaphorical meaning, the men's group, bibliotherapy, personal coaching, and the selective use of role plays. There are, of course, many other more helpful approaches for treating men that were discussed in prior chapters or are discussed in future chapters, including anger and stress management, cognitive therapy, couples therapy, and so forth, but because therapy with men enters uncharted waters for workers, the following might help in the process of building trust so that common male problems might be resolved.

PERSONAL COACHING

Although the distinctions between personal coaching, brief psychotherapy, and crisis intervention are often vague, for our purposes, personal coaching is a brief, goal-oriented way of problem-solving that generally works on a specific problem with healthy men for a short period of time. It is highly performance-oriented and is much less concerned than therapy with the development of insight or broader application to other areas of life. Clients are generally men who have intrusive problems requiring quick solutions. Work-related problems, job changes, divorce work, and relationship problems may all be issues that respond well to personal coaching.

Putting aside concerns about the professional credentials of coaches and the research on its effectiveness (which is limited), let's consider the elements of personal coaching that might be useful in work with men. Personal coaching focuses on "here and now" problems. It doesn't assume that a problem has its origins in the past, and it tries to find quick and logical solutions. Personal coaching is very practical. It uses advice, homework, and searching for answers in the literature and on the Internet. Personal coaches often suggest that clients keep logs or write down ideas that are then shared with the coach (or therapist). This technique seems efficient for many men who believe that taking personal responsibility for change will speed up the process. Personal coaching encourages the use of behavioral charting to analyze a problem and to track success. Charting is a way of problem-solving that is often familiar to men.

My daughter developed a chart to determine which graduate schools she should focus on when applying to schools in public health. I suggested four or five indicators to determine which schools were most likely to provide a good experience (national rankings, availability of assistantships, and program focus). By the time she sent the chart to me, she had over twenty indicators. When she was done filling in the information under each indicator, it was clear that four or five programs stood out. My daughter grew up with behavioral charting and feels very comfortable using it. She finds that it cuts down on extraneous efforts to problem solve and that it can be very efficient.

Continuing on with the elements of personal coaching, coaching assumes that clients are emotionally healthy and functioning well but just need some practical and supportive assistance with problem-solving. Compare this to therapy that assumes dysfunction, describes people in unhealthy ways, and often uses labels. Whether people are emotionally healthy is something no one can tell for certain at the start of treatment. It should soon become apparent whether problems need deeper and more long-term approaches as the client tries to use coaching and finds that it either doesn't help or the material focused on is difficult for the client to apply to his life. Coaching is very positive and optimistic. It believes that problems can be resolved in a short period of time and that the client has the necessary inner resources and skills to resolve the problem with just a little direction from the coach. Compare this to descriptions of therapy as an often long-term, painful, in-depth process and you can see why many men would prefer coaching. Coaching seems very much like the social encounters men have in their daily lives. Everybody understands the term *coaching*, while *therapy* is still a term with many misconceptions, and, among some cultures and men, negative connotations.

As an example of personal coaching, a friend of mine saw a coach because of concerns about his job performance. His most recent evaluation was mediocre to poor. Given the company's economic condition, my friend worried that he might lose his job. With a family to support and no other possibilities of similar work in his field in the community, my friend was very determined to improve his work performance. The coach looked at his written performance and saw three areas that definitely needed improving. Over two sessions, the coach and my friend worked together on practical ways of improving his performance. They also developed a way of measuring whether improvement was taking place. After the initial two sessions, the client sent the coach a weekly progress report by e-mail. Brief telephone calls augmented the reports. Several times my friend was clearly not following through on the strategies they had agreed to and the coach called him in for a chat. The coach and my friend also worked on a "360," a management technique used to get maximum feedback from important coworkers about my friend's work performance. With work evaluations coming every three months, they had less than three months to resolve the problem, and they did. The next evaluation placed my friend's performance in the low excellent range and his job was secure.

How did this differ from therapy? My friend had initially gone for therapy when he saw his work evaluations begin to deteriorate. The therapist felt that my friend was experiencing a mild depression in response to being passed over for a promotion. There were also some conflicts in the family that seemed to be troubling him that could have been responsible for his poor work performance. Therapy consisted of trying to find out more about his feelings regarding the promotion and his concerns about his family. There were some very good discussions and the therapist felt that therapy was certainly helping him until a quarterly evaluation suggested that his performance had deteriorated even more. Concerned that therapy wasn't helping, my friend sought out the personal coach on the advice of some coworkers who had used her in the past with good success. In comparing the two forms of help, my friend said the following:

> I liked both people. I thought they were very competent and caring. I think the therapist was helpful in getting me to talk about my reaction to not getting the promotion and my family problems. She was right in thinking that I was depressed, because I was. I just didn't know what to do about work and she wasn't overly helpful. When I went to the coach, all she talked about was work. I felt there were other things that needed dealing with but that work was the most important one. She helped a lot. She was very nice, in a no-nonsense way, and she knew her stuff. In no time, I was back on track at work but felt there were personal issues I needed to deal with before the same thing that happened at work started happening at home. So I went back to the therapist and I'm very happy with the work we're doing together. Why didn't I stay with the coach? I don't know. My personal life is a lot more complicated than work. I thought I needed someone who would listen and help me figure it all out. I don't think charts and 360's work well for personal problems, but maybe they do. I'd recommend a coach for very practical problems and a therapist for more complicated problems. That's my read on it, anyway.

In another example of personal coaching, a client who was having problems in his marriage went to a personal coach. He explained that he and his wife had been in marital therapy but they hadn't been able to resolve their problems and now, facing the prospect of a separation and divorce, he sought some short-term help to prepare himself for the divorce and his new life as an older single man. He shared the following with me:

> The coach was very supportive. He asked what I hoped to accomplish and when I told him, he went to the computer and wrote a contract that specified the problems we would try and resolve. I told him I wanted to feel a lot less stress than I was feeling then and to try and deal with the di-

vorce proceedings as calmly and objectively as I could. I said that my wife was trying to take me to the cleaners and I wanted to come out the divorce with some money and my ego intact. It was a very business-like experience; sort of like going to a lawyer, I guess. He wrote everything down and read it back to me. When he was done he asked me to read the contract and, if I agreed, to sign it. It spelled out what I wanted to change and what I had to do to make that happen. It was very logical and straight-forward.

I wouldn't say he was very warm but he was definitely confident and positive, and it sort of set the tone for our work together. I went 5 times and in that time we worked out an equitable divorce settlement and we worked on lowering my stress level. He encouraged walking and other activities and asked me to keep track of my blood pressure and pulse and, if possible, my cholesterol and blood sugars. He also got me to promise I wouldn't drink during this period when we were trying to figure things out. He said to think of it as if I were in training for a race. The better condition I was in, the better I'd do. And the truth is that I did very well with the settlement, better than I thought I would. I felt awful about being single and so we expanded the contract and worked on that. Everything had a solution, he said, I just had to think through the steps of finding the right solution.

It was all very logical, not very warm, but very successful. I think I went a total of 8 times, altogether. We went 20 times for marital therapy and we just got worse and worse. I can't say it was the most memorable experience I've ever had, but it was very successful. Maybe I'll consider therapy down the line if I have any adjustment problems to being single, and maybe I'd go back to see him. I'm just not entirely sure. What I *do* know is that I came out of this terrible time a lot better than I thought I would and I'd recommend coaching over therapy for the kind of problem I had. Maybe therapy is better for people who have serious problems, but for practical kinds of problems where you need some advice and direction, I don't think you can beat personal coaching.

THE USE OF STORIES

Allen and Laird (1993) suggest that one potential approach to treatment is to permit men to tell stories about their lives because sets of linked stories can help explain "paradoxes and contradictions" in a man's life. They describe the use of stories with men in the following way:

> Men have been denied their domestic stories. We know little of their private thoughts, their places in family life. In fact, men are frequently storied, in the media and on television, as incompetent buffoons when it comes to family life, understanding women, or parenting their children. If women's public stories have been limited and distorted and if women lack the "proper" language for public discourse, men's domestic stories are virtually unknown, and men are often at a loss for words in the intimate environs of family life. (p. 443)

The use of stories can be a powerful way of helping men find important themes in their lives. As Kelly and Hall (1994) suggest, "As long as we tell men what their behavior means instead of asking them to interpret their behavior for us, we do not yet understand men" (p. 482). Although reality is sometimes blunted when stories are told, they serve as an ideal way of helping men discuss important life events and to identify themes in their lives that may be continually repeated. Allen and Laird (1993) believe that the stories men tell are their interpretation of the way men are supposed to act in any given situation. A story represents the man's proximity to proscribed role expectations. In the following discussion by a woman about her father, male expectations of courage in a crisis and the impact of fear are discussed:

> When I was a teenager and away from school, there was a major gas main explosion in our community. Several homes blew up and others were threatened. My father rushed home to turn off the gas in our house. Several of the neighbor women, who had also rushed home, screamed at him to come to their homes and turn off the gas. He saved at least a dozen homes. In one of the houses, the floors were buckling. My father was a hero and I was terribly proud of him. I realized that my father never told this story, one of the few positive ones available in the family folklore, for he was much aligned and ridiculed. I asked him why he never talked about it and he said, "I didn't tell the story because I was afraid. I didn't want to go into those homes, and I'm ashamed." (Allen & Laird, 1993, p. 445)

This story is one that most men can easily recognize. A heroic act be-comes negated because the actor is fearful and has to fight feelings of cowardice. This paradox of acting bravely and feeling frightened would negate the heroic act for many men and it helps to understand the high standards men set for themselves.

It is common for men to tell stories that may have metaphorical meaning. Often, men fail to understand the broader implications of a story. This is where the therapist might help men find connections and themes in a story the client has chosen to tell. Men believe that stories are often safe ways of sharing feelings. The stories men tell may not be truth-ful or factual but they contain messages that may be unclear to the client but at some level have relevance. It's best to look at the subtext of the story to help the client see important connections. This is often the way men learn: by seeing and connecting disparate behaviors, themes, and life experiences.

THERAPEUTIC METAPHORS

Haley (1986) defines metaphors as a communication that has multiple meaning. Therapeutic metaphors, according to Hendrix (1986), help clients see similarities in situations and help clients connect events in their lives that may seem disconnected, but are not. Zuniga (1992) says that metaphors help clients overcome perceptions of events that inhibit dealing successfully with a problem. According to Martin, Cummings, and Hallberg (1992), metaphors may encourage new learning and help clients provide new meaning to important events in their lives. Heston and Kottman (1997) write the following: "The parallels between the cli-ent's situation, relationships, self-perception, and those of the protago-nist of the metaphor must be clear enough so that the client can make the bridge of personal connection" (p. 93).

Therapeutic metaphors can be very helpful with men because lan-guage often fails to adequately allow men to express inner feelings, and cultures have traditionally invented ways to transmit shared, highly per-sonal feelings thorough music, art, and literature, using metaphors to suggest implicit meaning. Although metaphors connect incompatible subjects, most people understand their implicit meaning. When metaphors are conveyed through humor, stories, poetry, literature, proverbs, and music, they have a power to influence men who might not otherwise understand connections between incompatible or misunderstood subjects. Penn (2001) believes that people in difficulty are surrounded by negative metaphors that suggest "dependence, poor genes, repressed personalities, weak constitutions" (p. 33). Our task in treatment is to replace negative metaphors with positive ones. People often think of metaphors as being spoken or written but Zuniga (1992) includes a number of additional ways in which metaphors are used and classifies therapeutic metaphors as:

> 1) Major stories that address complex clinical problems; 2) anecdotes or short stories focused on specific or limited goals; 3) analogies, similes or brief figurative statements or phrases that underscore specific points; 4) relationship metaphors, which can use one relationship as a metaphor for another; 5) tasks with metaphorical meanings that can be undertaken by clients between sessions; 6) artistic metaphors which can be paintings, drawing clay models or creations which symbolize something else. (p. 57)

HUMOR AS METAPHORICAL

The use of self-deprecation and gallows humor often strikes clinicians as dysfunctional, but generations of immigrant people, particularly Jewish immigrants, have learned to laugh at problems and to make fun of themselves as a way of coping with difficult life issues. Clinicians can use humor because it is a familiar way for men to convey subtle emotional messages. The humor used, however, must be constructive and insightful. It's purpose is to help people laugh at their behavior and to recognize that as bad as things are, there is still an opportunity to see the funny side of any situation and to feel a sense of shared identity with others having similar experiences. Humor can serve to solidify a feeling of collective purpose and a common bond.

An example of a joke with metaphorical meaning was used with a client who was losing his temper at the noise made by his next-door neighbors. Unable to just go over and talk to them, he was obsessing about the situation to the point of being continually upset. To help him better deal with the situation, the worker told him the following joke:

> A writer is sitting at his computer trying to write, when his parrot starts calling him names. "You're so stupid, you're lazy, you don't feed me enough, I hate you," the parrot screeches. The writer tries to calm the parrot down, but to no avail. Starting to do a slow burn, the writer threatens the parrot.
>
> "If you don't stop that noise, and I mean stop it now," the writer yells, "I'm putting you in the freezer, and I mean it."
>
> The parrot doesn't take the warning seriously and keeps up a steady flow of criticism. "You're a pet-hater, you have a thing against birds, my beak is bigger than yours," and so on until, in a rage, the writer puts the parrot in the freezer.
>
> Twenty minutes later, the writer takes the parrot out. Shivering and full of frost, the parrot apologizes. "I'll never do that again," he says. "I've learned my lesson. I know what I did wrong and I'll never interrupt you again while you're writing. But tell me," the parrot asks, "I'm curious. Just what did the chicken do?"

This joke, about going too far with anger and the fact that the person punished gets the last laugh, helped the client see how troubled his behavior had become. After listening to the joke and talking to the worker about its meaning, he was willing to go to his neighbors and talk to them in a calm and reasonable way. And if the noise level didn't decline, or if the neighbor was unwilling to comply, the client understood that there were legal options. However, the alternatives turned out to be unnecessary. When asked to lower the noise level, the neighbor readily agreed, apologizing in the process. The joke had held special metaphorical meaning for the client because it was the way his parents often spoke to him, preferring to tell stories or jokes about important issues rather than using direct statements with clear meaning.

Rosen (2003) describes his immigrant father's use of black humor to explain the immigrant Jewish way of making bad luck and misery seem somehow funny:

The humor and the odd link to more conventional elements of Jewish tradition (the Messiah, for example, has been about to not come for a long
time now) somehow saved these utterances from seeming like embodi-
ments of despair. They were, in a complicated way, an answer to despair.
Or at least they captured an aspect of Jewish tradition that has always fas-
cinated me—a wise pessimism that emphasizes the perpetuation of tradition rather than individual salvation. As Kafka memorably said, "There's
plenty of hope in the world—just not for us." (p. 87)

Humor should be linked to the presenting problem. It should also
help the client have an awareness of how the problem might be better resolved. Never assume, however, that what is funny to you might be
funny to your client. Before using humor with metaphorical meaning,
test out small bits of innocuous humor to gauge the client's sense of humor. And never tell ethnic jokes or you run the risk of offending the client. Use humor, but use it with caution and discretion.

BIBLIOTHERAPY: THE USE OF NOVELS, POETRY, FILMS, AND MUSIC

Bibliotherapy is the use of literature to facilitate the therapeutic process. Myers (1998) defines bibliotherapy as "a dynamic process of interaction between the individual and literature, which emphasizes the
reader's emotional response to what has been read" (p. 243). Pardeck
(1995) offers six goals of bibliotherapy: (a) to provide information, (b)
to gain insight, (c) to find solutions, (d) to stimulate a discussion of
problems, (e) to suggest new values and attitudes, and (f) to show clients how others have coped with problems similar to their own.
"Bibliotherapy provides metaphors for life experiences that help clients verbalize their thoughts and feelings and learn new ways to cope
with problems" (Myers, 1998, p. 246).

Novels, poetry, music, films, and videos can be particularly useful in
treating men because they often depict issues that men are trying to resolve in their own lives, including problems with children, problems at
work, relationship problems, and problems with fathers. Movies such as
"Prince of Tides" and "Forrest Gump" have had a positive impact on

men and help clinicians explain gender issues in ways that allow clients to open themselves to discussions of abuse, role confusion, intimacy, distant parents, and so forth. Novels such as *Bridges of Madison County* have clear meaning for many male clients because of its representation of romantic love and the hope it produces in all of us that love can happen spontaneously and unpredictably. Poetry can be particularly useful in helping men see a situation in a way that might elicit strong memories of prior events or powerful emotions. A poem used with a husband who could not accept the rape of his wife is a particularly poignant example:

The Two of Us

By

Jason Michael MacLeod

After six months,
I'm told about the oily green basement couch,
the muffled evening news upstairs,
and the two hands grabbing the back of her head,
forcing it down to his crotch.

And I can't hear this.
I just want to drink beer and talk
about the weekend or Raymond Carver
or any other damn thing, but here I sit
feeling my fingers rake flesh from my thighs.

She thought that if she just went along—
if she could have just made herself want to—
it wouldn't have been what it was. But no one
pulls that off and after walking past her parents,
she fell to her knees and vomited on their porch.

Then her voice trails off and I start in.
I stand up and say to her, *say* to her,
because I'm not yelling yet, what's his name?
But she shakes her head and she
just wants to forget. Forget it all.

We are not doing any forgetting tonight.
I punch the bookcase, knocking novels and poetry
to the floor. I take her arms so she can't ignore me
and yell things at her that I won't remember later and
I feel strong and goddammit, somebody is going to bleed.

Her look sobers me.
I shut up and let go.
Softly, she picks up her keys and walks out,
leaving me to melt deep into the cracks of the couch,
pale and shaking,
like him.

After reading the poem, the husband broke down and cried, telling the worker that it was just impossible for him to accept his wife's rape. Although he felt responsible to be loving and sensitive to wife, he also felt repulsed. These opposite feelings were driving him away from his wife. Although he knew these feelings were terribly hurtful to his wife, he also felt, irrationally, that his wife was to blame and that she had somehow encouraged the rape. The poem helped him get back in touch with the recognition that terrible things can happen to any of us, and it started a long, slow reconciliation with his wife who had felt rejected and demeaned by her husband's behavior since the rape.

Interestingly, it wasn't so much the content of the poem that prompted the client to reevaluate his feelings about the rape, but rather the suggestion of powerlessness in the phrase, "Leaving me to melt deep into the cracks of the couch." The poem didn't touch the client at a literal level but instead described, through the metaphor of melting into the couch, the client's feeling of powerlessness at not being able to cope with the rape. The client felt that he should be an understanding and sensitive husband and support his wife, but what he actually felt was anger, self-recrimination, and the urge to blame her. The confusion over this collision of feelings made him feel powerless, and the metaphor in the poem allowed him to discuss these significant feelings with the clinician.

In an application of metaphors to a research study, a former graduate student of mine was doing his master of social work (MSW) research project on the reasons gay and bisexual Latino men fail to disclose their

HIV Positive or AIDS status to family members. I suggested that he include questions about *dichos* (a Spanish word for wise sayings or proverbs) that expressed the reasons for the failure of the men to inform their family members (chapter 14 on work with Latino men describes dichos in much more detail). Almost without exception, the dichos provided by the men focused on feelings of uncleanliness and getting what they deserved because of their behavior. We found these metaphorical responses the most significant part of the study because they explained why men in such a family-oriented culture would be so unwilling to share vital health information. In effect, they had internalized negative stereotypes of gay and bisexual men, something we would not have known had we not asked for *dichos*, and something that helped us reconcile the men in the study with their families.

I'm also reminded of a Native American client whose brother died, unnecessarily, of hepatitis, and the rage he felt at his brother's death. His brother's death triggered long held feelings of fear about death that he began to discuss three months into treatment following a chance occurrence. The client was driving home from a job he held on a reservation in Arizona. He was listening to the radio when an erratic driver almost hit his car at a cross section. While the accident was in progress, he remembered clearly that he was listening to a song whose lyrics were, "You left me, just when I needed you most." The song and the accident in progress brought back powerful feelings of the fear he had as a child of driving on the reservation with his family and the concern everyone had that they would die from alcohol-related accidents. Before his brother's death, the client went on a business trip and when he returned, his brother was in a coma. The client felt deep unconscious responsibility for his brother's death and the song and the potential accident helped him understand his current feelings.

However, it wasn't the words of the song that helped the client progress, or the potential accident, or even the combination of the two. What the client said was that as he looked at the oncoming car, the driver made a nonverbal sign of forgiveness. He had all but forgotten that the shrug and the raising of hands in futility was what his brother did before he died. It was the passive acceptance of death that had always made him feel such anger at his people and which he now felt for his brother. The lyrics of the song and the sadness of the melody had not touched him literally but had prompted unconscious memories that helped put him in touch with his anger at his brother's death. In this way, the song and the potential accident acted as a catalyst for his conflicted feelings of powerlessness and rage at the death of his brother.

As many of us have discovered, literal interpretations of a client response to seemingly random events often fail to recognize that they have deeply personal and metaphorical meaning. As Franklin (1992) states in his work with Black men, insights should be approached gently and should not appear magical or outrageous, but should convey,"… knowledge, understanding, and empathy, all of which will strengthen the client's sense of trust in the therapists humanity and competence" (p. 354). Metaphors can do just that. They provide a slow, safe, but meaningful way to help the client understand hidden or fearful material that may be at the root of his problem and may offer the key to his progress.

THE MEN'S GROUP

One way to deal with male patterns of behavior is to help them understand how men assume roles in life. An effective way to promote this process is through the use of men's groups. Eisikovits and Edelson (1989) indicate that treatment success in men's groups where violence is an issue has been as high as 65%. Salloum, Avery, and McClain (2001) used a ten-week group therapy experience with Black adolescents who had lost a loved one to homicide. They concluded that both young women and young men benefited from the group experience at roughly the same levels and that, "On completion of group therapy, the adolescent participants reported an overall significant decrease in traumatic symptoms on an index of posttraumatic stress, especially in the areas of re-experiencing and avoidance symptoms" (p. 1125). Writing about the power of the group experience in what certainly describes men's groups, Scapillato and Manassis (2002) report that groups encourage powerful feelings with an emotional intensity that takes the group and the actor by surprise. Such events provide a further emotional and social learning experience, as group members have the opportunity to master strong feelings within a social situation. (p. 740)

Men's groups help men understand common male themes that sometimes result in troubled behavior. They also provide men with a reference group to help them view their current behavior in new ways and to test out new behaviors. For this to take place, the following conditions should first be met (Glicken, 1995): (a) an accepting environment where bonding and social interaction are emphasized; (b) a therapeutic environment that emphasizes the strengths and positive behaviors of group members and where men experience full acceptance for their emotional problems; (c) a nurturing and safe therapeutic approach that allows men to feel that being vulnerable may lead to important change; (d) an emotional outreach by the leader and by participants that helps men feel wanted, accepted, and valued; and (e) a reframing of men's issues where life problems are not explained by using a pathology model but are understood to exist in a social context which emphasizes the roles that men are often asked to assume and the problems that might occur as a result.

Groups where men participate, including a number of alcohol and drug-related treatment groups, are sometimes led by nonprofessionals and might best be thought of as self-help groups. In men's groups, participants are allowed to discuss highly emotional and often hidden issues that resonate with the experiences of other men. In one men's group, a member talked about his father:

My father was a very sarcastic man with my brother, sister, mother and especially with me. He took pleasure in ridiculing us. He always seemed to know what really bothered us about ourselves and he could be deadly with his comments. He reserved for me, his oldest son, particular attention. When I started dating, he kept talking about my pimples, how I sometimes slouched, and how shy I was around girls. He said that I had a "nothing personality" and that girls would find me boring. These were all things that I worried about anyway and when he started talking about them, it made me more self-conscious than ever. He did this until I left home and once I was on my own, I let him have it back with the same meanness and condescension that he'd used with me. I knew his weaknesses and I was prepared to say anything that would hurt his feelings. It was complete role reversal. The more I criticized him, the more he praised me. What was this all about? In some strange way, I think he associated being critical with being loving. It got to a point as he aged where I couldn't stand the sight of him and I tried to avoid him as much as I could. Of course, he was very hurt. As he aged he seemed to just dry up like a dying bird, and when he passed away, he was almost invisible. I've hated myself for doing that to him and I find that I've been depressed since he died last year.

Many of the men in the group had similar experiences with their own fathers and spoke to the client about their feelings of guilt and recrimination at treating their fathers so badly after their fathers had done the same to them. One man in the group finally said,

You try your best to be a good person, even when people hurt you. As a way of trying to get healthy, all of us struck out at our fathers. I don't feel good about it but you learn from the experience and if you feel remorse now at what you did, it makes you a much better father with your own children. My father couldn't accept a truce and he went to his grave fighting with me. I regret it and I wish I could have changed things between us before he died, but you learn from those experiences and if a father wants to continue treating you with a great deal of meanness, you suck it up, make the best of it, and get on with your life. The thing is you don't have to believe what he says about you anymore. That's the difference between being a kid and being a grown up. You have control over your feelings now because you know a lot more about yourself.

Another member of the group said,

My father was abusive, an alcoholic, and a very mean drunk. When my mom died he came to live with me and my wife and kids. I hated him and treated him very badly. It embarrassed my kids the way I was acting and we had a family meeting where they told me how they felt. They said it was affecting my relationship with them. So we had another family meeting with the old man present and we talked a lot of things through. The fact is that my father has changed over the years and he's become a very decent person. I can't forgive him for what he did when I was growing up but I'm being much better with him and the kids comment about how nice it is to have a peaceful family again.

These types of exchanges typify men's groups and have a particularly positive impact on the way men see themselves and the way they problem solve common life issues. Getting feedback from other men often has a powerful impact. Another member of the group said:

When I heard about this group, I thought it was a lot of crap. It wasn't even led by a therapist, just a bunch of guys shooting the breeze. I thought it would be like the women's groups I'd heard about where they whine and complain and nothing ever changes. But this group's had a really big effect on me. I trust everyone and I feel safe saying what I say. We respect each other's privacy and we don't get real confrontational, even when guys are starting to lose it. What we do is listen, sympathize sometimes, and give advice and a lot of support. We feel comfortable accepting the advice or turning it down, and we feel O.K. about not talking when it feels right to keep quiet. I really care about these guys.

It was interesting to see how long it took us to talk about real stuff instead of being phony. Once we got past that point, the spigot opened and we were talking about some pretty heavy stuff: Impotence; attraction to other women than our wives; drinking; our feelings about gays; the kids we have who don't like us much; working; just a lot of things. I wouldn't say it's like therapy. It's more like a bunch of guys being honest with each other. It doesn't happen often that men are honest with other men, but when it does, it's pretty powerful.

ROLE PLAYS

One effective way of resolving ambivalence toward important people in a man's life is through the use of role plays. The following dialogue demonstrates how the approach helped an immigrant Black man work through confused feeling about his father.

Client: (Looks down at his hands. Pauses) "You know I just came back from England where I saw my son for the first time since he was born five years ago. (Pause. Rubs his hands. Tears form in his eyes.) "I am very sad for myself. I feel very guilty and angry." (Client wipes tears from eyes.)

Therapist: "Whose voice do you hear inside when you feel guilty?"

Client: "My father's voice."

Therapist: "Describe your father. How does he look and sound?"

Client: "He is a warrior, a chief of my people. He is powerful and strong, with a deep voice. He has a scar on his cheek from a spear wound. He lived to be 103 and he was strong and powerful when he died. I loved him, but I am still afraid of him."

Therapist: "Let's move a chair in front of you where your father can sit. Can you imagine him in front of you? His face and expressions? Yes? Good. Tell your father why you haven't seen your son in five years."

Client: (Looks uncomfortable. Clears his throat. Rubs his hands.) "Father, my wife was unfaithful to me. She went with other women to bars and she left me at night." (Wipes tears away.)

Client—As Father: (Switches chairs.) "So, you do not tell me of this and you abandon your son? You are a disgrace to me." (The client's voice is appreciably lower. His body seems more powerful and larger.) "You do not do these things."

Client—As Self: (Switches chairs.) "I could not tell you, father, you were ill. I was afraid to discuss it with the family. I did not want you to be ashamed of me."

Client—As Father: (Switches chairs.) "Ashamed? I am ashamed of you and I will never stop being ashamed until you have your son with you in America. A father and son should be together. It is against nature to be apart." (The voice continues strong and deep and the power of the body continues to grow.)

Client—As Self: (Switches chairs. He tries to explain the complexity of the immigration laws and his attempts to have a reconciliation with his son. And then suddenly he says in a strong voice): "Father, I am still the warrior I was when I returned home from the army. You were proud of me then. You told me so. I will do the right thing, father. I will make you proud of me once more."

Client—As Father: (Switches chairs.) "It is something you do for your-self and for your son. We are a chain. We are warriors. When the chain breaks, we lose our power."

Client—As Self: (Switches chair. Begins to speak and cries. When he is finished crying, a look of calm appears on his face.) "I am done. I am *not* irresponsible!" (The voice he spoke in when he assumed the role of father is now the same voice he uses when he finishes this piece of work.)

This confrontation with the father is an element of all work with men, although it is a subject that makes many men aware of the depth of anguish they feel whenever they are asked, or forced, to confront the troubled relationships they've often had with their fathers. In fact, it is often the possibility of exposing the private arena of feelings that makes therapy such a threatening experience for many men and role plays, with their immediate emotional impact, so useful in treating the male client.

SUMMARY

This chapter offers some suggested treatment approaches that may be particularly useful with male clients. Included in the alternative approaches suggested in this chapter are personal coaching, the use of stories, bibliotherapy, the use of humor and metaphors, men's groups, and role plays. All of these approaches should be used with caution by making certain that male clients understand the purpose of each approach and agree, beforehand, to use them.

Self-Help Groups With Men

This chapter discusses the use of self-help groups in the treatment of male health and mental health problems. Because there is such passion for self-help groups in the absence of supportive data, the chapter considers the available research information on the treatment effectiveness of self-help groups with men and the reasons that self-help groups have become so popular in America. The chapter also provides a case study showing the use of a self-help group with a man trying to cope with alcohol abuse and depression.

DEFINING SELF-HELP GROUPS

Wituk, Shepherd, Slavich, Warren, and Meissen (2000) define self-help groups as "individuals who share the same problem or concern. Members provide emotional support to one another, learn ways to cope, discover strategies for improving their condition, and help others while helping themselves" (p. 157). An estimated 25 million Americans have been involved in self-help groups at some point during their lives (Kessler, Mickelson, & Zhao, 1997). Positive outcomes have been found in groups treating substance abuse (Humphreys & Moos, 1996), bereavement (Caserta & Lund, 1993), caregiving (McCallion & Toseland, 1995), diabetes (Gilden, Hendryx, Clar, Casia, & Singh, 1992), and depression (Kurtz, 1990). Riessman (2000) reports that, "More Americans try to change their health behaviors through self-help than through all other forms of professional programs combined" (p. 47).

Kessler, Frank, Edlund, Katz, Lin, and Leaf (1997b) report that 40% of all therapeutic sessions for psychiatric problems reported by respondents in a national survey were in the self-help sector, as compared to 35.2% receiving specialized mental health services, 8.1% receiving help from general physician's medical sector, and 16.5% receiving help from social service agencies. Wuthnow (1994) found that self-help groups are the most prevalent organized support groups in America today. The author estimated that 8 to 10 million Americans are members of self-help groups and that there are at least 500,000 self-help groups in America.

Fetto (2000) discusses a study done by the University of Texas at Austin which found that approximately 25 million people will participate in self-help groups at some point in their lives, and that 8 to 11 million people participate in self-help groups each year. Men are more likely to attend groups than women and Whites are three times as likely to attend self-help groups as Blacks. This number is expected to be much higher with the full use of the Internet as a tool for self-help. Male participants most likely to attend self-help groups are those diagnosed with alcoholism, cancer (all types), diabetes, AIDS, depression, and chronic fatigue syndrome. Those least likely to attend suffer from ulcers, emphysema, chronic pain, and migraines, in that order (Fetto, 2000).

Many of the attributes of self-help groups are consistent with the developmental model discussed in chapter 7. Riessman (2000) suggests the following common attributes: (a) Members share a similar condition and understand each other as no one else can; (b) members determine activities and processes, making self-help groups highly democratic and self-determining; (c) helping others is therapeutic; (d) self-help is built on the strengths of the individual members, the group, and the community; (e) self-help groups usually charge no fee and are not commercialized or sold as a product; (f) the social support that exists in self-help groups allows participants to cope with traumas because of supportive relationships between members; (g) self-help groups project values that help define the intrinsic meaning of the group to its members; (h) self-help groups use the expertise of the members, all of whom are coping, in various ways, with a common problem; (i) seeking help from a self-help group is not as stigmatizing as it may be from a health or mental health provider; and (j) self-help groups use self-determination, inner strength, self-healing, and resilience as part of the group experience. These attributes are consistent with male socialization and often have a very positive impact on male participants.

Wituk, Shepherd, Slavich, Warren, and Meissen (2000) studied the characteristics of self-help groups and report the following: (a) The groups studied had been in existence an average of eight years and 30% met weekly with an average attendance of thirteen participants; (b) on average, twenty new people became group participants in the prior year; (c) participants were almost evenly balanced between men and women and minorities, something one can't say about therapy; (d) group outreach was generally done by word of mouth, but some groups used newspaper ads and radio and television spot ads; (e) thirty-four percent of the groups were peer led with some professional involvement, 28% were led by professionals, 27% had no professional involvement, whereas 86% of the groups responding had two or more members acting in leadership capacities; (f) the primary function of the groups was to provide emotional and social support to members (98% of the groups reporting), whereas 32% provided information and education, and 58% provided advocacy services for members and their families; (g) seventy-seven percent of the groups felt that networking with the larger community was important. To do this, they had guest speakers, buddy systems, training seminars open to the public, and social events open to the community; (h) almost all of the groups studied held meetings in very easily accessible places. Many offered child care during meetings, transportation, and bilingual meetings for non-English-speaking participants; (i) more than half of the groups had national affiliations with groups such as the National Multiple Sclerosis Society. Groups reported a great deal of help from these organizations by way of brochures, newsletters, conferences and workshops, but very little help with finances or information related to advances in research; (j) seventy-five percent of the groups had local affiliations with hospitals, churches, and social service agencies; and (k) the authors found self-help groups to be surprisingly well connected to the professional community. As Reissman and Carroll (1995) suggest

Certainly, it is useful for a self-help organization to facilitate the inner strengths of its membership and to remain self-reliant. But not to be ignored is the value of outside resources as well—outside knowledge, advice, expertise, and financial support. (p. 185)

THE INDIGENOUS LEADERS OF SELF-HELP GROUPS

Men often find that involvement in self-help groups may result in leadership roles and a recognition that they have skills in facilitating change in others. What are the attributes of self-help leaders? Patterson and Marsiglia (2000) report similarities in the characteristics of two cohorts of natural (or indigenous) helpers from two very different geographic locations in the United States. The similarities include offering assistance to family and friends before it was asked for, an attempt to reduce stress in those helped, and a desire to help people strengthen their coping skills. Lewis and Suarez (1995) identify the primary functions of indigenous helpers as buffers between individuals and sources of stress, providers of social support, information, and referral sources and lay consultants. Waller and Patterson (2002) believe that indigenous helpers strengthen the social bond holding communities together which increases the well-being of individuals and communities.

Patterson, Holzhuter, Struble, and Quadagno (1972) found that natural helpers used one of three helping styles: (a) active listening, encouragement, emphasizing positives about the client, and suggesting alternative solutions to problems; (b) direct intervention by doing something active for the client that had an immediate impact; and (c) a combination of a and b in a way that fit the client's needs. However, Memmott (1993) found little difference between natural helpers and professionals, although natural helpers were more inclined to advocate and intervene on behalf of clients, tended to think much less about causal reasons for a client's problems, and used direct methods of help that were atheoretical but often sound.

Robert Bly (1986) suggests that we seek out others in the community for advice and support. He calls these natural helpers "People of Wisdom" because they listen well, are empathic and sensitive, and are known for their expertise in solving certain types of problems. Men often gravitate to these people because they help us in unobtrusive and informal ways that are often profoundly subtle because the lack of formal training by natural helpers is offset by their kindness, patience, common sense, and good judgment.

SOME EXAMPLES OF MEN WHO ARE NATURAL HELPERS

Sam Glicken (my father) was involved in the union movement in North Dakota and Minnesota, and then nationally, for over 50 years as a railroad worker. He believed in reaching out to his co-workers and helping them in times of need. His weekends, when many of the men in the union drank to excess, were often spent helping the men who came to our home to discuss their serious personal problems. My father didn't believe in counseling or psychotherapy, but what he did looked very much like therapy, in a rough and unorthodox way. He listened well, offered advice when it was needed, and knew where men could get specialized help if they had addictions or family violence problems. He could be supportive and encouraging as well as confrontational and very direct. Before he died, my father had the following to say about helping people on the job:

> Most counselors I know never tell people that a lot of what they've done in their lives is good. They never praise people for their hard work or their support for families. They never use humor. All they do is criticize. I see a lot of immature young people at work. It's taken them a long time to grow up. You can't help people grow up over night, it takes time. You've got to listen carefully to what they say, praise them for what they do well, and offer some advice and support for what they don't do so well. Most of all, you can't give up on people. They all change, everyone of them, even the worst ones, and I've learned to bide my time and let nature take its course with people. None of the men who got into trouble on the job, or with families, or with the law that I've helped are still in trouble. They all saw the light and they're good people now. I'd say the best thing we can do is to believe in the goodness of men to change and to be their cheerleaders when they need help. But you, Morley, being a social worker when you could have been a lawyer or better still, a doctor ... now that makes no sense to me at all. Let me do the helping. You should make the money. [He really said that, too.]

Sam Goldfarb, another natural helper, was a retired manager of a large accounting firm. He is now deceased. Sam was originally from Russia but lived in Minneapolis for 40 years. His synagogue suggested a talk with Sam because he'd spent his working years informally helping his co-workers as well as the members of his synagogue. When Sam was interviewed, at the age of 83, he was helping to transport an elderly member of the congregation to a doctor's office.

You don't go around with a sign on your head that says to come see you if anyone wants to talk, but you let yourself be around the people who are in trouble. You can tell from their faces and the way they're acting that they're in some trouble in their life. Pretty soon they talk. People love to talk, but only if they feel you won't criticize them. I just listen ... an old man with an ear and a heart to offer. And when they're done talking, I give them advice, an old man's advice. Sometimes they take it, sometimes they don't. That's life. But most of the time they're grateful to get their problems off their chest.

Young men and men in their 40's are the worst. They got so much to prove to themselves and their just starting to learn that they won't be the big machers (successes) they thought they'd be. They have big dreams but they won't be met. It's a terrible thing when a man realizes that his dreams are really pipe dreams and that they'll never be achieved. That's when they come to me. Maybe they think I've been through it and I'm OK, but men are never OK with accepting their limits. They want the sky and the moon and the stars, and when they have it, they want more. This pressure makes good men a little crazy and my job is to let them know that their dreams are worth having and they should try and have every dream come true while understanding that what they've got now, their families and friends and jobs, they're not so bad. Maybe they're even great. Coming from an *alta cocker* (old man) like me, they listen and in time, they're OK with it. Maybe I've helped save a marriage, or some good accountant taking off and playing guitar at some commune for a year. Maybe I've encouraged the poet to write, or the ambitious person to take the extra step toward promotion. It seems to me that most of the help men get in their lives comes from men like me at jobs over lunch and coffee. I haven't known many men who go to see a counselor, but guys like me, they beat the door down and are always hanging around the office waiting to talk to

me. This idea that men can't talk about their problems is idiocy. They talk
and they want someone who cares to listen. And they love advice. So I
don't know, with all this male bashing, it seems people like me are doing
more and more everyday to keep good men from giving up. I'd say that's
important work, wouldn't you?

THE EFFECTIVENESS OF SELF-HELP GROUPS

Although the research is somewhat limited on the subject of the effectiveness of self-help groups, Kessler, Mickelson, and Zhao (1997) report that

> the little available data suggest that self-help groups are sometimes able
> to promote emotional recovery from life crises (Emrick & Tonigan, 1993;
> Lieberman & Borman, 1991; Videcka-Sherman & Lieberman, 1985), [al-
> though] methodological limitations make it impossible to draw firm
> conclusions. (Levy, 1984; Humphreys & Rappaport, 1994) (p. 30)

With those limitations, here are some data on the effectiveness of self-
help groups with men.

Substance Abuse

In an evaluation of a large study by *Consumer Reports* on the effectiveness of psychotherapy with both male and female clients, Seligman
(1995) concluded that, "Alcoholics Anonymous (AA) did especially
well, ... significantly bettering mental health professionals [in the
treatment of alcohol and drug related problems]" (p. 10). Humphreys
and Moos (1996) found that during a three-year period of study, male
alcoholics who initially chose Alcoholics Anonymous (AA) over professional help had a 45% ($1,826) lower average per-person treatment
cost than those receiving professional treatment. Even with the lower
costs, AA participants had reduced alcohol consumption, had fewer
days intoxicated, and experienced lower rates of depression when
compared to alcoholic clients receiving professional help. In follow-

up studies, these findings were consistent at one year and three years after the start of the study. Humphreys, Mavis, and Stoffelmayr (1994) report that Black male participants ($N = 253$) in Narcotics Anonymous and AA showed improvement over twelve months in six problem areas (employment, alcohol and drug use, and legal, psychological, and family problems). Participants had much more improvement in their medical, alcohol, and drug problems than did nonparticipants. Emrick and Tonigan (1993) did a meta-analysis of more than 50 studies involving male and female participants and report that AA members who were also professionally treated alcoholic patients were somewhat more likely to reduce drinking than those who do not attend AA. Membership in AA was also found to reduce physical symptoms and to improve psychological adjustment.

Christo and Sutton (1994) report that male members of Narcotics Anonymous who stayed off drugs for three years or more as a result of their involvement in the group had the same level of anxiety and self-esteem as a random sample of people who had never been drug addicted. Hughes (1977) studied male and female adolescent members of Alateen, a self-help group for children who had an alcoholic parent. They report that Alateen members had significantly fewer negative moods, more positive moods, and higher self-esteem than adolescents who were not members and didn't have an alcoholic parent. McKay and Alterman (1994) reported on Black male participants in self-help groups for substance abuse after a seven-month follow-up. Participants with high rates of attendance at group meetings reduced their use of alcohol and drugs by half as much as those who were poor attenders of meetings. Both groups were similar in their use of substances prior to the start of their group involvement. Pisani and Fawcett (1993) studied male and female alcoholic patients admitted for a short hospital treatment program who were referred on release to AA. In an 18-month follow-up study, the more days group members attended AA meetings, the longer their abstinence lasted. Interestingly, AA involvement was seen as a more powerful way to continue abstinence than use of medication to treat the addiction. Men did as well as women in the group. Walsh, Hingson, and Merrigan (1991) report that male employees of a company who were assigned to AA or face the loss of their jobs lessened their drinking over a two-year period. AA members did as well as clients involved in mandatory in-patient treatment in terms of job-related performance. Tattersall and Hallstrom (1992) report on a study involving a British self-help group offering telephone counseling and a support group experience formed to help members reduce their reliance on tranquilizers. Members had been addicted to tranquilizers on average for more than twelve years. Most members of the group reported that the symptoms for which tranquilizers had initially been prescribed had lessened and that 65% were at least moderately satisfied with their withdrawal from tranquilizers as it affected their quality of life.

Medical Problems

Riessman (2000) reports on a project to use self-help groups with primarily male patients suffering from heart disease. At first, the project used patient-led self-help groups to help keep patients on their diet and exercise regimens, but Reissman says that it soon became apparent that "participation in the groups themselves was one of the most powerful interventions" (p. 48). Nash and Kramer (1993) studied 57 Black patients who were involved in self-help groups for sickle-cell anemia. Those involved the longest had the fewest psychological symptoms and the fewest problems from the disease, particularly in work and relationships. Hinrichsen and Revenson (1985) compared scoliosis patients in a self-help group who had undergone bracing or surgery with patients having the same treatment who were not in a self-help group. Participants had a more positive outlook on life, better satisfaction with their medical care, fewer psychosomatic symptoms, better self-esteem, and fewer feelings of "shame and estrangement." Simmons (1992) evaluated members of a self-help group of diabetics for blood sugar levels and knowledge about diabetes. Members attending the group twice or more during a year had a significantly greater drop in blood sugar levels and an increased knowledge about diabetes than nonparticipants. The group emphasizes education, support, knowledge sharing, and social activities. Men and women benefited equally from the group.

Bereavement

Caserta and Lund (1993) found that widows and widowers participating in a bereavement group for at least eight weeks experienced less depression and grief than nonparticipants. Lieberman and Videka-Sherman (1986) followed widowers and widows involved in a self-help group for bereavement. Over a period of a year, the group members experienced better social relationships, less emotional distress, and better emotional functioning than did nonmembers. Men and women benefited equally. Marmar and Horowitz (1988) found that self-help groups worked as well as therapy in reducing symptoms of grief and in overall psychological functioning for both men and women.

Emotional Problems

Edmunson and Bedell (1982) report that after ten months of participation in a patient-led support group, half as many former male psychiatric inpatients ($N = 40$) required rehospitalization as those not participating in the support group ($N = 40$). Members of the patient-led group had average hospital stays of seven days as compared to 25 days for nonparticipants. Kurtz (1990) reports that 82% of 129 members of the Manic Depressive and Depressive Association coped better with their illness after becoming members of a self-help group. Eighty-two percent of the sample required hospitalization before joining the support group. This number fell to 33% after becoming members of the group. Men and women benefited equally from the experience. Kennedy (1990) studied the benefits of a self-help group for 31 participants with chronic psychiatric problems and found that members of the self-help group spent far fewer days in a psychiatric hospital over a 32-month period than did 31 former psychiatric patients matched by similar age, race, sex, marital status, number of previous hospitalizations, and other factors. Group members also experienced an increased sense of security and self-esteem and an improved ability to accept problems in their lives without blaming others. Galanter (1988) studied 356 male and female members of a self-help group for former mental patients. Although half of the members of the self-help group had been hospitalized before joining the group, only 8% of the group leaders and 7% of the recent members had been hospitalized since joining. Gender was not a factor and men and women benefited equally from the experience.

CASE EXAMPLE: A MALE SELF-HELP GROUP ASSISTS A MALE ALCOHOLIC TO STOP DRINKING

John Holmes is a 63-year-old retired executive of a large corporation. Although John was a heavy drinker throughout his career, he had a long and successful career moving up the ladder in his company to one of its most important and highly paid executive positions. Since John retired three years ago, his drinking has increased and he was recently told by his doctor that his cardiovascular system was in jeopardy if he didn't stop drinking. John has few friends and although he's still married, he and his wife seldom see each other and live in separate communities. John has two grown children but he sees them seldom and believes that they dislike him. He isn't sure why and can't remember a time the family sat down as a unit and had a meal together. He hasn't seen his children in over a year and feels that he's been a failure as a father and as a husband. He thought he would travel after retiring and spend more time with his children and grandchildren, but his attempts to be with them have failed. So John sits alone at the bar in his club from 4 P.M. to closing and slowly drinks two bottles of Scotch every night. He is also very depressed and has active thoughts of suicide.

After a minor car accident where his license was suspended for a DWI violation, John was ordered by the court to attend an educational group to learn more about his drinking. At first he thought the group was silly and regressed back to elementary days by drawing pictures of his teacher and passing the picture around. The picture showed the teacher drinking from a gallon jug of Scotch. As John attended the group, he began to have active thoughts of suicide and decided to share this with his teacher who immediately referred him to a therapist. The therapist worked with John but felt that he might benefit from a group experience and suggested a self-help group for people with alcohol problems and chronic depression.

The therapist arranged for John to meet the group leader, who also suffered from alcohol-related depression but had successfully learned to cope with it. The leader invited John to attend a meeting and asked participants to stay after so they could honestly discuss their feelings about the group and to answer questions John might have about the group's effectiveness. After the first meeting he attended, the men in the group spoke about how the group had helped them stop drinking and to feel better about themselves. Following the meeting, John shared his positive sense of the group with the therapist and his surprise at how strongly the members felt about the group experience. He began attending sessions on a regular basis while also seeing his therapist weekly. After six months as a participant, John summarized the experience as follows:

> It's very supportive. Everyone there is like me. They're all struggling with alcohol and depression and they've all been successful men who are now retired and feel they've made a mess of their personal lives. Because of the group, they've been able to get on with their lives. That's what I've begun doing. I've been assigned a guy my age as a mentor whom I call when I feel so down that I can hardly function. We've begun walking together and it's helped. I feel positive acceptance from the other people, and that helps. We have speakers who talk about alcohol and depression and who keep us informed about the latest research. I've been assigned as a mentor to a new member and surprisingly, he seems to find a lot of solace from our contacts.

> I've stopped drinking but I'm still a bit depressed. My personal life is better and a bright spot is that I've made some wonderful male friends through the group. My wife and I have decided to divorce and I've written my children informing them of our decisions. So far, no one's written back or called. It's frankly very hurtful. I guess I forgot to mention that I met a female colleague of one of the guys in the group, someone a little younger than me who's a ranking executive in a company doing very similar work to my own company. We see plays together and share meals, and while we're not on intimate terms, we have a lovely friendship and I don't feel so lonely. She doesn't drink and so we're not around alcohol at all. I still crave a drink. Sometimes it's more than I can stand and I've gone off the wagon a few times. It's an addiction and you can't know how bad it is until you've had it. I think of it as the devil trying to tempt me and sometimes he does. Overall, I'm much better. I think the group helped an awful

lot and I have a great therapist who's an ex-alcoholic and knows the demons inside of me. She's a wonderful, warm, supportive lady who gives me hugs and holds my hands when I'm down. At first I thought, how inappropriate, but believe me, all of us drinkers long for comfort and she knows when to give it. She can also kick me in the butt when I need it and does so regularly.

I think I'm less depressed than I was before I started the group. The support, the camaraderie, the loving environment, and the sense that we're all experts on drinking and depression and have something to say worth listening to about how to handle depression, that's what helps the most. I've made a couple of good friends from the group and instead of staying home and being lonely, I go out to movies or have dinner with my friends. Do I feel better than I did six months ago? Yes. Is it because of the group? I think some of it is, but I have to admit that because of the group, I'm using therapy better. So overall, yes, I give it high marks. I'll stay with it as long as I need to and maybe because I have something to offer, maybe after I'm OK, I'll stay so I can offer my little bit of wisdom and can help the others who are struggling with loneliness, feeling like failures, and waiting to die alone.

SUMMARY

This chapter on self-help groups offers some hopeful evidence that self-help may provide assistance to a variety of male clients experiencing problems with addictions, health, mental health, and other social and emotional problems. Self-help is generally supportive in nature and usually provides an affirming and positive approach to problem solving. Although self-help groups may not be effective for everyone because they sometimes have an unacceptable religious ideology or encourage people to believe that recovery is a lifelong struggle, the weight of findings provides a reason for optimism.

PART III

Clinical Work With Violent Men

Clinical Work With Violent Male Youth

As I noted in a volume I wrote on violent young children (Glicken, 2004a), most youth-related violent acts are committed by boys. Less than fifteen percent of the acts against persons (violent acts) are committed by girls, according to Scahill (2000), and those acts usually don't involve the degree of violence found in male violence. Wolfgang (1972, 1987; see also Briscoe, 1997) report that six to seven percent of all boys in a given birth year will become chronic offenders, indicating that they will have five or more arrests before their eighteenth birthday. These same six to seven percent will commit half of all crimes and two thirds of all violent crimes committed by all the boys born in a given birth year by age 18. Briscoe (1997) confirms Wolfgang's studies and predicts that an increase in the numbers of adolescent boys does not bode well because it increases the number of boys in the six to seven percent category who will become violent perpetrators. Consequently, the following discussion relates to boys who commit violent acts, although some of the discussion may sound generic to boys and girls.

VIOLENCE IN BOYS UNDER 18

Trends in juvenile crime are not encouraging. Although overall violent crime decreased after the peak years of 1983 to 1993, the number of juvenile arrests for serious crimes has continued to increase (Gramckow & Tompkins, 1999). Currie (1993) attributes much of the increase in violent juvenile crime to a weakening of traditional socializing institutions of the community—the family, schools, and churches. However, social conditions have also changed. Schools increasingly deal with problems of misbehavior in the classroom and the easy availability of dangerous drugs and guns has significantly changed the juvenile justice landscape. After a period of relative stability in the rates of violent crime committed by juvenile offenders, the growth in juvenile violence that began in 1985 was accompanied by a steady growth, from 1985 to 1995, in the use of guns by juveniles "... leading to a doubling in the number of juvenile murders committed with guns" (Blumstein, 1995, p. 5).

Using data from the Federal Bureau of Investigation's (FBI's) Uniform Crime Reporting Program and the National Juvenile Court Data Archive, Butts and Snyder (1997) show that the 1995 arrest rate for "Violent Crime Index offenses" was 89 per 100,000 for juveniles twelve and under, 460 per 100,000 for youth ages thirteen and fourteen, and an astonishing 979 per 100,000 for older youth. Commenting on the increase in juvenile crime, Osofsky and Osofsky (2001) write the following:

Put simply, youth violence in the United States has reached epidemic proportions. The homicide rate among males 15–24 years old in the United States is 10 times higher than in Canada, 15 times higher than in Australia, and 28 times higher than in France or Germany. (p. 287)

Herrenkohl et al. (2001) report that children involved in early onset violence are at very high risk of committing violent crimes during adolescence and adulthood. The risk for later violent behavior increases the younger the violence begins. Elliott (1994) found that 45% of the children who commit violent offenses by age eleven go on to commit violent offenses in their early twenties. The older the age on onset of violence, the less likely children are to commit violent offenses in adulthood. According to Thornberry, Huizinga, and Loeber (1995), almost twice as many children committing violent acts before the age of nine commit violent acts in adulthood as compared to children between the ages of ten and twelve. In a study of early onset violence, Herrenkohl et al. (2001) report four primary indicators of future violent behavior in children at the age of ten: hitting a teacher, picking fights, attacking other children, and a report by parents indicating that a child fights a great deal at home or in the neighborhood.

Sprague and Walker (2000) report the following: "Early starters are likely to experience antisocial behavior and its toxic effects throughout their lives. Late starters have a far more positive long-term outcome" (p. 370). Walker and Severson (1990) indicate that diagnostic signs of "early violence starters" include disobedience, property damage, conduct problems, theft, the need for a great deal of attention, threats and intimidation, and fighting. Mayer (1995) suggests that certain environmental factors may correlate with the potential for violent behavior. The most prominent environmental factors include inconsistent and harsh parenting styles, disorganized or badly functioning schools, and the availability of drugs, alcohol, and weapons.

Hamburg (1998) considers youth violence to be a public health concern and reports the following data on victimization:

• Intentional violence accounts for one-third of all injury deaths in the United States.

• Intentional interpersonal violence disproportionately involves young people as both perpetrators and victims.

• Among minority youth, particularly African Americans, violence has struck with unique force in recent years. Homicide has been the leading cause of death among African American males and females between the ages of 15–24 for more than ten years.

• Firearm-related deaths among African American youth have particularly increased. Between 1984 and 1993, gun-related deaths of young African American males tripled, with the most dramatic rise among those 13 to 18 years old.

• In recent years, weapon carrying by students in schools has become a growing source of violence and threat of violence. A study by the Centers for Disease Control and Prevention (1995) found that nearly one-fourth of students nationwide had carried a weapon to school during the month preceding the survey. (pp. 31–54)

In another area of violence, sexual violence, Zolondek, Abel, Northey, and Jordan (2000) found that in self-reports by almost 500 juveniles undergoing evaluation by the police for possible involvement in sexual offenses, including voyeurism and exhibitionism, over 60% reported they'd molested a child. The average age of onset for the sexual offenses was between ten and twelve years of age. Of the boys who reported never having been accused of molesting children, 41.5% reported that they had molested a younger child. The authors suggest that between 15% and 20% of all sexual offenses are committed by youth younger than eighteen, and as many as 50% of all child molestations may be committed by youth younger than eighteen. Commenting on the very early age of onset of various sexual behaviors in their sample (9.7 to 12.4 years of age), the authors indicate that the average age of onset in their sample was considerably earlier than has been reported by other researchers. The authors believe that adolescents begin their sexual offending prior to puberty and that many of the offenders in their sample were molesting younger siblings or close friends of the family. The authors believe that very early deviant sexual behavior is a strong predictor of later predatory sexual offending.

Groth, Longo, and McFadin (1982) report that juveniles have been identified as the perpetrators in more than 25% of all child sexual abuse cases. Caputo, Frick, and Brodsky. (1999) note that, although it is assumed that juvenile sexual offenses are merely exploratory and will not be repeated in adulthood, Groth, et al. found that half of all adult sexual offenders report committing their first sexual offense as teenagers. The authors further report that patterns of sexual offenses as defined by the age and characteristics of the victim, the amount of force used, and other aspects of the assault, appear to have first developed in adolescence and continue into adulthood.

Berliner (1998) indicates that half of all adult sexual offenders began having deviant sexual thoughts in adolescence or during preadolescence. Berliner believes that juvenile sex offenders have very similar characteristics to adult sex offenders and that, "They may engage in serious sexual crimes, have multiple victims, exhibit deviant sexual preferences, have comparable cognitive distortions, and lack victim empathy" (Berliner, 1998, p. 645). Because the characteristics of juvenile sexual offenders are similar to those of adult offenders, Berliner reports that treatment programs for juveniles have also been similar to those of adults without any strong evidence that an adult treatment model is necessarily the correct model for young offenders.

Veneziano, Veneziano, and Legrand (2000) studied the sexual behavior of adolescent sexual offenders. The authors believe that youthful offenders relive their own sexual molestations by the choice of victims and the circumstance in which they were molested and found the following:

1. Adolescent offenders generally molested children near an age when they'd been molested.

2. Adolescent male offenders molested by a male were more likely to molest a male.

3. Adolescent offenders generally victimize children who are related to them in the same way that they were related to the person molesting them.

4. Adolescent offenders use the same sexual behavior on victims that was used on them.

PREDICTORS OF EARLY VIOLENCE

Murray and Myers (1998) report that conduct disorders in childhood are frequently predictive of later delinquency and adult criminality. By age six, family dysfunction is a strong indicator of delinquency. At age nine, the child's antisocial and aggressive behavior further predicts delinquent tendencies. Sprague and Walker (2000) believe that we have the diagnostic tools to identify children at risk of violence as early as age five. Fagan (1996) and Hawkins and Catalano (1992) report that antisocial behavioral patterns coupled with high degrees of aggression early in a child's life are strong predictors of future violence. Although many of these children will cause major acts of violence, many more will experience problems with domestic violence, substance abuse, unemployment, mental health problems, and a host of social and emotional problems that, if identified and treated early, may be lessened, if not completely eliminated (Sprague & Walker, 2000).

There appears to be a relation between violence and school disciplinary problems. Six to nine percent of the children referred for disciplinary problems in elementary and middle schools (almost always boys) are responsible for more than 50% of the total disciplinary referrals and practically all of the serious offenses, including possession of weapons, fighting, assaults on other children, and assaults on teachers (Skiba, Peterson, & Williams, 1997). Early disciplinary problems in school are accurate predictors of future and more serious problems (Walker, Colvin, & Ramsey, 1995). According to Walker et al. (1995), students with ten or more disciplinary referrals per year are seriously at risk for school failure and for other more serious life problems. Many of the children who are frequently referred to principals for disciplinary action are defiant and disobedient and may often be involved in bullying and intimidation of other students. They are, according to Sprague and Walker (2000), likely to move on to more serious offenses, including "physical fighting, and then ultimately rape, serious assault, or murder" (p. 370).

One of the strongest reasons for violence in childhood and adolescence is child abuse. In a volume I wrote on violence in children twelve and younger (Glicken, 2004a), I found that the primary reason for early onset violence is child abuse, which not only creates rage but also suggests a chaotic and badly functioning home where values and acceptable conduct are not taught. The combination can be combustible.

TREATING EARLY MALE VIOLENCE

Studer (1996) suggests that children with behavioral problems may benefit from learning anger management techniques, assertiveness training, problem-solving techniques, and conflict mediation. These techniques are described by Studer as follows:

1) *Anger Management*: Anger management is a cognitive therapy approach in which children learn to identify situations that lead to angry responses, recognize their physical reactions to anger (clenched fists, sweaty palms, heightened heart rate), and learn to rationally perceive their role in the situation so that the anger can dissipate or be dealt with appropriately.

2) *Assertiveness Training*: Assertiveness training is a way of helping children learn to have their needs met without violating the rights or feelings of others. In distinguishing aggression from assertiveness, Baer (1976) believes that the purpose of aggression is to have needs met by violating the rights of others, while assertiveness helps the child

achieve those needs without disregarding the needs of others. Huey & Rank (1984) report that a class in assertiveness training was given to disruptive 8th grade urban male students. The class met one hour a week for 4 weeks for a total of 8 hours. The students in the class showed decreased aggressive behavior and increased assertiveness. Mathias (1992) supports the use of assertiveness training for elementary students and notes that assertiveness training programs get overwhelmingly positive evaluations from children, teachers, and parents.

3) *Problem-Solving Training*: Problem-solving training helps children learn to think their way through difficult social situations and to increase empathy and sensitivity for others. Rundie (as cited in Goldstein & Glick, 1987) reports that when 5th grade students were allowed to process actual life situations that affect most 5th graders (issues such as cheating, stealing, using drugs, and lying to parents), they did much better on group tasks than children who were not involved in problem solving discussions.

4) *Conflict Mediation*: Conflict mediation helps children learn to resolve conflicts with others by actually negotiating solutions. Schrumpt, Crawford, and Usadel (1991) outlined the following basic steps in the mediation process: Step 1: Explain the ground rules and describe the conflict. Step 2: Gather information. Each person is permitted time to tell his or her story without interruption. Step 3: Focus on common interests. The purpose of this step is to help those in conflict identify common goals and to find out what each person views as a suitable resolution of the problem. Step 4: Create options. People in dispute are permitted to think the problem through, offer solutions, list possible options, and provide a venue for joint problem resolution. Step 5: Evaluate options and choose a solution. Those in conflict are encouraged to agree on the list of options that come from step 4. Step 6: Write an agreement and close the mediation session. A written agreement is presented that all parties sign spelling out the conditions of the conflict resolution and each party's responsibility to abide by the agreement. As a further aspect of strengthening the agreement, the parties are asked to shake hands. Lane & McWhirter (1992) report that mediation improves the behavior of potentially troubled children, helps children improve their listening skills, and enhances the climate of the school.

Mental health professionals have implemented a wide variety of treatment approaches in an attempt to address one or more of the many psychosocial risk factors associated with youth violence. The primary approaches include cognitive-behavioral skills interventions with seriously aggressive or violent youth, cognitive restructuring techniques, role plays, therapist modeling, and behavioral assignments. All of these approaches attempt to reduce violent behavior in children by directly addressing risk factors within a child, such as ineffective problem-solving skills, deficits in moral development, incorrect or illogical perceptions of others, and feelings of insecurity and low self-esteem, to mention just a few of the at-risk behaviors that might lead to violence in children.

Overall, mental health treatments have been most effective with younger, nonviolent, or mildly aggressive youth (Sechrest, 2001). However, they have been largely ineffective in reducing or preventing further violence with more serious or chronically violent offenders. As a result, many mental health professionals and policy analysts are skeptical about the ability of the juvenile justice system or the mental health profession to rehabilitate violent children. It has been argued that the approaches previously reviewed have not been successful for two main reasons. First, they have included interventions that focus on only one or two psychosocial risk factors associated with youth violence (e.g., individual cognition, family relations) and have failed to simultaneously address the many other factors (i.e., peer, school, and neighborhood factors) that contribute to youth violence. Second, these interventions take place in only one location, such as a mental health clinic or a juvenile incarceration facility, and fail to address other influences on violent behavior such as home life, school, or neighborhood.

This sense of pessimism is widely noted in the literature. For example, Rae-Grant, McConville, and Fleck (1999) write,

> Because exclusive individual clinical interventions for violent conduct disorders do not work, the child and adolescent psychiatrist must seek opportunities to be a leader or team member in well-organized and well-funded community prevention efforts. (p. 338)

Sprague and Walker (2000) complain about poorly matched treatment approaches that deny the severity of the problem. Elliott, Hamburg, and Williams (1998) believe that counseling has no effect on the problems of antisocial and predelinquent youth.

Steiner and Stone (1999) also report widespread pessimism among clinicians regarding effective clinical work with violent youth, but believe that this pessimism is unwarranted. The authors indicate that treating childhood violence requires clinicians to practice with flexibility and to be cognizant of the need to develop treatment approaches that permit clinicians to offer interventions in many different settings, including schools, juvenile detention centers, prisons, and homes, as well as in the consulting room. Patterson and Narrett (1990) believe that there is strong evidence to support the effectiveness of family and parent-based interventions in the elementary grades to reduce violence and related pathology. Myles and Simpson (1998) argue that because aggressive and violent children often experience a range of problems, we should provide services to meet the children's academic and social needs. Those services should include the use of counselors, psychologists, social workers, and treatment interventions that meet the social and emotional needs of aggressive and violent children.

In writing about therapeutic approaches in work with gang members, a unique subset of violent children, Morales (1982) provides the following reasons why clinical interventions often fail to work with gang members, and, by extension, with violent youth in general: (a) a belief by many clinicians that antisocial behavioral problems are untreatable; (b) therapists often fear violent people and assume that all gang members are violent; (c) a belief by many therapists in the incapacity of poor people to possess psychological insight; (d) an overappreciation of the benefits of therapy and a belief that everyone can benefit; and (e) an opposite belief that gang members can't be treated because they are manipulative and dishonest.

Morales (1982) believes that gang members have complex issues regarding treatment that must be understood by therapists before they can be effective. Those issues include the following: (a) a distrust or dislike of authority figures, often the result of prior negative experiences with parents, teachers, and police; (b) a strong resentment to being forced into treatment involuntarily as the result of the juvenile justice system; (c) a feeling of discomfort with therapists who might be of a different

ethnic or racial group; (d) a sense of a generational, cultural, and perhaps language gap with the therapist; and (e) the anticipation of winning yet another struggle with a social control agent, or the notion of the
therapist as a "Freudian cop" (p. 143).

Although there are undoubtedly many reasons for youth violence,
one of the most widely supported reasons is the link between youth violence and child abuse and neglect. Longitudinal studies by Widom
(1999) and by McCord (1999) support the linkage between early life violence and child abuse and neglect. Glicken and Sechrest (2003) note that
youth violence often begins in childhood as a result of early physical and
sexual child abuse and family violence. Many of the children who experience child abuse and family violence have already begun to show the
complex signs of future violent behavior in the fire setting, sexual abuse,
theft, cruelty to animals, and distorted thoughts that often precede adolescent and adult violence.

Because many of the children who become violent come from abusive
homes, it is interesting to note the lack of effectiveness in current approaches to work with abused children. Lukefahr (2001), in a book review of *Treatment of Child Abuse*, edited by Robert M. Reece (2000),
writes,

> Although there is a very strong effort throughout to base findings and rec-
> ommendations on the available evidence, these chapters highlight the re-
> ality that this young, evolving specialty remains largely descriptive. A
> common theme of several authors is the prominent role of cognitive-be-
> havioral therapy for child abuse victims, but therapists may be disap-
> pointed in the lack of specific protocols for implementing CBT.
> (Lukefahr, 2001, p. 36)

Kaplan, Pelcovitz, and Labruna (1999) report that the effectiveness of
treatment of physically and sexually abused children, "has generally not
been empirically evaluated. In a review of treatment research for physically abused children, Oates and Bross (1995) cite only 13 empirical studies between 1983 and 1992 meeting even minimal research standards" (p.
1218). Steiner and Stone (1999) suggest that whatever we may say about
large-scale programs and the ineffectiveness of clinical work, violent cli-

ents, particularly children, almost always see a clinician at some point in their lives. Steiner and Stone believe that juvenile delinquency is a problem which presents a high probability of multiple pathologies, all requiring well-researched treatment approaches, and argue that without effective interventions, we will be unsuccessful in curtailing future relapses and continued violence throughout the life cycle.

Ellickson and McGuigan (2000) note that because early deviance and poor grades are useful predictors of later violence, violence intervention should begin as early as elementary school and should focus on issues of self-esteem, life choices, drug and alcohol abuse, and peer choices. These are issues that clinicians routinely deal with when treating children and adolescents. More significantly, Steiner and Stone (1999) write,

> Our understanding of how to help these children and adolescents is far from complete. We need better tools to mitigate the human suffering of perpetrators and victims alike. By involving our profession, which has a long and distinguished history of standing up for those who cannot do so for themselves. (p. 234)

VIOLENCE PREVENTION AND TREATMENT PROGRAMS

Rae-Grant, McConville, and Fleck (1999) report that a number of programmatic interventions have been tried with youthful offenders with some success. For a child with multiple risk markers to develop violent or antisocial behavior, many programs target specific aspects of the child's family life. Olds, Henderson, Tatelbaum, and Chamberlin (1988) provide an example of how an early infancy project for economically disadvantaged mothers with poor prenatal health, self-damaging behaviors, and poor family management skills, can (a) improve maternal diet, (b) reduce smoking during pregnancy, (c) result in fewer premature deliveries, (d) increase the birth weight of babies, and (e) result in significantly less child abuse.

Johnson (1990) reports that providing social, economic, and health-related services to preschool children and their families with multiple risk markers improves academic success, reduces behavioral problems in at-risk children, improves parenting skills, decreases family management problems, and lowers the subsequent arrest rates for children in families provided services. However, Johnson (1990) cautions that some of these positive outcomes are only effective for several years after follow-up because of diminished services to at-risk families, poor school experiences for children, and the many serious social problems experienced by the families served. Zigler, Tussig, and Black (1992) believes that preschool services to at-risk families coupled with programs such as Head Start may actually help prevent antisocial behavior in young children.

Rae-Grant, McConville, and Fleck (1999) suggest early intervention because in elementary grade school children, "interpersonal cognitive problem-solving programs gave rise to better problem-solving skills and fewer behavior problems in children with economic deprivation, poor impulse control, and early behavioral problems" (p. 338). Hawkins et al. (1992) report that a social development program in Seattle for similarly at-risk grade school children demonstrated positive results. Preschool and elementary school programs may be one proactive approach to preventing future violent behavior.

Izzo and Ross (1990) found that programs using a cognitive theoretical base were twice as effective as those using other theoretical bases. Effective programs, according to Izzo and Ross, have a positive impact on the way youthful offenders think about their behavior. Andrews et al. (1990) found that programs using cognitive-behavioral approaches providing anger management and conflict and substance abuse treatment were more effective than programs using other approaches. Tate, Reppucci, and Mulvey (1995) report that the most effective treatment approaches were "child-focused, family-centered, and directed toward solving multiple problems across the numerous contexts" (p. 779).

Guetzloe (1999) suggests that youth violence should be treated as a public health concern and that prevention of youth violence may be seen as primary, secondary, or tertiary, depending on the progression of the problem. Primary prevention tries to reduce the rate of certain problems and to keep those problems from occurring. Secondary prevention involves the early location of youth violence with appropriate interventions. Tertiary prevention concerns itself with youth who are chronically violent.

Primary prevention attacks youth violence at its point of origin and believes violence may be caused by any number of problems, including brain injury, mental illness, chemical abnormalities, availability of weapons, exposure to media violence, and the acceptance of violence in a particular society or culture (Guetzloe, 1999). Secondary prevention may be achieved by approaching home, school, and community issues that may contribute to youth violence. Guetzloe (1999) gives the following examples of secondary prevention: (a) providing resources and services to ensure the physical and psychological safety of all youth, (b) making certain that all students develop the skills necessary for academic and social achievement, (c) working cooperatively with parents and community agencies, (d) providing effective training for everyone involved in preventing and treating violence, and (e) making appropriate referrals to provide youth with the best possible intervention based on the problems they are experiencing. Tertiary prevention provides protection of the population from violent behavior and may include prison sentences or other "containment" approaches to maintain a healthy community. In justifying tertiary prevention, Guetzloe (1999) writes,

> Regardless of the specific origins of their behavior, the prognosis for chronically violent individuals is generally poor, and provisions must be made for interventions such as imprisonment and incarceration as well as rehabilitation. The primary goal of incarceration is to isolate violent individuals to protect the rest of the population. Young people who feel pleasure—or nothing at all—in the slaughter of other human beings need a complete emotional overhaul. The only hope for many violent offenders lies in changing their thinking, a process that requires a lengthy period of time and total supervision. (p. 22) ♦

Alexander (2000, p. 216) found that the best candidates for treatment programs are youths whose offense resulted from a situation of conflict with friends, family, or classmates. Alexander notes that Aggression Replacement Training (ART), as developed by Goldstein and Glick (1996), has been found to be effective with highly aggressive children. ART consists of three components, which are taught weekly: skill streaming, anger control, and moral education. "Skill streaming involves the teaching

174

CHAPTER 10

of fifty skills characteristic of pro-social behaviors taught in group counseling [groups of] about six to eight juveniles [through] modeling, role-playing, performance feedback, and transfer training" (Alexander, 2000, p. 217).

Anger control techniques are incorporated into ART in a ten-week period designed to teach responses to anger-provoking incidents. Principles of moral education stress the development of an increased sense of justice, fairness, and concern for other's rights. However, Goldstein and Glick (1996) do not see this aspect as effective in reducing aggressive behaviors without skills training. Alexander (2000) also found that programs which rely on positive and negative reinforcement generally accelerate the development of prosocial behaviors. These types of therapies are now beginning to appear under the rubric of strength-based approaches and are sometimes called "cultural competence" programs. They can result in strength-based courts, "such as the drug courts used mostly with adults" (Alexander, 2000, p. 7).

CASE EXAMPLE: TREATING A CONDUCT DISORDER

This case first appeared in somewhat modified form in Glicken (2004a).

Jeremy is a nine-year-old boy who has been diagnosed with a severe childhood-onset conduct disorder. The diagnosis was made after five years of acting out behavior in class, progressively more severe lying, stealing from classmates, cruelty to family and neighborhood animals, and a volatile temper that often results in physical aggression to members of his family, neighborhood children, and classmates at school. Jeremy is presently suspended from school because of his violent outbursts and is being seen by a clinical social worker as part of Jeremy's school's requirement that something be done about his behavior before he can return to class.

Jeremy has many of the classic signs of a conduct disorder. In treatment, he is grandiose about his accomplishments, highly manipulative, attacks the therapist verbally when he doesn't get his way, and sulks when the therapist suggests that he might be wrong about the way he views the world. Jeremy externalizes blame for everything and can only see malicious intent in having to see a therapist. He frequently talks about getting back at the teacher and principal who, he thinks, were responsible for his suspension from school.

The therapist has been using cognitive therapy with Jeremy. Cognitive therapy focuses on helping clients rationally think through solutions to social and emotional problems. It also helps clients analyze their thought processes as they critically evaluate irrational self-sentences about situations that often result in dysfunctional behavior. Jeremy has resisted therapy and tends to respond to the therapist in an exaggerated voice in which he mimics everything the therapist says. Nonetheless, the therapist has maintained his treatment plan and at every session, Jeremy is encouraged to view his behavior as logically and as honestly as possible. This process of rationally reviewing his behavior is having a demoralizing impact of Jeremy. After three months of treatment, he has begun to show signs of depression and regression. He often sits on the sofa curled up in the fetal position, sucking his finger and crying. Jeremy's defenses are beginning to break down. Instead of the angry and aggressive child he presented initially in treatment, he has begun to show a frightened and troubled side that suggests the cognitive and emotional functioning of a much younger child.

The therapist believes that Jeremy suffered a trauma when he was a very young child, but there is no evidence of child abuse or any of the other problems one associates with a developmental shutdown. The therapist thinks it's possible that the birth of a sibling when he was five and the subsequent loss of his role as an only child may be partially responsible for the change in his behavior. After five months of treatment, Jeremy is miserable and doesn't want to talk to the therapist. He complains to his parents that the therapist hurts his feelings and that he hates him, but changes are taking place in his behavior at school and at home.

He has stopped acting out, is more thoughtful in his responses to others, and has begun to see his role in the interactions with others that end in painful confrontations.

After eight months of treatment, the therapist began to see real changes in Jeremy's behavior. He is more animated, engaged in treatment, and is more willing to discuss his behavior. His anger has also begun to diminish. Jeremy is acting in a more age-appropriate way. He can now discuss feelings and concerns. It is difficult to know why the change has taken place because conduct disorders are often felt to be as difficult to treat as antisocial personality disorders in adults. The therapist now believes, after meeting Jeremy's parents on a number of occasions, that Jeremy lacks consistent parenting and that the birth of his sibling ushered in a degree of chaos in the family that Jeremy deeply resents. He also thinks that the therapeutic relationship has provided Jeremy with a source of intimacy that has been missing in his life. The consistent, structured therapy he is receiving provides a caring substitute for his chaotic family life.

The changes in Jeremy have been dramatic. He exhibits few of the symptoms he initially presented. After a year of therapy, he is progressing well in school and shows good social and emotional progress. But is he cured? The therapist hopes so but is inclined to wait and see. He told me the following:

> Therapy doesn't produce miracles, and when you treat acting-out children like Jeremy, you hope for the best, but you temper it with reality. Jeremy is still a troubled child who is about to enter the turbulent years of adolescence. His underlying issues haven't changed although his adaptation to the world has improved, probably as a result of the structure and consistency provided by therapy. Jeremy has shown amazing progress and you always want to be optimistic with children. I suspect that the more treatment is able to help Jeremy, the more he will progress as he enters adolescence. I would strongly recommend continued therapy for quite a long time to come, and a good deal of help to his family. He has a troubled and disorganized family. To be sure, they're loving and non-abu-

sive, but they haven't much skill in setting limits or in providing consistent affection and support. All Jeremy can see in his family is chaos and disorganization, and it makes him angry and resentful. Like most children, Jeremy craves consistency. You can't really expect him to maintain his improvement in functioning without a similar improvement in the family. We have already begun to provide family therapy and parent education classes with excellent results. Jeremy doesn't live in a vacuum. His family environment affects his behavior. As the family improves, so, I hope, will Jeremy.

SUMMARY

This chapter discusses diagnosis, treatment, and social programs to help violent children and adolescents. A great deal of the reason for early violence stems from child abuse and neglect in highly dysfunctional families. Unfortunately, we are still at an early stage of knowing the best treatment approaches to use with abused and neglected children. A distinction is made between early violence starters who often cycle on through life with serious social and emotional problems as opposed to late starters whose violence often diminishes or completely goes away in early adulthood.

Chapter *11*

Clinical Work With Physically and Sexually Abusive Men

Two major problems facing men is their use of physical and sexual violence against women. This chapter discusses the dynamics of male abuse and offers suggested treatment approaches. Some of the material in this chapter was first reported in modified form in three prior volumes I wrote or cowrote (Glicken, 2004, 2005; Glicken & Sechrest, 2003). The reader may wish to review those works for a more comprehensive discussion of the material.

DOMESTIC VIOLENCE

Domestic violence is a deeply disruptive and dangerous problem that not only creates physical and emotional injuries to adult victims but also increases the probability of troubled behavior in the children who observe domestic violence. Jacobson (1998) says that over 3 million children a year witness acts of domestic violence and that 50% to 70% of the men who abuse women also abuse the children in the home. In homes with four or more children, this amount increases to 90%. Although rates of domestic violence by men have decreased during the past ten years, it still remains a serious problem and one that many clinicians feel unprepared to treat. Men who commit physical violence to intimates often respond to treatment. Even limited success suggests that men who change their behavior as a result of treatment will no longer abuse, a finding all clinicians should find encouraging.

THE AMOUNT OF MALE SPOUSAL AND PARTNER ABUSE

Tjaden and Thoenner (1998) report that approximately 1.5 million women are sexually or physically assaulted every year in the United States. In a number of studies, a third to a half of all women seeking therapy as adults have been abused by men, many before the age of eighteen (Bagley, 1990; Hale, Duckworth, Zimostrad, & Scott, 1988). Dewhurst, Moore, and Alfano (1992) note that sexual and physical assaults are the two major crimes committed by men against women in our society. Victimization rates for both types of offenses have been estimated at between 10% and 30% of all women.

The actual amount of domestic violence is confused by methodological differences among researchers. Neuman (1995) says that many researchers confuse domestic violence (violence between loved ones) with general violence. The result is that the absolute amount of domestic violence has become subject to conflicting sets of data. Neuman (1995) indicates that some researchers consider domestic violence to be the occasional bad acts that many men and women are guilty of in relationships, including such less violent acts as the bumping or light contacts between people when they're arguing. To further confuse the picture, Neuman believes that violence by women to men and violence between same-sex partners has been grossly underestimated, resulting in a belief that almost all domestic violence is committed by men to women. Rates of violence among lesbian women have been estimated at almost 60% as compared to rates of violence of 27% to 33% between heterosexual couples (Neuman, 1995). Rates of violence to men by women, always felt to be low, are now beginning to show levels almost as high as those of men abusing women. In a National Family Violence Survey from 1975 to 1985, Straus and Gelles (1986) found that women initiated violent acts at rates similar to that of men. In a later report, Straus and Walsh (1997) maintain that female to male violence in relationships parallels that of male to female violence, but when underreporting by men is included, it may actually be higher. Police reports, which rely on the actual number of people arrested for domestic violence, show a significant increase in female to male violence but at rates that are still much lower than arrests made for male to female violence. The Los Angeles Police Department in

1995 (1997) noted a 14.3% arrest rate for women accused of abuse to an intimate adult, a 100% increase over arrests for women in 1987.

THE DYNAMICS OF MALE ABUSE

Roy (1982) found that although abusive men are not distinguished by a history of criminal arrests, over 80% of the men who abuse women and children have witnessed or experienced abuse as children. Waldo (1987) believes this finding suggests that battering is a family pattern transmitted from one generation to the next. Kalmuss (1984) reports that a disproportionate number of men who engage in physical aggression against their partners learn their behavior as a direct result of witnessing abuse between their parents. Murphy, Coleman, and Haynes (1986) indicate that men who are prone to the use of violence in their relationships with women have a generalized belief in the use of violence as a way of controlling others. These men are frequently unable to separate seductive from friendly behavior, or hostile from assertive behavior. The authors also believe that aggressive, hostile, emotionally labile men who lack empathy are likely to physically and emotionally abuse women and children.

Wiederholt (1992) reports that abusive men are likely to batter when they have minor doubts about their partners, particularly when partners criticize their competency and integrity. This loss of trust sometimes leads to an inability to control impulsive violence and results in an emotionally chaotic condition similar to a presuicidal state. Hotaling and Sugarman (1984) report that alcohol use is a disinhibitor of the constraints against the use of violence. Waldo (1987) reports that abusive men imitate their father's abusive behavior as a way of exerting authority and control over family members.

Peterson (1980) suggests that husband to wife violence is highly related to past exposure to violent role models and often has its origins in the way role models treated mothers and sisters. The desired impact of the abuse was the emotional surrendering of women in the abuser's life to his violent and abusive behavior. As a result, generations of violence may be perpetuated by a single angry man with poor skills at containing rage. Dodge and Richard (1986) believe that children who have witnessed abuse and have developed aggressive behaviors see more malevolent intentions in accidental or ambiguous aggressive acts and retaliate more often than nonaggressive children.

Many researchers report the tendency of abusive men to feel remorse after an episode of abuse. The term *Honeymoon Period* is used to define the remorseful period during which the abuser becomes warm, loving, and tender. Abuse victims describe this period as the time in which their lives are the happiest. Giles-Sims (1983) suggests that violence may be rewarding to the abusive man. In addition to relieving tension, it often results in pleasing changes in the spouse's behavior. For many abusive men, this is a moment of power and control that is unique in their lives. Having temporarily satisfied his esteem needs, the abusive man may become guilt-ridden and afraid that he will lose the relationship on which he is so dependent. During this period, the abusive man tries to win back his spouse's heart by being overly solicitous and intimate. During this honeymoon period, Waldo (1987) suggests that abusive men experience a heightened sense of intimacy and commitment, which acts as a reward for having been violent, a condition that reinforces the cycle of violence.

Commenting further on the honeymoon period, Waldo (1987) suggests that it is a time of fragility where the abusive man is less willing to be assertive about his needs. But when the same relationship problems reoccur, they are more powerfully felt because they touch on old wounds. Eventually, the anger shows itself again in violent incidents, completing the cycle and starting it over again. Although the violence is repetitive, it is likely to become more frequent and severe because it takes stronger abuse to get the same effect from the spouse. The fundamental problems in the relationship, which are set aside during the honeymoon period, remain unchanged.

Adams (1988) reports that intrapsychic problems often lead to violent behavior in men. The list of potential problems include poor impulse control, low frustration tolerance, fear of intimacy, fear of abandonment, dependency, and underlying depression. Adams believes that abusive men are emotionally fragile and overwhelmed by uncertainty and confusion, often feeling as if they've been victimized and that their abusive behavior may be absolved by what was done to them by their partners. Scher and Stevens (1985) found that violence to women and children is rooted in cultural and historical folkways and mores that define men as caretakers who are necessarily tough and aggressive. Because the abuser has systemically reduced the abused woman's ability to feel independent and to seek autonomous work and relationships, the abuser has significant financial and emotional power which permits continued abusive behavior.

PREDICTING POTENTIAL FOR ABUSE

Jacobson (1998) reports a study funded by the National Institute of Mental Health in which batterers and their partners were brought into a laboratory setting and were videotaped during arguments (no physical violence was permitted). From this study, the researchers found two distinct types of abusers, who were subsequently called "Pit Bulls" and "Cobras" by the researchers.

Cobras were seen as cold-blooded and deliberate with long histories of antisocial behavior. Cobras had high potential for violence outside of their marriages, often abused drugs and alcohol, and frequently grew up in violent homes. They demanded complete control in their relationships and expected and got immediate self-gratification. Their violence was quick and ferocious, making it difficult for battered spouses to anticipate when the violence would occur or to physically separate themselves from husbands for fear of retaliation. The researchers found that the danger period when spouses leave Cobras is shorter than previously thought because Cobras may soon stop pursuing their spouses and move on to other relationships they can better control.

Pit Bulls seldom have criminal records and are usually violent only in their homes. Many Pit Bulls have been battered by their fathers. Like Cobras, they must have total control of their marriages, fear abandonment, and often experience jealous rages that lead to more control of their spouses. The researchers found the following:

> Pit Bull violence is marked by a slow burn that explodes into violence.
> They may be easier to leave initially, but can be more dangerous in the

long term because some of them are likely to become obsessed with their spouses, stalking and harassing them. (Jacobson, 1998, p. 11)

Jacobson (1998) is concerned that we know so little about the treatment of batterers and whether Cobras and Pit Bulls respond to treatment in different ways. He provides a cautionary note on the effectiveness of treatment: "It is difficult to believe that someone [a batterer] who has been raised for 10 or 20 years not to respect women and has treated them as chattel, will suddenly change after a 16-week group treatment class" (p. 11).

Hotaling and Sugarman (1984) reviewed the literature on the risk markers in predicting abuse. These markers indicated six characteristics of male abusers, five characteristics of the women whom they victimize, and eight characteristics of the marital relationships in which violence to women and children were most likely to occur: (a) characteristics of the abusive men themselves revealed lower self-esteem than nonbatterers, lower levels of income and lower occupational status, higher probability of abusing alcohol, and a higher probability than nonabusers to having been abused as children and to have seen parental violence while growing up; (b) battered women were also likely to have lower levels of self-esteem, to have more traditional sex-role expectations, to use drugs more often, to have been abused by parents when they were children, and to have seen more parental abuse while growing up; and (c) the marital relationships in violence-prone families were marked by conflict and maladjustment, higher levels of educational and religious incompatibility, lower family incomes, higher levels of verbal abuse, and the increased likelihood that separation or divorce would occur in the marriage.

Schuerger and Reigle (1988) explored the personality markers of violent men and found the following: most of the men studied had a DSM–III diagnosis of explosive disorders (312.34, 312.39). More than 60% of the men were chemically dependent, mainly on alcohol. Twenty-four percent of the sample were more severely disturbed and could be diagnosed as schizoid, schizophrenic, or borderline personality. Twenty-five percent of the men studied had depressive disorders. Interestingly, aside from violence toward women and children, about 25% of the abusive men studied had no discernable or significant disorders. Although it is often difficult on psychological tests to distinguish violent from nonviolent men, the authors note that abusive men often tend to be more withdrawn, compulsive, rigidly tough minded, and anxious, than nonviolent men. Although a significant number of the men in the sample were substance abusers, the authors indicate that resolving the substance abuse did not lead to a lessening of violence.

Wolf-Smith and LaRossa (1992) report that abusive men tend to continue the use of excuses and apologies in the aftermath to episodes of violence, but as time progresses, the excuses used are more frequently characterized as ones that blame the victims for the abuse. Dewhurst, Moore, and Alfano (1992) found that abusive men are more hostile to women than nonabusers and that often the abuse is coupled with alcohol use and "… situational intolerance and general frustration coupled with a thinking pattern that tends toward pessimism, suspicion and catastrophizing, particularly about their partners. These negative ruminations may be the motive for their behavior …" (p. 44).

Bernard and Bernard (1984) believe that because of a lack of ego strength, abusive men choose spouses on whom they can be dependent. The dependence stems from an inability to develop other sources of emotional intimacy and validation. Consequently, the abusive man expects his wife to understand all of his thoughts and feelings without hesitation. When the spouse is unable to anticipate and satisfy the man's needs and desires, Waldo (1987) reports that the man becomes outraged and resorts to violence. Waldo believes that abusers have low self-esteem, which makes them highly vulnerable to criticism and overly reactive when they feel threatened. In time, abusers may become hypervigilant to threats to the relationship and their behavior toward women may become increasingly defined by jealousy and lack of trust.

Jourad and Landsman (1969) believe that many abused men grow into adulthood emotionally disconnected from significant experiences in their lives and become socially isolated. Not surprisingly, these men often come to psychotherapy to try and cope with the dysfunctional consequence of isolation and the inability to understand repetitive behaviors that may be consistently troublesome. Symptoms related to an emotional disconnect from prior abuse as a child include the following: silence and nondisclosure, intellectualization and hypermasculine identification, dependency, identification with aggressors, and difficulty connecting current behavior with early life experiences.

In national surveys, Dutton (1994) reports that 72% of all men surveyed are not violent in their homes and that the remaining 28% use violence occasionally to frequently. Of those who do use violence, Dutton indicates that 55% are stifled men who have poor impulse control and have problems controlling their anger, whereas 20% of those surveyed have

> Borderline personalities and are prone to intensive anger in intimate relationships. A quarter of the remaining abusers are so entrenched in their violent behavior that they are considered untreatable by current technologies to help reduce abusive behavior. (p. B16)

Widom (1989) notes that individuals who have been identified by juvenile courts as abuse victims as children are 42% more likely than controls to perpetuate the cycle of violence by committing violent acts as adults. Strauss and Gelles (1990) report that the character traits of abused children become increasingly organized to ward off the anxiety inherent in their family relationships. Children from highly abusive families exhibit depression and cognitive deficiencies, including poor ability to abstract, and suffer from limitations in self-awareness and problems with the identification of feelings. Strauss and Gelles (1990) indicate that many abused children reveal almost paranoid-like hypersensitivity, which results in distorted interactions with others and often evolves into adult suspiciousness and manipulativeness.

TREATING ABUSIVE BEHAVIOR

Mandatory Arrest and Treatment

In the early 1980s, Lerman (1984) began to argue for a set of policies that required a more specific role for the police and the courts in abuse cases. She recommended the following: (a) a policy for prosecutors not to drop domestic violence charges once they were filed; (b) providing advocacy services for victims; (c) charging perpetrators whether or not they were related to victims; (d) releasing perpetrators only if restraining orders were issued; and (e) taking the victim's desires into consideration when sentencing the perpetrator.

Additional attempts to modify the legal consequences of abuse have been developed in many cities, including Duluth, Minnesota, where advocates are provided to victims whose function is to (a) provide battered women and children legal information and assistance, (b) educate and evaluate judges, police officers and prosecutors, (c) advocate for conviction as well as mandated treatment of perpetrators, and (d) monitor perpetrators to make certain that the conditions of sentencing are completed.

How successful is mandatory arrest and sentencing? In the initial phase of the Minneapolis, Minnesota study, which used mandatory arrest and compared its effectiveness with on-the-spot counseling by the police and a cooling off period where perpetrators left the home for eight hours, Sherman and Bark (1984) found that arrests of perpetrators reduced by half the likelihood of continued violence as compared to mediation by the police or asking the abuser to leave the home for eight hours. Later studies by the authors found that in 15% to 25% of the arrests for domestic violence, the level of future assaults increased in frequency and severity and that mandatory arrests actually led to more murders of intimates. Fagan et al. (1983) found that mediation and victim assistance by the police tended to be as effective as police arrest. But as Eisikovits and Edelson (1989) note, "Outside of a few studies in the criminal justice system, it remains unclear what actions are taken by the various actors, professions, or organizations that react to domestic violence and what influence, if any, these actions have on ending violence" (p. 406).

Davis, Smith, and Nickles (1998) found no evidence that mandatory prosecution for domestic violence reduced the likelihood of recidivism in domestic violence misdemeanor cases. Furthermore, they found mandatory treatment in diversion projects for men and women found guilty of misdemeanor abuse to be unrelated to additional abuse following treatment: "The likelihood of recidivism was indistinguishable for cases resulting in nolles, dismissals, probation with batterer treatment program, and jail sentences" (Davis, Smith, & Nickles, 1998, p. 440). The authors go on to say that domestic violence cases are "messy" and involve children, property, and emotional bonds that may not be affected by the punishing aspects of the courts. People stay together for reasons that may override the violent aspects of their relationships and they are often less than truthful with researchers and therapists regarding the discontinuation of violence in the relationship after any treatment input, including incarceration and therapy. Although the justice system may help in protecting people, it does poorly in resolving complex interpersonal relationships among people involved in domestic violence. As Davis et al. (1998) note, "Habitual behavior that occurs in the privacy of people's homes and out of the public eye is likely to be highly resistant to change in many instances" (p. 441).

Mandatory Treatment

Hamberger and Hastings (1993) reviewed 23 outcome studies conducted between 1984 and 1991 on the efficacy of treatment with perpetrators of domestic violence and found no significant difference in recidivism between those who had completed treatment and dropouts up to one year later. However, Gondolf (1997) found that only four percent of those treated were found to be recidivists as measured by re-arrests for domestic violence. Untreated batterers had a 40% re-arrest rate over a three-year follow-up period. Rosenfeld (1992) found that men who completed treatment had only slightly lower rates of recidivism than men who rejected treatment, were dropouts, or remained untreated. Gondolf (1997) also found that when husbands entered treatment, wives were more willing to return to the relationship after being in shelters. The author concluded that treatment programs may increase the risk of being battered by providing a false hope that husbands had actually benefited from treatment and wouldn't be abusive again.

Considering the relation between substance abuse and domestic violence, it might be logical to assume that treating the substance abuse would lower abuse rates in male batters. However, Babcock and Steiner

(1999) found that abuse rates were unchanged for men who had successfully completed programs for substance abuse although they did find a
strong relation between completing treatment for domestic violence
and much lower recidivism rates. However, treatment in lieu of incarceration had no positive impact on recidivism rates and incarceration
actually increased the antagonism of some perpetrators toward treatment and the resistance to changing their abusive behavior. Interestingly, the authors found that many of their participants completed
treatment after one or more bench warrants were issued for noncompliance with court-mandated treatment. The authors suggest that the de-
termination of the court to maintain a commitment to treatment may
actually be necessary to change abusive behavior in men who reject
treatment. They call for a community effort that includes coordinated
handling of all abuse cases.

Perpetrator groups are often mandatory in lieu of incarceration and
emphasize the following: (a) self-assessment techniques including the
use of logs and diaries that help male abusers analyze a series of events
and behaviors which may have ended in violence; (b) developing plans
to deal with volatile situations which are likely to result in violence,
also called "safety plans"; (c) understanding the cycle of violence, the
legal ramifications of violence, and the underlying reasons for violence. This is also called a "reeducation" approach in the literature; (d)
teaching nonviolent skills to help in conflict resolution. These skills
may include teaching clients to remove themselves from stressful situations and to take "creative time-outs"; (e) other nonviolent skills include helping the client develop language to express feelings and
opinions about situations which may lead to violence, helping change
rigid role expectations of others, and relaxation techniques to help remove stress from the client's life; (f) techniques that encourage clients
to examine early life situations which may underlie and explain abusive behavior; (g) consciousness raising and empathy training; and (h)
learning to confront group members about their behavior and to accept the opinions of others.

In determining the effectiveness of perpetrator groups, Grusznski
and Carillo (1988) reports that the use of cognitive-behavioral therapy, social skills training, and problem-solving skills training, by

themselves or together, were more effective than self-help approaches, but when these approaches were combined with a self-help group, the combination was quite effective in reducing violent behavior and had the most long lasting results. The authors report that twelve-week groups were helpful in immediately reducing the violence and self-help groups were most effective in maintaining the reduction over time. However, a review of the literature on treatment of abusive men suggests such a wide range of interventions with a number of borrowed treatment approaches and theories that Eisikovits and Edleson (1989) wrote the following:

> Overall, however, it can still be said that the intervention literature (on abusive men) is quite often atheoretical or it has borrowed its theoretical grounding from other areas. There is an urgent need to develop theory grounded in the experience of men who batter and battered women rather than theory borrowed from others. (p. 407).

CASE EXAMPLE: A PERPETRATOR IN TREATMENT

Dale Jordan is a 26-year-old White male who badly beat his girlfriend after a party when he thought she was flirting with another man. Dale has a history of abusive behavior and this is his second sentence for abuse. The first sentence required community service but no therapy. He is now expected to attend up to a year of treatment under state law. If he hasn't progressed after the year, the therapist can recommend more therapy or that he be remanded back to court for jail sentencing. Dale must pay for his treatment and has been required to pay for his girlfriend's medical bills related to the assault and for her ongoing therapy for symptoms of PTSD (posttraumatic stress disorder).

Dale attends a cognitive-behavioral group run by a master's-level counselor. The group uses a concept known as the "Power Wheel" to show group members how they view their girlfriends and spouses and the behaviors that define healthier attitudes. There is a great deal of processing and self-disclosure with homework assignments. Group members are expected to practice new behaviors whenever they feel they might be abusive. Dale has been asked to practice a frequently used technique called a "time-out." Whenever Dale hears his voice getting louder or when his hands begin to rise to a point of peril where he might hit, he has been told by the group to remove himself from the situation and to "cool off." He has also been asked to "freeze-frame" the situation that made him angry to see if it actually happened the way he described it and to develop strategies for dealing with potentially abusive behavior that exclude emotional or physical abuse.

After six months of nonproductive therapy, Dale finally took a "time-out" from an argument with his girlfriend. During the time-out, he was able to think about what the group said about nonviolent strategies and decided that he'd try explaining his anger to his girlfriend in the most rational way he could. Much to his surprise, he was able to resolve the situation without battering her or being verbally abusive. Later he told the group, "I didn't believe in any of this crap until I finally tried it and I could see that it works. I suggest that you guys try it sometime. I'm sick of myself beating my girlfriend up when you can talk things through instead."

This initial success led to other successes, and although Dale can still be verbally abusive, his girlfriend has made gains in her own therapy and won't put up with it. The continuation of emotional abuse has led to several major breakups, but, feeling that they have deep affection for one another, they return to the relationship and have progressively done better. In the course of their treatment, both Dale and his girlfriend were able to better understand the relation between their own abuse as children and their behavior as adults. They understand that the attraction they feel for one another and the continuation of abusive behaviors are long-held behaviors that require ongoing help and vigilance if their relationship is going to work. Even after the perpetrator group officially ended, Dale asked to continue his work in the group. He also sees a therapist weekly in individual treatment.

In evaluating his gains in treatment, Dale told me the following:

I have a serious problem with my temper. It's not only with my girlfriend but it's at work, when I drive, and lots of other places. I don't have patience to stand in line or for anything that doesn't go my way. I know I have a problem and the best thing to do is get help. My doctor also put me on a drug to help control my temper and it's really helped a lot. He also has me on fish oil because he read a study saying that fish oil is good for bad tempers. Whatever is helping, I'm a lot better. In my home, my dad hit us until we were bloody. He said things about me and my sisters and brothers that you wouldn't ever say to a kid. He made us have sex together in front of his friends. I used to think that a real man could take it and be OK, but it's left me pretty messed up and angry. I go to the group, see my therapist, and take my meds. The thing I learned is that being mad all the time and beating up my girl friend is an illness, just like if I had cancer. In order to get better, I have to get help. But it took a long time for me to feel that way and like a lot of guys I know, going for help about head stuff means you're weak and like a woman. I don't believe that anymore and I tell my friends that if they want to think that way it's OK with me but it's not OK with their wives and kids and the people who love them. They're going to hurt those people and it makes them think. I'm not cured, but I'm getting there and that's saying something.

SEXUAL ABUSE

In 1998, The U.S. Census Bureau (1998) estimated that during a woman's lifetime, there was a 17.6% possibility of her being raped (a 14.8% completion rate and a 2.8% attempt rate). In actual terms, the data indicate that 302,091 women were raped in America, but when nonreported rapes were added to that figure, the estimate increased to 876,000 rapes and 5.9 million physical assaults (U.S. Census Department, 1998). When the data considered only an intimate partner (current and former spouses, opposite-sex cohabiting partners, same-sex cohabiting partners, dates, and boyfriends or girlfriends), it was predicted that 8% of all women will experience rape by an intimate and 22% will experience some form of physical assault during their lifetime. To make the assault data more vivid, women are seven to fourteen times more likely to have been beaten, choked, threatened with a gun, or actually had a gun used on them by intimates than men. Women are stalked eight times more often than men. Of the 18% of women facing a probability of being raped in their lifetime, 54% will have been raped before the age of 18. Women raped before the age of 18 are significantly more likely to be raped as adults (U.S. Census Department, 1998). Greenfeld (1997) reports that the group most at risk of being raped are women sixteen to nineteen years of age, of low-income, and urban residences. There is no significant difference defining rape by race or ethnicity. A 2001 National Institute of Alcohol Abuse and Alcoholism (NIAAA) report (2001) estimated that there were 70,000 cases of sexual assaults and acquaintance rapes on American campuses alone, many related to binge drinking by perpetrators.

Dating and Acquaintance Assault

A study by Frinter and Rubinson (1993) at a large Midwestern university indicated that 27% of the college women in the study had experienced sexual assault, attempted sexual assault, sexual abuse without penetration, or had been subjected to battery, illegal restraint, or intimidation. Eighty-three percent of the women knew the person who assaulted them. Fifty-six percent of the victims and 68% of the offenders had been drinking at the time of the assault. Regarding the perpetrators, Malamuth (1989) indicates that male sexual perpetrators have high scores on scales measuring dominance as a sexual motive. They also have hostile feelings toward women, condone the use of force in sexual relationships, often have an inability to appraise social interactions, and have experienced prior parental neglect or physical and or emotional abuse early in life. Drugs and alcohol are commonly associated with sexual aggression. Of the men identified as having committed acquaintance rape, 75% had taken drugs or alcohol just prior to the rape (Koss & Dinero, 1988).

A University of Nebraska (1996) report indicates that many sexually violent men "stalk" victims or follow them to prove that the woman is being faithful and as a means of controlling the other person through intimidation. The report indicates that "Stalking can be very frightening particularly when the victim thinks the other person is following them but isn't able to verify it" (p. 4). When the stalker frequently shows up wherever the victim finds herself, this is often a "clue" that the victim is being stalked. Perpetrators might deny the use of the word "stalk" and in its place, "indicate that they end up in similar locations because they share many of the same interests" (p. 4). The stalking may increase when the victim is trying to leave the relationship. It is at this point when sexual violence is most likely to occur, although from the many reports of women who experience date and acquaintance sexual violence, "there may have been prior instances where the victim has forced the client into sexually compromising situations that fall under the definition of rape" (p. 4).

Victims often define their willingness to have sex as semiconsensual, indicating that they may have sex to reduce the risk of serious physical violence. Again, it should be noted that sexual violence among intimates and acquaintances frequently occurs when both the victim and the perpetrator have been drinking and boundaries are often blunted and full intent may be difficult for both the victim and the perpetrator to define. Restraining orders may be necessary when stalking begins, although to be fair to victims, the police seldom enforce restraining orders unless there is actual physical contact where some form of assault has taken place. This makes restraining orders something of an absurdity to many women who are stalked and frightened by former boyfriends, husbands, or friends.

Dynamics of Sexual Perpetrators

Yang (1992), writing about rape, reports the work of G. N. Hall (uncited in the article), who believes that there have been two primary explanations of rape: anger at women, and becoming sexually excited by the wrong stimuli. Hall argues, "for a long time, these two approaches dominated the thinking on why men rape, which is understandable; it would be great to be able to pin sexual aggression on a single cause" (Yang, 1992, p. 6). Hall doesn't believe either theory explains why men rape and describes four primary types of rapists:

> Type 1 is influenced by deviant sexual arousal, which occurs when he has thoughts of violence against women. This type is likely to be extremely impulsive.

> Type 2 is motivated by cognitive distortions, or thinking errors; he mistakenly interprets events or information differently than other men would. He believes that some women enjoy being raped, or want to be raped. For this type, rape is part of a conquest, a way of demonstrating masculinity. Most date rapists are Type 2's.

> Type 3 is motivated by anger or emotional discontrol. These men are so angry, especially at women that the only way for them to deal with their anger is to act out sexually toward women. Not surprisingly, this type is the most violent and most dangerous.

> Type 4 is the repeat offender. He is most likely to have been physically or sexually abused as a child. He has difficulty establishing enduring relationships, and a history of chronic problems in schools or in his family. Type 4 men break a variety of rules, both sexual and nonsexual. (Yang, 1992, p. 46)

Treating the Perpetrators of Sexual Violence

A number of treatment approaches have been used with male perpetrators of sexual violence including those molesting children and perpetrators of rape of intimates and strangers. The literature suggests that the primary approaches used in various treatment settings include the following traditional and less traditional approaches: insight-oriented individual psychotherapy, group psychotherapy, family therapy, psycho-educational skills training, behavioral treatments, chemical castration, sexual addiction twelve-step recovery programs, relapse prevention programs, Parents United, and several model approaches that combine each of these approaches. Several of the therapies used with sexual predators are explained in more detail.

Chemical Castration. This controversial treatment is used to decrease sexual obsessiveness by significantly lowering libido, erotic fantasies, erections, and ejaculations. One commonly used drug is Depo-Provera, a testosterone-suppressing agent. Side effects of the drug include weight gain, lethargy, cold sweats, nightmares, hot flashes, hypertension and elevated blood pressure, high blood sugars, and shortness of breath. Berlin (1982) reported an 85% effectiveness rate in eliminating deviant sexual behaviors, "as long as the medication was taken on a regular basis. It is not a cure and relapse often follows discontinuation of medication and is not recommenced as an exclusive treatment" (p. 93).

Psycho-Educational Skills Training. Because sexual offenders as a group tend to be uninformed about human sexuality (Groth, 1978) and often have difficulty expressing their feelings, skills training groups teach offenders "... multiple aspects of assertiveness skills, including making eye contact, duration of reply, latency of response, loudness of speech and quality of affect" (Groth, 1978, p. 14). Rosen and Fracher (1983) recommend teaching tension reduction and anger management to those offenders who may experience anxiety and anger before the assault. Groth (1978) believes that the majority of offenders have very little awareness of the physical and emotional impact of sexual assault on their victims and suggests the use of empathy training to help offenders understand the impact of the offender's behavior on the victim.

Behavioral Treatments. These treatments include covert sensitization, electrical aversion, odor aversion, chemical aversion and suppression, and satiation techniques. Covert sensitization is a procedure in which the therapist describes a deviant sexual scene followed by an aversive scene. The aversive scene may include going to jail, blood, odors, community responses, and other aversive stimuli the therapist has determined effective in a screening interview. Scenes last about ten minutes and two scenes are presented at each session (Mayer, 1988). This same concept can be used with the addition of unpleasant odors or electric shock with the aversive scene. In satiation procedures, the offender is told to masturbate to nondeviant fantasies and then ejaculate. The client is asked to continue masturbating to deviant fantasies for 45 minutes. Throughout, the client is asked to verbalize his fantasies which are then recorded and monitored for client compliance. Satiation procedures attempt to destroy the erotic nature of the deviant urges by boring the client with his own fantasies (Johnson, Hudson, & Marshall, 1992).

Treatment Effectiveness With Sexual Offenders

Looman, Abracen, and Nicholaichuk (2000) report that the most common treatment techniques for work with sexual offenders are confrontation, role plays, supportive psychotherapy, and empathy training, usually provided for about six months. When considering the effectiveness of these techniques, the authors found that the treated group in their study had a sexual recidivism rate of 23.6%, whereas the untreated group had a sexual recidivism rate of 51.7%. However, when it came to recidivism for non-sexually-related offenses, both groups had high recidivism rates. Treated sexual offenders had re-arrest rates of 61.8% compared to 74.2% for the untreated group, raising questions about the overall treatment effectiveness of the therapeutic techniques used.

Loza and Loza-Fanous (1999) report that many correctional facilities require that inmates attend anger management programs. This is particularly true of rapists because of the assumption that anger at women is a primary cause of violent criminal acts. However, when the authors (Loza & Loza-Fanous, 1999) tested this assumption by reviewing the effectiveness of anger management programs in reducing violent behavior, including the violent behavior of rapists, they found

> ... no differences between violent offenders and nonviolent offenders and between rapists and non-rapists and nonviolent offenders on anger measures [even with] a prevalence of the belief among correctional professionals that there is a link between anger and violence, rape, and recidivism. This situation exists despite the (a) supporting evidence against a link between anger and violent behavior among non-criminal populations and criminal offenders in particular; (b) lack of relationship between anger and criminal recidivism, and; (c) shortage of researches

examining the role of anger in violent behavior and crime. (Loza & Loza-Fanous, 1999, p. 497)

CASE EXAMPLE: USING THE STRENGTHS PERSPECTIVE
WITH A SERIAL RAPIST

This case first appeared in modified form in a volume I wrote on the strengths perspective (Glicken, 2004). Most clinicians believe that rapists are among the most difficult clients to treat because of the severe nature of their antisocial personality disorders. Accordingly, the belief is that men who rape women feel little compassion for their victims, act out their sexual impulses when they feel like it, and enjoy the pain inflicted on female victims. That may all be true, but this case shows that some rapists do respond to treatment and particularly to a form of treatment that focuses on positive behavior.

THE CASE

John is a 28-year-old serial rapist who has raped and physically and emotionally assaulted more than 100 women by his own count. The authorities believe it's more than that because John has been raping and molesting children and women since he was ten. Like many sexual offenders, John began molesting his own sister when she was five years old. By any standard, John is a violent, devious, and emotionally labile man who has been in and out of jail for sexual assaults and drug-related crimes. The authorities who supervise John dislike him intensely, not only because of the crimes he's committed but because he often brags about his crimes. In a prison full of unlikable people, John stands at the very top of the list.

Because the state John lives in requires treatment for all felons convicted of sexual assault, John is being seen by a clinical psychologist in individual and group treatment. The prospects for improvement are not very promising and John dutifully goes for treatment twice a week and attends a sex offender group once a week. He is cynical about therapy, having been in some form of treatment since he was ten. Most therapists are easy to manipulate and John has set out to "con" his therapist which, by his early assessment, should have been easy.

The clinician is unlike anyone John has ever worked with before, and he has seen many therapists over the years. At first, John thought he was manipulating the therapist because, in addition to being genuinely nice to John, the therapist let John talk. Often, John lied and the therapist didn't seem to call him on anything. But in time, John got tired of lying and despite his best attempts to never tell the therapist the truth, John found himself telling the therapist everything. At first, he did this to get the therapist's sympathy, which never seemed to happen. Then he began telling the therapist the truth because it felt good to unburden himself. When John was truthful, there was a shift in the therapist so subtle that John missed it at first. But after a time, John could feel the therapist becoming so in tune with him when he was truthful, that it felt to John as if the therapist was reading his mind and he could feel John's emotional pain.

Truthfully, John is disgusted by his behavior. The fact that he can't control his impulses causes him to be full of self-loathing. To be so generally disliked by everyone is often too much for John to contain and sometimes he breaks down and cries in the therapist's office. It felt terribly feminizing to cry and yet, it felt wonderfully freeing. John began to realize that unlike other therapists he'd seen, this one never focused on his sexual offending. Instead, he seemed to focus on what John did well and on his dreams and aspirations in life, his regrets, and his feelings of disgust and guilt. When John shared these feelings with the therapist, a change began to take place in him that others noticed. He became open in his group treatment and spoke for many of the men in the group about the way he felt about himself. He sought men out in prison for advice. He helped a sick prisoner get treatment. As John began to change, so did the reaction to him by the people around him.

When John was released to go to a supervised halfway house after serving seven years for rape, he promised the therapist that in exchange for the help he'd received, that he would never rape or molest anyone again. After eight years, he has kept his word. When asked about the help he received in prison, John said the following:

No one thinks that people like me have feelings. We do. I began molesting my sister when she was 5. She's a drug addict today. I did that to my own sister and God only knows the pain I brought to many women and children. I'm full of regret over what I did. I don't want pity and I don't want anyone to think I didn't enjoy what I did, because I did enjoy it. Rapists have free rein to satisfy their needs for sex anytime they feel like it. Don't think that's not a powerful feeling, because it is. Any rapist who says they don't get off on it is a liar. At the same time, it's a disgusting feeling to think about what I'd been doing to people. I saw one of the women I'd raped in a store six months after I'd raped her and this beautiful woman of 20 looked like an old haggard witch. I couldn't sleep for days. Gradually, I couldn't get it up when I raped, and then I couldn't rape anymore. People think that once a rapist, always a rapist. It's not true. Like any sick behavior, you start to feel repulsed by it.

Gary, my therapist, seemed to understand what I was feeling right away. He never lectured me or told me how many lives I'd ruined. He knew I already knew that. What he did do was to listen, give me suggestions when I asked for them, tell me good things about myself that no one had ever said before, and he was patient. He didn't fall for my cons and he didn't push. He said we had lots of time and we could go at a pace that was comfortable for me. I had a lot of unburdening to do and I had a lot of sorrow inside. Gary listened, he was supportive, and I think more than anything, he genuinely liked me. Rapists are treated like scum in the "joint" and to have someone like Gary helping me, made me feel loved. I'd never felt that way before unless it was early in my life when I thought of my child molesting as a form of love. Rapists tell themselves lies all the time and Gary just seemed to expect the truth. In time, so did I.

Have I changed? Yes, I think I have. Will I ever be able to make up for the pain I've caused or help those poor women and children I molested? I'm sure I won't be but I try everyday to do something good. It'll never be enough but, like Gary said, you can only try and you're only human. He said that a lot.

SUMMARY

This chapter discusses the effective approaches for work with men who are physically and sexually abusive. Although we are at a very early point in our development of effective treatment approaches for male perpetrators, the promise of even some men discontinuing abusive behavior is reason for optimism.

Treating Male Sexual Harassment and Workplace Violence

Many men believe that sexual harassment and workplace violence are always about men and that women who misbehave are generally not punished. Although we know that men often act badly in the workplace and that women suffer from their bad behavior, one of the problems with treating men sent for help is that they are often in denial about their behavior. This chapter provides examples of men accused of sexual harassment and workplace violence and offers suggestions on how best to work with them.

HOW MEN VIEW SEXUAL HARASSMENT

Men often believe that what they've said or done is harmless and that women are overreacting when they accuse them of sexual harassment. The immediate problem this raises for the clinician is that one may see men clinically who either deny that sexual harassment took place or who see the harassment as not substantially different from the behavior of women toward men.

Leo (1994) believes that highly negative statements about men, although hurtful and offensive to men and often having a small following, "are being voraciously employed by university administrations and corporate offices that fear being called sexist" (p. 24). These policies often place men in difficult and sometimes indefensible positions. In my own experience, a university at which I formerly taught, California State University, San Bernardino, had an undergraduate foundation course on gender. Perhaps they still do. The course was really about women, not gender, and there was a great deal of male bashing by the female faculty members who taught the course. Although there were numerous complaints to administration about the course from students and male faculty members, nothing was ever done and the course was known around campus as "Male Bashing 101." I'm certain that a similar course taught by men that bashed women would have led to major grievances and that the male faculty would have been severely reprimanded and punished. I also know of several occasions when male students were asked to leave class by female faculty members for making, in their judgment, anti-female statements. What would happen to a male faculty member who did the same thing to women who bashed men? I can promise you, unquestionably, that the male faculty member would have been disciplined. In fact, the union representing faculty in the huge California State University system has made a point of not representing union members accused of sexual harassment, assuming, one supposes, that an accusation inherently indicates guilt.

As an example of the way men believe they are treated in the workplace, a colleague in social work told me the following story about the way he was treated when he applied for a position at Boise State University:

> You always hear that universities are so fair when it comes to sexual harassment polices, but schools I know of continually deny men even a modicum of respect and often treat men as 3rd class citizens. Let me give you an example.
>
> I was teaching part-time at Boise State University and I was encouraged by several faculty members to apply for a vacant full-time position in the department of social work. I had a very positive telephone interview with 2 members of the social work search committee and was told that I would be contacted by the search committee to set up a personal interview on campus.
>
> After almost a month of not hearing from the committee, the search committee chair called me late one Sunday evening to tell me that although I'd been recommended by the department, the dean of the college had

turned me down for an interview. The reasons he gave were a supposed incident on the elevator with his secretary and phone calls he'd made indicating that I was not a team player, but was instead, a trouble maker.

Needless to say, I was deeply offended by what the dean said. I have no memory of anything happening on an elevator and no one on the search committee was able to tell me precisely what happened since the dean refused to share this information. I'm very cautious when I'm on elevators and, like most people; I tend to look at the floor indicator. I don't even know his secretary. One of the social work faculty members told me that he asked the dean's secretary if she'd ever had a problem with me and she said she never had. If his secretary felt that I acted inappropriately, why wasn't something said so that I could have discussed it and resolved any difficulties? I mean an incident on the elevator? That sounds either sexual or violent. Regarding the phone calls he made, I wonder who he talked to, what he asked, and what answers he received. And if I was such a troublemaker, why did the dean approve me to teach 3 courses the next semester, two of which were new courses I developed for the social work program?

Would any of this been said about a woman? Never. The implication of sexual misconduct or violence always involves men. And you really have no defense. You're automatically assumed to be guilty by reason of gender bias. After racking my brains trying to remember if anything happened on an elevator, I remembered that I was waiting for the elevator door to close months before when a woman stopped the door from closing. She said it would only be a few minutes. After waiting 2 or 3 minutes, I took another elevator. That was the incident. That's what made all my colleagues at BSU think I was some sort of monster. People I'd been friendly with actually stopped talking to me because of what the dean said.

The Amount of Sexual Harassment

Katz (2003) reports that studies of sexual harassment indicate that between 40% and 70% of women and 10% and 20% of men have experienced sexual harassment in the workplace. Almost 15,000 sexual harassment cases were brought to the attention of the Equal Employment Opportunity Commission (EEOC) last year indicating a tripling of complaints filed by men and representing fifteen percent of all claims filed against female supervisors. A telephone poll conducted by

Louis Harris and Associates on 782 workers revealed that 31% of the female workers claimed to have been harassed at work whereas 7% of the male workers said they'd been harassed at work. Sixty-two percent of the victims took no action. One hundred percent of the women polled claimed the harasser was a man, whereas 59% of men claimed the harasser was a woman, and 41% of the men said the harasser was another man. Of the women who had been harassed, 43% were harassed by a supervisor, 27% were harassed by an employee senior to them, 19% were harassed by a coworker at their same work level, and 8% were harassed by a junior employee.

REASONS FOR SEXUAL HARASSMENT

Kim and Fiske (1999) suggest that whatever form it takes, sexual harassment is always about male dominance and superiority. MacKinnon (1979) says that the frequently inferior position of women in the workplace is a cause and sometimes a consequence of sexual harassment. According to Grauerholz (1989), men in inferior social and economic roles often harass women, another consequence of male dominance. Tangri, Burt, and Johnson (1982) write that the

> ... function of sexual harassment is to manage ongoing male–female interactions according to accepted sex status norms, and to maintain male dominance occupationally and therefore economically, by intimidating, discouraging, or precipitating removal of women from work. (p. 40)

To reinforce this view of sexual harassment, Burgess and Borgida (1997) report that women view unwanted sexual attention as more harassing, threatening, inappropriate, and uncomfortable than do men, raising the unpleasant question about comfort rather than accuracy of the perception of harassment (Cochran, Frazier, & Olson, 1997; Fitzgerald & Ormerod, 1991; McKinney, 1990).

Matchen and DeSouza (2000) studied perceptions of sexual harassment in a university setting and found that "professors may be victims of sexual harassment from students and that male professors, with the exception of unwanted sexual attention, appear to experience sexual harassment from students at about the same rate as females" (p. 27). The authors suggest that future studies should look at men harassed by women and other men but who do nothing about it (Waldo, Berdahl, & Fitzgerald, 1998). Matchen and DeSouza also suggest that "it might be advisable to include clear policies discouraging any sexual (romantic) relationships between faculty and students and letting faculty members know that they can complain if a student is harassing them on the basis of their gender" (p. 28).

One of the difficulties in clinical work with men accused of sexual harassment is that the term itself has become quite unclear. Although the courts have a thirty-year history of trying to define the legal definitions of sexual harassment in organizational settings, whether the actual behavior meets the legal definition of sexual harassment is highly subjective (Gutek, 1995). This gives rise to concerns that local customs define sexual harassment and that a man in one situation may have wider or lesser latitude than a man in another situation. Obviously, the definition of sexual harassment should be clearly stated and enforced in all work and academic settings alike. Although physical harassment and unwanted attention are usually defined in similar ways, men are often concerned that women who use behaviors that would be clearly harassing were they done by a man, are seldom if ever accused of sexual harassment, and that organizations give women far more latitude to harass than is given to men.

SEVERAL EXAMPLES OF MEN ACCUSED OF SEXUAL HARASSMENT

Organizations are responsible for having thoughtful sexual harassment policies and procedures to investigate sexual harassment complaints. They are also responsible for having mandatory training for all employees which clearly explains the policies and procedures for investigating complaints. Most training programs give examples of what many people would clearly identify as sexual harassment: quid pro quo for sexual favors, unwanted attention, direct unwanted physical contact, and repeated efforts to ask people out on dates when they've repeatedly said no. In some organizations, there are clear policies which state that supervisors and subordinates or faculty members and students can't date. In other organizations, pictures, jokes, and making personal statements about how someone looks or smells might also be considered sexual harassment because the implication might be that the person making the remark is doing it to gain sexual favors. The result is that even with training and policies, many people feel very uncomfortable with anything other than business contact with one another. But the lines get blunted, as the following two cases demonstrate.

CASE 1

A group of faculty members in a private midwestern university met every Friday afternoon at a local bar for what they called "choir practice." Although the atmosphere was generally jovial, one of the men with a drinking problem became sexually offensive. His department chair was present during these times but said or did nothing to modify or eliminate behavior the women who were present found offensive. One of the women complained to the department chair who said nothing to the offending male faculty member. Although the meetings were not mandatory and were held off campus, one of the junior-level female faculty members complained to the university provost who investigated. The university was in the midst of developing its sexual harassment policies but hadn't gotten very far. The woman who complained said that although the meetings were informal and she didn't have to attend, as a junior member of the department, she worried that if she didn't attend she would be denied tenure because she wouldn't be seen as "one of the guys." The men countered that what they did off campus was private and that the woman not only wasn't required to attend but that she was doing so poorly in her work that she would have been denied tenure and was using the accusation as a self-serving way to get tenure she didn't deserve.

The provost granted the junior faculty member tenure rather than face an embarrassing public accusation, removed the chair from his position, and placed the offending faculty member on three years probation with mandatory counseling that he attended, but was too unmotivated to actually change his behavior. "Why should I?" he said. "She used the incident to get tenure and to ruin 2 lives. Why should I go for therapy when what she did was a lot worse than what I did?"

DISCUSSION

Was the male faculty member wrong in this case? Clearly he was. His department chair should have spoken to him immediately when his behavior became offensive. Waiting for someone to complain suggests that he wasn't really on top of the situation. In fact, at the first sign of unwanted sexual behavior, the group should have disbanded with apologies to everyone present. The department chair should also have gone to his superior and discussed the problem. Although the situation developed off campus, the meetings were quasi-department meetings and the misbehavior of the faculty member was no more acceptable there than had it taken place at a meeting on campus. Bribing the female faculty member with early tenure she may not have deserved gave a clear message to everyone on campus that accusations of sexual harassment could be used for purposes of self-promotion. However, both the offending faculty member and his chair were incorrect in their behavior and would have been punished in most organizations. Bad feelings will persist in the department that a thoughtful policy and adequate training would have made unnecessary. Holding informal gatherings in bars that people think they need to attend is a relic of the past and a prescription for conflict.

CASE 2

In another example of an accusation of sexual harassment, Bernstein (1994) documents a University of New Hampshire case where a tenured professor was placed on leave without pay for making several statements considered sexually offensive. The sexual harassment charges against the faculty member, whose name was Silva, began in a technical writing class early in the spring of 1992 when Silva was trying to explain the concept of "focus" to his students:

> "Focus is like sex," he said, trying, he told me later, to capture what he perceived to be the student's flagging attention. "You zero in on your subject. You seek a target. You move from side to side. You close in on your subject. You bracket the subject and center on it. Focus connects experience and language. You and the subject become one.... Several days later, Silva said, "Belly dancing is like Jell-O on a plate with a vibrator under the plate." (Bernstein, 1994, p. 11)

Bernstein (1994) quotes a student in the Silva case who said, "Those women who made complaints have gone on to live their own lives, and they haven't been affected by this at all. But they practically ruined a man's life" (p. 14). A faculty member who was involved in the case said,

> The meaning of the Silva case is not that a bunch of zealots got together and packed the hearing. The meaning of the case is that a perfectly decent group of people, because of climate, or the way they were trained, or something, made this terribly unjust decision. Even the good people can't see clearly anymore. (p. 14)

DISCUSSION

Was Silva wrong? Absolutely. The statements he made were entirely inappropriate and he needed to be told, in no uncertain terms, not to make them anymore. Was the punishment just? Probably not. A more appropriate response might have been some cognitive therapy to help him see connections between what he said, why he said it, the consequences of his conduct, and what might have been a more appropriate way of handling the concerns raised by the students with a clear understanding that continued use of inappropriate sexual imagery would result in a forced leave of absence and mandatory treatment.

CLINICAL WORK WITH MEN WHO SEXUALLY HARASS

Returning to the faculty member who made sexually inappropriate comments at an off-campus gathering of faculty, the clinician who saw him (let's call him Ed) recognized early on that he had a serious drinking problem. This became clear when he came to sessions drunk and when several students complained that he smelled of liquor in the classroom. Another issue the clinician recognized was that he had a long history of verbal abuse in past and current intimate relationships with women. The clinician also realized that Ed was a deeply insecure man who felt that his lack of academic preparation (he didn't have a doctorate and had no publications or research studies in his background) locked him into a junior rank for the remainder of his career. According to his therapist, much of his offensive behavior was an attempt to compensate for feelings of insecurity and jealousy that women in his department were all surpassing him.

The clinician used a cognitive-behavioral approach frequently used with abusive men where irrational thoughts are challenged and in their place, more rational perceptions of situations are encouraged. In addition, Ed was sent, reluctantly, for alcohol counseling and was told to join an AA group in the community. He went faithfully to both, was completely unmotivated to change, and although he stopped his offensive behavior with women and didn't drink while he was working, he was arrested and charged with domestic violence in the battering of his wife. The university had a clause in its contract giving it the right to fire any employee, including tenured faculty, for morally offensive behavior (the university had a religious affiliation). Because domestic violence was a behavior that fell within the definition of morally offensive, Ed was fired. In discussing her work with Ed, the therapist said the following:

> Ed doesn't think he's done anything wrong. He sees women as inferior and thinks he can do whatever he wants to them. He has a long history of

abusive behavior toward women and believes that they have no place in professional settings. I tried to find out about abuse in his childhood and I'm reasonably certain that his mother abused him, but he never admitted it. In our sessions, he was charming, witty, insightful, and completely phony. He repeatedly said that he was making great strides in understanding women and in controlling offensive behavior. In reality, he was playing mind games with me. It was very tedious and when the university asked me to summarize my work with him, I had to tell them that after 6 months, I saw absolutely no progress. His behavior at work had changed so the university could do little to force him to be more involved in his treatment. He was told to continue on in treatment and to try harder, but after a year of no progress, he abused his wife and was fired from his job.

He talked to me after his arrest and told me he was fighting the charge and his dismissal. Apparently, he and his wife had been fighting and he claims he was just protecting himself when he struck her. When I saw him last, the charges had been dropped and the university had to reinstate him. Most people would have tried to do something about their behavior after what he'd been through, but Ed thinks sexual harassment is a joke and that given the opportunity to do it and get away with it, he'll continue. I saw him in town with a very young woman whom I assume is a student. They were in a restaurant holding hands. I think Ed will keep the harassment up and that he's too clever to have anything serious happen to him. It's awfully discouraging.

In another case where sexual harassment proceedings were brought against a man for continually asking a female worker out on a date when she had repeatedly told him she wouldn't go out with him and not to ask anymore, the man was transferred to a different department and was told that if he was accused of another incident of harassment, he would be fired. He was also told to go for counseling as a condition of his continued employment. The client readily accepted these conditions.

The worker who saw him used a cognitive-educational approach in his treatment. She went over the sexual harassment policies of the workplace to fully explain each policy to him and to see if he understood them. She asked if he understood the female worker's growing discomfort with his repeated attempts to go out on a date with her and showed him videotapes of other women workers who had gone through similar experiences. Many of the women felt frightened and described the conduct by men as similar to being stalked. This approach was used as a type of empathy training with the client. The worker then asked the client to describe his behavior, explain his motivation, and share his thinking when he asked his coworker out, although she'd repeatedly said no. He said the following:

> I didn't get it. I don't know much about women and I haven't dated much. When she said no, she was always so nice about it and I thought she was being a little encouraging. She'd always have excuses why she couldn't go out but I had the feeling that once those reasons went away, that she'd go out with me. I don't remember her saying no and being forceful about it. When I was called in by my supervisor with the complaint she'd made against me, I was flabbergasted. I'm not denying her perception, but it sure wasn't mine.

When reminded that he'd asked her out over 30 times, the client scratched his head and said, "Really? That much?" The worker showed him a log the woman had kept with dates, times, and statements made by both parties. The client was appalled. "I just had no idea I was being so persistent, none at all."

As the treatment continued, the worker found three other examples of the client repeatedly asking women out although they'd given him no encouragement, or had said no in very clear terms. All three women started hanging up on him when he called for dates and one woman called the police, who investigated, told him to stop, and let the complaint go with a warning. Why was he doing this, the worker wondered? After discussing his behavior several times, the client told her, "I don't get it with women. They give me the come on and then when I ask them out, they keep encouraging me. Once I'm hooked, they don't want anything to do with me." The worker then focused, through role plays and by testing his ability to correctly understand cues women were giving him, his ability to accurately gauge the interest women had in him. What she found was that he actually could not differentiate positive messages that were encouraging from negative messages that were discouraging. The worker helped him increase his differentiating abilities. She also explained that many women have been socialized not to hurt the feelings of men who ask them out. Sometimes, as a result of not wanting to hurt a man's feelings, they use certain excuses that most of us understand mean that a woman really isn't interested. Gradually, he was able to see how his misperception of the situation led to his problem on the job and through homework assignments and involvement in a treatment group, he was able to successfully learn more socially appropriate behavior. He has had no problems on the job since counseling and is now dating successfully, but continues on in therapy and told me,

> I guess most people think that what I did was harassment. I didn't see it that way. I thought she was a sweet person and if she wanted to go out with me, she'd be shy at first, but encouraging. That's how I read her behavior. It makes me a little angry that she wasn't more truthful since I would have taken "no" for an answer, but she never said no. I guess asking her out 30 times was pretty sick of me but I had this idea that she really liked me and that she really wanted to go out but that she was just breaking things off with her ex-boyfriend. Sooner or later, I thought, she'd say, yes. I was certainly wrong and I've learned to be very careful about the way I interpret the things women say and to check them out by asking clear questions about their intentions. I also think that I must be a little dense not to have known that before. My grandmother raised me and I didn't start dating until my twenties. The things I should have learned along the way, I never did. It's an excuse because I should have known better. In fact I *did* know better because at my job they showed a video of a guy doing exactly what I was doing to Glenda. I was raised by a grandmother who never answered any questions. You had to keep asking and asking. But like someone said in group, "You're not talking to your grandmother anymore, you're talking to adult women." I guess that's true and I've had to make a lot of adjustment in the way I behave around women. I hope I'm doing better.

ACCUSATIONS OF CO-WORKER VIOLENCE AGAINST MEN

Although the number of workplace homicides by co-workers is relatively small, workplace violence between co-workers also includes a great number of fights, assaults, threats, sexual attacks, and other dangerous behaviors. As an example of the impact of co-worker violence on other workers, 500 managers were surveyed at an American Management Resources Conference (65th Annual American Management on-site survey, 1994). The managers reported that 43% of the workers they supervised experienced reduced morale as a result of workplace violence in the prior four years, whereas 39% experienced lowered productivity. There was an 8% increase in workers filing disability claims citing workplace violence as a contributor to stress and emotional difficulty, whereas companies with workplace violence experienced a 10% increase in litigation against those companies for not containing workplace violence. Clearly, workplace violence has a negative impact on organizational life and on workers who experience the end result of violence.

Men are often accused of behavior that is intimidating and which, if unchecked, may lead to violence. Many of the perpetrators of workplace violence are disgruntled employees who were terminated or downsized. Twenty-five percent of the perpetrators of workplace homicide commit suicide after the violent act. Some of the similarities in the employees who have committed acts of violence at work as reported by Robinson (1996) from Federal Bureau of Investigation and U.S. Department of Labor data, include the following: (a) a history of violence; (b) fascination with the military or being a survivalist; (c) White men; (d) over the age of 35 years; (e) a loner or an extremist; (f) someone who carries a grudge; (g) someone who has difficulty accepting authority or reality; (h) a history of violence toward women; and (i) may have substance abuse problems or mental health problems.

The following indicators of potential for workplace violence by co-workers have been identified by the Federal Bureau of Investigation's National Center for the Analysis of Violent Crime, Profiling and Behavioral Assessment Unit, in its analysis of past incidents of workplace violence (Bureau of Justice Statistics, 1998, p. 4):

a) Direct or veiled threats of harm to others in the workplace;

b) intimidating, belligerent, harassing, bullying, or other inappropriate and aggressive behavior;

c) numerous conflicts with supervisors and other employees;

d) bringing a weapon to the workplace, brandishing a weapon in the workplace, making inappropriate references to guns, or fascination with weapons;

e) statements showing fascination with incidents of workplace violence, statements indicating approval of the use of violence to resolve a problem, or statements indicating identification with perpetrators of workplace homicides;

f) statements indicating desperation (over family, financial, and other personal problems) to the point of contemplating suicide;

g) drug and or alcohol abuse;

h) very erratic behavior with serious mood swings.

Each of these behaviors is a clear sign that something is wrong and none should be ignored. Some behaviors require immediate police or security involvement whereas others constitute misconduct and require disciplinary action or an immediate referral to an employee assistance program. It is not advisable to rely on "profiles" or "early warning signs" to predict violent behavior. "Profiles" often suggest that people with certain characteristics, such as "loners" and "men in their 40s," are potentially violent. Stereotyping of this kind will not help predict violence and may lead to unfair and destructive treatment of employees. The same must be said of the use of "early warning signs," such as assuming that anyone in therapy or those experiencing marital difficulties may be at risk of workplace violence. Most of us experience emotional turmoil but very few of us become violent.

Co-worker violence may also be suggested by the following indicators of potential for workplace violence:

1) the expression of irrational beliefs and ideas;

2) high levels of stress outside of work because of marital, personal or financial difficulties;

3) an unusual fascination with weapons; angry and unwarranted outbursts; an inability or unwillingness to take criticism; and

4) disregard for the safety of others.

Jossi (1999) believes that it is unlikely for most people to exhibit all these risk factors and suggests that an astute manager should be able to identify workers who "give off" at least several of these behaviors and determine when it's time for professional intervention. When employee assistance programs (EAPs) were used to deal with early signs of workplace violence in the U.S. Postal Service, Jossi reports that although assault rates dropped from 757 in 1994 to 538 in 1997, the EAP caseloads in the Postal Service went from 24,299 in 1994 to 33,800 in 1997. Professional intervention with early signs of workplace violence decreases threats of violence, leads to a reduction in actual violence, and motivates workers with personal problems to seek help. At a yearly cost of $30 per worker and a 98% approval rate, the approach used by the Postal Service has considerable potential for other organizations experiencing workplace violence.

Workplace threats need to be taken seriously. Organizations should have written policies outlining the procedures for reporting all threats of violence. Those procedures should also describe the actions that will be taken in cases of workplace violence. Threatened employees have a right to know what an organization will do to protect them and what measures they need to take to protect themselves. Because it is impossible to know whether a threat is going to be carried out, the organization should always treat threats in a serious manner and act as if the person may carry out the threat.

Glicken and Ino (1997, p. 6) describe the progression in the development of violent co-worker behavior as follows.

Level 1: A preoccupation by the worker that he has been mistreated. A tendency by the worker to blame others for his lack of success on the job and to obsessively complain about how badly he has been treated by someone specific or by others in the workplace. At this stage, the problem should be evaluated and an attempt should be made to try and resolve the worker's concerns with supervisors, other workers, or personnel departments. A worker's concerns, if voiced irrationally or if illogical, are particularly problematic and need to be dealt with in a proactive way by encouraging counseling or by trying to help the worker develop a more accurate perception of the problem. Employee assistance programs or mediators can help at this early point in the worker's preoccupation with his maltreatment on the job. If the worker is unwilling to become involved in counseling, mediation, or some other form of dispute resolution, the worker needs to be clearly told about the organization's "no-tolerance for violence" rules. There must also be an agreement from the worker to accept a "no-violence" contract so that any future concerns will be dealt with in a violence-free atmosphere. It may also be wise to provide the worker with an advocate or an ombudsman to help in future disputes. The advocate represents the interests of the worker in any dealings with the organization and is recognized as the worker's ally.

Level 2: Obsessive thoughts begin to develop with a plan to pay others back for the way the worker believes he has been treated. The plan may be vague and non-specific, or it may be elaborate. The plan is often shared with others on the job who may incorrectly think that the person is just venting anger and don't take the plan seriously. This is a serious mistake often made by organizations since it is at this point in time that workers begin to obsess about revenge and when the plan they've devised becomes more firmly fixed in their minds. The reason for the progression to level two is that the organization has not handled the worker's earlier concerns described in level one. The way the worker is dealt with initially can have significant meaning for the progression, or the lack of progression of violent impulses. All threats, plans, indications of payback, obsessive thoughts and preoccupations with unfairness should be seen as problematic by the organization, and every attempt should be made to deal with the problem through the use of an EAP, mediation, or some conciliatory process to logically resolve the problem. If the worker is being laid off, it should be done with notice, with respect, and with some semblance of concern for the worker's long-term well being. Stories of the way organizations lay people off, in cruel, insensitive and often rude and disrespectful ways, suggest reasons for the development of anger in workers and dramatically increase the risk of violence.

Level 3: The plan is now articulated to those in the workplace who need to respond. Generally, pre-violent workers will confide their plan or make specific threats to supervisors they trust or find sympathetic. At this stage, if threats are not taken seriously and if nothing is done to deal with them, the anger grows and workers become victims of their own inability to control emotions that are now clearly out of control. Most perpetrators of workplace violence have discussed their plan, to the extent that it is now clear, with others in a position of authority. Some managers act on the information, but all too many others ignore it thinking it best not to make problems for the worker, or they worry that any report of the plan might end in a court action by the worker. For whatever reason, most workplace assaults and homicides have been articulated clearly by perpetrators and it often doesn't come as a surprise when perpetrators actually end up killing or badly assaulting someone. When one hears about a workplace killing, it is almost always followed by statements from co-workers saying that they didn't take the worker's threatened violence seriously, or that they misjudged the degree of his anger. This is the moment in time to make formal reports to the police or to company security so that action can be taken to protect other workers.

Level 4: Actual threats are made to people on the job. The worker's anger is now increasingly more difficult to control since he has made a decision to confront others as a release for intense feelings of anger at the organization. At this point in time, the worker has clearly lost control. Co-workers begin to complain to superiors who often do nothing to control the behavior or who may terminate the worker without necessary professional help or police involvement. The worker, at level 4, is now ready to commit an act of violence. In almost all cases of workplace violence, supervisors, personnel departments and union stewards were forewarned about problematic employees but did nothing to ensure that help would be given or that the problem would be resolved. When threats are made, it may be necessary to bring in the police and to file charges against a violent employee. While this may end in a trial or in a prison sentence, it may also end in mandatory treatment and the safety of a number of innocent people. Remember that many perpetrators of workplace violence injure innocent bystanders who just happen to be in the vicinity and who may not be part of an organization. They may also kill their own family members, often in despair over what they intend to do at work.

Level 5: The worker commits violent acts on the job. When workers say they are going to kill someone or commit an act of violence to co-workers, take it seriously. Threats are more than words. They are acts about to take place and are often the worker's attempt to have the act stopped. When a threat is made and nothing constructive is done to help the worker, violence is very likely to follow. The violence may be directed at specific people but more often than not, it is random and affects people who have nothing to do with the worker's grievances against the organization.

It shouldn't surprise us that many workers move to level 5 in the development of violence. Far too managers and supervisors worry about lawsuits or union actions if they intervene, and they become immobilized when violent behavior begins to show itself. It should also not surprise us if workers show none of the levels noted above and act out without seeming provocation. These are the anomalies of the workplace and the individual workers within the workplace. By and large, however, workers give advanced notice of potentially dangerous behavior. When that behavior is poorly dealt with by organizations, violence is likely to result. In the next section, we will see how intervening in all work-related problems is a much more effective way of dealing with unhappiness on the job than avoidance.

INTERVENTIONS IN WORKPLACE PROBLEMS INVOLVING CO-WORKERS

When problems in the workplace begin to surface, managers should meet with the worker and find out what is bothering him. If the problem is beyond their ability to resolve, professional help should be sought. Many problems, however, can be dealt with by the organization. Work assignments can be varied to prevent burnout. Promotional and salary decisions can be made equitably to ensure that all workers feel treated with dignity and respect. References of workers can be checked carefully with the added protection of having potential workers undergo careful screening and evaluation before they are hired to identify those applicants with obvious emotional problems or histories of violent behavior on other jobs. Disputes between workers can be mediated informally before they become serious problems. When workers feel diminished and no longer believe that the organization cares about them, the potential for workplace problems grows in severity.

When companies are responsive to their workers, many of the problems that lead to workplace violence can be resolved. In these companies, EAPs are used to offer workers an alternative way of resolving problems that may be difficult to resolve by managers and supervisors. Companies using EAPs offer a variety of alternatives to workers. Some EAPs are located in the organization and are readily available. In these organizations, managers, workers, and treatment personnel work closely together to resolve the problem. In other organizations, the worker might go to a social agency or counseling center with which the organization has contracted. The services provided may be time-limited and supportive, or they may be longer-term and designed to meet the individual needs of the client (Glicken, 1988, 1996).

Often workplace problems have their origins in the personal lives of workers. Resolving personal problems is important, but keeping the worker employed supersedes the resolution of a personal problem. Organizations often correctly complain that workers do not improve on the job after treatment is provided. This complaint is valid but organizations also need to be made aware of how long it may take for the worker to improve. Problems such as addictions are slow to respond to treatment and may take months to improve, with the added possibility of a need for residential treatment. Just as employers give workers time to heal after an illness or surgery, employers need to give workers time to heal when they have emotional problems (Glicken, 1988, 1996).

Helping professionals can also function in other roles to identify and prevent workplace violence. The following roles are noted in the literature as those most likely to help angry and potentially dangerous workers:

1. *Ombudsmen*—Ombudsmen are employed by an organization and use a variety of strategies to resolve workplace disputes, including counseling, mediation, conciliation, and fact-finding. An ombudsman may interview all the parties involved in a dispute, review the history of the problem and the organization's personnel policies to see if they've been correctly applied, and might offer suggestions and alternative ways of resolving the dispute to the workers involved in a disagreement. An ombudsman doesn't "impose" solutions but may offer alternative strategies to resolve it. Workers involved in a dispute may refuse options offered by the ombudsman and are free to pursue other remedies or strategies, including legal ones.

2. *Facilitation*—The facilitator focuses on resolving the dispute and is most helpful when the level of emotions about the issues is fairly low. Facilitation is most effective when the people involved trust one another and are more likely to develop acceptable solutions.

3. *Mediation*—Mediation uses a third party who is not a member of the organization and is free of bias in the situation. The mediator can only recommend, although some organizations accept binding mediation as a way of resolving disputes with the mediator placed in the role of decision maker. Mediation may be helpful when those parties involved in a dispute have reached an "impasse" and the situation is potentially dangerous. A mediator may offer advice, suggestions, and options to help resolve the problem. The authority the mediator brings to the dispute is neutrality and expertise. Hopefully, those involved in the dispute will accept suggestions made by someone in this capacity. Care must be taken to bring someone in with a very fair and unbiased track record in mediating disputes.

4. *Interest-Based Problem Solving*—Interest-based problem solving attempts to improve the working relationship between the parties in dispute. Techniques used in interest-based problem solving include brainstorming, creative alternative solutions to a problem, and agreed-on rules to reach a solution.

5. *Peer Review*—Peer review involves the evaluation and possible solution of a problem recommended by fellow employees. Because these suggestions come from peers, they may have more impact on the involved parties. However, peer reviews are fraught with concerns about objectivity, composition of the review panel, dual loyalties, and conflicts of interest, and are usually only helpful if done with the complete confidence of all parties involved. Review panels in sexual harassment cases might be a good model to explain this approach. Sexual harassment review panels have a mediocre to poor record of objectivity and recommendations to upper management are often rejected because of due process issues and concerns regarding objectivity. On the other hand, courts have been reluctant to overturn decisions made by organizations when review panels are used in sexual harassment investigations.

6. *Employee Training*—All employees should understand the correct way to report potentially or actively violent and disruptive behavior ob-

served in other workers. Robinson (1996, p. 6) suggests that the following topics be included in all workplace violence prevention training:

    a) Discussion of the organization's workplace violence policy;

    b) a willingness of employees to report incidents;

    c) suggested approaches to preventing or coping with potentially violent and hostile behavior;

    d) conflict resolution training;

    e) training in managing stress and anger;

    f) Understanding the various programs offered by organizations including employee assistance programs, the ombudsman, and mediation.

    7. *Supervisory Training*—Special attention should also be paid to effective training of supervisors so that they know how to identify, evaluate, and resolve workplace problems that may lead to violence. This includes the use of personnel policies to provide accurate evaluations of performance and reports that correctly identify the worker's behavior with just and organizationally correct disciplinary actions provided. Skills necessary to prevent workplace violence by managers may include the ability to screen applicants for potential for violence, crisis management and conflict resolution skills, and encouragement of other workers supervised by the managers to share incidents of observed violence or potential violence in co-workers.

    8. *Preemployment Screening*—Before a worker is officially offered a position, the personnel department should be contacted to find out what preemployment screening techniques (such as interview questions, background and reference checks, and drug testing) are permitted by federal and state laws and regulations for the position.

CASE EXAMPLE: WORKPLACE VIOLENCE

This case first appeared in a volume on the role of helping professionals in treating the victims and perpetrators of violence (Glicken & Sechrest, 2003).

Jim Kennedy is a 45-year-old engineer working in the aerospace industry in Southern California. For the past two years, Jim and his supervisor have had a running battle over the quality of

Jim's work. Jim thinks that his work is fine, as do his colleagues, but the supervisor believes that Jim doesn't follow directions and that his work wanders off into areas that aren't related to his assignments. On several occasions, they've almost come to blows.

Jim was referred to the company's EAP and was told by his supervisor that he either enter counseling or he'd be fired. Jim has a wife who doesn't work and two children in college. His salary barely covers his expenses and many months, he lives on credit cards and loans. Quitting isn't a realistic option because a weak business market in the aerospace industry limits his work opportunities. The opportunities to transfer to a different department at work are also limited because what Jim does is highly specialized. At 45, he doesn't want to ruin a very good pension plan. He feels stuck and resents going for counseling. He believes that his problems at work are the supervisor's fault and thinks the supervisor should be in treatment, not him. He is becoming surly and difficult at work. On several occasions, he's written derogatory remarks about the supervisor in the men's rest room or on the company elevator. Although no one can prove that Jim is guilty, everyone knows that he is to blame.

In the past six months, Jim has begun to deteriorate physically and emotionally. He often comes to work looking haggard and unkempt. People have begun to find his body odor offensive and wonder if he bathes. His EAP counselor suspects that Jim is drinking heavily and has ordered a random alcohol test.

Jim has made several indirect threats against his supervisor that co-workers have heard but have not reported. They believe that Jim has a grievance and they feel obligated to protect him. Jim's co-workers feel that Jim is going through a midlife crisis but on closer examination, Jim is deteriorating badly. His thoughts, which he confides to his wife and family, have increasingly become violent. He purchased a gun and shoots it in the basement of his home and outside in the desert. The feel of the gun and the sound of the bullets give him a sense of power that he finds intoxicating. He has also begun to drink heavily and has a driving while intoxicated (DWI) charge that resulted in the removal of his license and the impounding of his car. He drives anyway, using a second car he purchased in his wife's name.

He feels invincible and doesn't think anything will happen to him. Because of his sophistication with the Internet, he has begun sending e-mail messages to everyone at work which imply violence to certain people in upper management. He never mentions the name of the supervisor he hates so much and his e-mails are untraceable. In a company with thousands of people, it's difficult to pinpoint who has made the threats or how seriously they should be taken, but the messages unnerve everyone at work and there is a sense of foreboding in the company that something awful will happen.

Jim's EAP counselor believes that Jim's deteriorating condition is reason to worry about potential violence and has warned the company that Jim may be at risk. The company fears a lawsuit if it fires Jim. The company believes that he will do something serious enough, but not dangerous enough to fire him. The EAP counselor disagrees. He sees concrete signs of potential for serious workplace violence. Those signs include a highly intelligent man who is emotionally deteriorating and who also demonstrates increasing paranoia and an obsession for getting revenge. The drinking and fondness for guns add to the counselor's sense of potential violence. If the counselor knew of the verbal threats Jim has shared with his co-workers and the fact that Jim is the one making e-mail threats, the counselor would be absolutely certain that Jim's volatile behavior would end in a violent act.

Jim has always been eccentric. His aloofness from people, his disdain for others he considers to have lesser ability, and his angry feelings at management for not recognizing his abilities, all suggest his potential for workplace violence. As an unsupportive supervisor thwarts his ambitions and as he suffers the indignity of having to go for counseling, Jim has begun to have fantasies of violence. They include going into the management side of the company and randomly killing every manager in sight, starting with his own supervisor. The fantasy is so clear and appealing to him that it has almost taken on sensuous overtones. It is likely that although Jim seems troubled, but functional, that he is having moments of irrationality and severe emotional dysfunction that make him highly dangerous.

The EAP counselor is concerned about Jim's potential for danger and has asked Jim to take a leave of absence. He has also warned the company. Unfortunately, he cannot pinpoint a specific threat or act to concretely suggest that Jim will be violent at work. Although Jim seems to be going through a rough stretch, his co-workers aren't seeing the dangerous side of his behavior and believe that, like all eccentric people, Jim has a side to him that is different from the rest of the engineers with which he works. That side, aloof, uncomfortable with people, egocentric, also makes him a good engineer, probably the best engineer in the group. For these reasons, his co-workers haven't accurately evaluated his level of increasing danger.

A day after a particularly degrading and offensive meeting with his supervisor where Jim was placed on administrative leave without pay because of the deterioration in his work, Jim took his guns to work and shot and killed three managers, including his supervisor. He wounded four others, including several people who were just there to deliver packages. The security guards assigned to the company shot and killed Jim in a struggle, and the company is left to sort out the reasons it took so long to take remedial action and to correctly determine his level of violence. Everyone interviewed believed that Jim was going through a patchy time and that he would eventually snap out of it. No one felt that he was excessively dangerous or that he had potential for violence other than the EAP counselor whose warning to the company went unheeded.

DISCUSSION

I asked the EAP counselor about the incident. He told me the following:

I wrote 5 memos to the company outlining my concerns about Jim's potential for violence. He took 3 tests showing elevated signs of alcohol usage. I urged Jim to seek inpatient help to protect himself and others from his growing anger. I spoke to company security. Everyone thought I was over-reacting and that what I was predicting was a joke. Highly educated people like Jim don't kill others, they'd say. And so it went for many months. Jim was absolutely unmotivated for help and resented seeing me. When he *did* share his angry feelings with me, he'd immediately take back whatever he said and tell me he was "funning me" to make me feel that I was helping. It was a big joke and unfortunately, the joke ended with lost lives and a workplace where every one of the engineers in Jim's group has either left the firm or gone to other departments. No one feels safe on the job and from what I hear, the company has lost some major contracts and is in bad financial shape. It was one of the most frustrating professional experiences I've ever had.

I'm happy to know that it helped other companies take threats of violence much more seriously. As a result of what happened with Jim, most companies we work with have instituted "no violence" policies and use EAP workers to help mediate grievances. It's had a very calming effect on the workplace in my community. Not a single person we've seen in the last year for potential for workplace violence has lost his job or had his anger at a company develop into violent behavior. Counseling is only as successful as the workplace takes violent behavior seriously. And believe me, after what Jim did, it's a serious issue.

SUMMARY

This chapter discusses treatment approaches with men accused of sexual harassment and workplace violence. Men often believe that they are unfairly accused of both behaviors and may be very resistant to treatment, believing that women get away with the same behaviors and that the playing fields in certain educational and corporate organizations are unfair.

PART IV

Clinical Work With Men of Color:
Special Concerns

Clinical Work With African American Men

African American men continue to feel the impact of racism, violence, and poverty. Data for Black men continue to show high rates of involvement with crime. Slater (2003) reports almost 900,000 Black men in prison as compared to 600,000 Black men in college. By 1995, DiIulio (2001) said that the death rate by violence for Black men living in urban areas was ten times the national average. Inner-city Blacks experience much higher rates of rape, robbery, burglary, and aggravated assault than do Whites. By 2001, half of the homicide victims in America were Black and a third of the perpetrators of homicide were also Black (FBI Uniform Crime Report, 2001, 2002). Robert Froehlke said, of the disproportionate number of Black victims of homicide, "If this were a disease and that disease had increased 40% in four years ... there would be a substantial public health effort to eradicate it" (Christian, 1990, p. A.3).

Harris (1990) said that for men of color, the stress of living in unsafe, often violent, unhealthy, economically insecure environments with high rates of unemployment and minimal future opportunities, "create(s) a situation where these men have higher death rates, higher rates of major fatal diseases, and higher levels of institutionalization than any other sector of the population" (p. 228).

Black men have lower levels of education than White men and although the data are improving, more Black men fail to finish high school than White men. Commenting on his level of educational preparation, the professional fighter, Mike Tyson (Hamill, 1996) said,

I never learned percentages and decimals before. It's a small thing, maybe, something I should of learned in grammar school. But you come from a scrambled family, you're running between the streets and school, missing days, fucking up, and you end up with these *holes*. One thing never connects to another, and you don't know why. You don't know what you didn't learn. Like percentages. I just never learned it, it was one of the holes. I mean, later on I knew what a percentage was, you know, for a ten million dollar purse, but I didn't know how to do it myself. That was always the job of someone else. One thing now, I can figure out how to leave a tip. There's restaurants out there where I should eat for free for a couple of years. (Hamill, 1996, p. 101)

The availability of jobs to those who don't have a high school diploma is limited and usually falls within the category of low-status service jobs with minimum wages paid. More Black men hold low-status service jobs than White men. Also, White men are more likely to be fully employed. Low-status service positions include front-line cook, security guard, fruit picker, day laborers, or gardeners. These jobs usually do not guarantee 40-hour work weeks, offer no health insurance benefits, and do not have such luxuries as merit raises or cost-of-living increases. Low-status service jobs have more on-the-job safety and health risks than many other types of occupations. As Staples (1986) writes, "The jobs most typically offered to uneducated and young Black males is that of the minimum guard, an occupation that entails protecting the prosperity and person of the affluent whites from other Black males of the underclass" (p. 436).

A great many Black men in America seek help from the state in the form of welfare, but as Marin (1991) argues

It is not surprising that many African American men see welfare as an extension of slavery that destroys families, isolates women and humiliates men according to white bureaucratic whim. Or is it accidental that in poor communities family structure has collapsed and more and more children are born outside marriage at a time when disenfranchised men are flooding the streets? (p. 86)

Although Black men are socialized to internalize the masculine roles of dominance and aggression, as are other men in American society, they are also taught the limitations of their skin (Aboramph, 1989). Considering the lack of work opportunities for Black males, Aboramph (1989) suggests that they are often unable to serve as family providers and are consequently perceived as being weak:

> The security derived from one's employment has a bearing on one's sexual behavior. The extent to which a relationship can be satisfactory depends, in part, on the extent to which one enters the relationship without having to worry about economic support. In other words, a successful relationship depends partly on the extent to which partners are economically self-supporting. (p. 324)

Lawson and Sharpe (2000) indicate that the structure of the Black family has changed dramatically in the past 30 years. Two thirds of all Black marriages end in divorce. Two out of three Black children will experience the dissolution of their parents' marriage by the time they reach age 16. In 1970, 68% of Black families had both the husband and wife present. This number dropped to just 50% in 1990, a decrease of 18 percentage points over 20 years, compared with a 6-percentage-point decrease over the same time period for White families. The impact of divorce on Black men is considerable. In their study of Black men following divorce, Lawson and Sharpe found that 85% of the men reported the following after their divorce: loss of appetite, anxiety or depression, impulsive behavioral problems, irritability and angry outbursts, and an inability to concentrate. The authors also report a 90% depression rate with 20% of the sample experiencing strong thoughts about suicide or actual suicidal attempts. Physical reactions to their divorce included stomachaches, headaches, dental problems, asthma, and problems serious enough to require emergency room treatment. The authors conclude,

> One additional stressor of divorce for black men was the belief that a stable marriage counteracted the cultural stereotypes that black men often abdicate family responsibilities. Indeed, studies have shown that black men confront discrediting stereotypes, institutional racism, and economic marginality, which have a profound effect on their relationships with women. One consequence of divorce for black men is increased psy-

chological and physical distress. The men who fared the worst were those who believed that their ex-wives had had intimate relationships [with other men] before finalization of their divorce. These men felt hurt, humiliated, and rejected, which led, in some cases, to suicide attempts. (Lawson & Sharpe, 2000, p. 24)

TREATMENT ISSUES AND BLACK MEN

Diagnosis

A number of studies have examined the relation between racial bias and psychiatric diagnoses. Adebimpe (1981) found that a high number of Black male patients were misdiagnosed as schizophrenic, a finding, according to Laszloffy and Hardy (2000), supported in subsequent studies that examined White, Black, and Latino patients. According to the authors, although the symptoms were the same, male Black and Latino patients were often diagnosed as schizophrenic whereas White patients were almost always correctly diagnosed with emotional or affective disorders (Garretson, 1993; Solomon, 1992). Laszloffy and Hardy (2000) believe that underlying the misdiagnosis is a "subtle, unintentional racism" (p. 35). In defining racism, the authors write that "all expressions of racism are rooted in an ideology of racial superiority/inferiority that assumes some racial groups are superior to others, and therefore deserve preferential treatment" (p. 35), a definition that makes unintentional or subtle racism difficult to imagine.

Flaherty and Meagher (1980) found that among Black and White male schizophrenic inpatients who had similar global pathology ratings

African American patients spent less time in the hospital, obtained lower privilege levels, were given more p.r.n. medications, and were less likely to receive recreation therapy and occupational therapy. Seclusion and restraints were more likely to be used with black patients. (p. 679)

Although the authors avoid suggesting a direct relation between racial bias and the treatment of minority patients, they conclude that it is an important intervening variable.

In a report on race and mental health, the U.S. Surgeon General (Satcher, 2001) wrote that the cultures of clinicians and the way services are provided influence diagnosis and treatment. Service providers, according to the report, need to be able to build on the cultural strengths of the people they serve. The Surgeon General concluded that, "while not the sole determinants, cultural and social influences do play important roles in mental health, mental illness and service use, when added to biological, psychological and environmental factors" (Satcher, 2001, p. 1). In trying to understand barriers to treatment that affect ethnic and racial minorities, the Surgeon General said that the mental health system often creates impediments, which lead to distrust and fear of treatment, which deter racial and ethnic minorities from seeking and receiving needed services. Importantly, the Surgeon General added the following:

> Mental health care disparities may also stem from minorities' historical and present day struggles with racism and discrimination, which affect their mental health and contribute to their lower economic, social, and political status. (Satcher, 2001, p. 1)

In an earlier report on mental health, the Surgeon General (Satcher, 1999) wrote,

> Mental illness is at least as prevalent among racial and ethnic minorities as in the majority white population. Yet many racial and ethnic minority group members find the organized mental health system to be uninformed about cultural context and, thus, unresponsive and/or irrelevant. With appropriate training and a fundamental respect for clients, any mental health professional can provide culturally competent services that reflect sensitivity to individual differences and, at the same time, assign validity to an individual's group identity. Still, many members of ethnic and racial minority groups may prefer to be treated by mental health professionals of similar background.

Whaley (2001) believes that White clinicians often see Black men as having paranoid symptoms that are more fundamentally a cultural distrust of Whites because of historical experiences with racism. He argues that the diagnostic process with Black men tends to discount the negative impact of racism and leads to diagnostic judgments about clients suggesting that they are more dysfunctional than they really are. This tendency to misdiagnose, or to diagnose a more serious condition than may be warranted, is what Whaley calls "pseudo-transference." Cultural stereotyping by clinicians who fail to understand the impact of racism leads to "more severe diagnoses and restrictive interventions" (p. 558) with Black men. Whaley's work suggests the subjective nature of the diagnostic process in general, and the *DSM–IV* in particular.

Laszloffy and Hardy (2000) believe that as long as racism occupies such a significant role in our everyday lives, it cannot be completely eliminated without carefully examining what we say to clients, what we do with clients, and what we really believe. In validating the need for cultural and racial sensitivity, Pena, Bland, Shervinton, Rice, and Foulks (2000) suggest that:

> In work with African-American patients, the therapist's skill in recognizing when problems do or do not revolve around the condition of being black could have serious implications for the acceptability of treatment, the development of the treatment alliance, and in psychotherapy, the accuracy of interpretations. (p. 14)

The authors report that each of these variables has a significant impact on treatment outcomes, and that therapists with limited awareness of the significance of race in their interactions with clients may experience problems in "listening empathically" and actually understanding client conflicts that are directly related to race.

Forming Therapeutic Relationships

Franklin (1992) acknowledges that Black men have very low participation rates in therapy for reasons that may primarily have to do with notions that therapy indicates weakness and that it is not a traditionally Black or male outlet for resolving problems. Franklin believes that trust is often difficult for Black men to develop because relationships with wives and girlfriends are frequently based on the woman's perception of the man as a provider. When that perception is affected by unemployment or underemployment, Black men often view their spouses as untrustworthy and likely to dismiss them as men of value.

Franklin (1992) believes that although Black men may seem to be intimately involved in treatment, particularly group treatment, where concern and interaction with others is so important, "... doubts and inadequacies of the inner self are tightly guarded secrets. African American men are not likely to share personal vulnerabilities" (p. 351). Franklin goes on to say that:

> Masking true feelings or thoughts and being guarded has unique consequences for both African American men and women. Learning to trust is difficult to achieve in a climate of racism. Seeing a therapist is perceived as an abdication of a man's fundamental right and ability to solve his own problems. (p. 352)

Franklin (1992) believes that all therapy must recognize the invisible factor of racism, which provides messages from childhood that Black men, "... lack value and worth and deny Black males full access to life's amenities and opportunities" (p. 353). Franklin suggests that a Black man's sense of invisibility damages self-esteem because of constant messages that he is unacceptable and of little worth:

> Constant assaults on his self-esteem lead, in turn, to feelings of anger and internalized rage. To cope with these indignities, African American men devise various strategies and behaviors [including] immobilization, chronic indignation, acquiescence, depression, suicide or homicide, and/or internalized rage. (p. 353)

To deal with these complex issues, Franklin (1992) suggests that therapists must go slowly with Black men, allowing them to gradually develop trust. He also suggests that therapists must keep in mind the need to frame black male clients in a positive way by approaching them with respect and positive reinforcement. Insights should be approached gently and should not appear magical or outrageous but should convey "... knowledge, understanding, and empathy, all of which will strengthen the client's sense of trust in the therapist's humanity and competence" (p. 354).

Williams (1992) is concerned about the "sparse" literature on the treatment of Black men and argues that mental health workers must be sensitized to Black culture before working with Black men. He provides the following information for effective work with Black men:

1. *Confronting negative and acknowledging positive behaviors*— Black men must be recognized for their many strengths, and, although distorted or negative behavior needs to be confronted, it must be remembered that the client is doing well in many aspects of his life and that positive behavior must be considered when confronting negative behavior.

2. *The influence of labels*—Williams (1992) believes that Black men want to see themselves as "partners in treatment" and resent labels which suggest pathology. Labels send up signals to Black men who have had to deal with other labels that subtly or overtly suggest racism.

3. *Addressing sexism and racism*—Williams (1992) notes that Black men are particularly sensitive to sexist notions which berate or bash men and that they are likely to increase violence. We must be particularly careful not to generalize male behavior and we must be aware that Black men are very sensitive to racist notions which may include negative attitudes toward Black men.

4. *Cultural congruence*—William (1992) suggests the need to value the Black experience and approach Black men with respect, concern, and an awareness of the many factors that create tensions in the lives of Black men that may not be true of other men.

5. *Working with the Black community*—As important as treatment might be, Williams (1992) believes that it is equally important to work with Black institutions, including the church and the client's extended family. Black institutions are particularly important in the lives of Black men and they can be used effectively to deal with serious family and relationship problems, including domestic violence.

6. *Love and intimacy*—Issues of love and intimacy are very complex in the lives of Black men. Because of poverty and lack of mean-

ingful employment, Bell (1978) believes that many Black men are unable to provide for their families. Although Black women understand the resulting powerlessness of Black men and the social sources of this powerlessness, Bell indicates that the discrepancy between White and Black male status causes "… unconscious resentment that manifests itself in stresses and strains in black male–female relations" (p. 21). Bell (1978) goes on to say that:

> Black men are not allowed to be real men, at least according to the white male definition of manhood. They are frustrated at their inability to provide in the same way that white men support their families.… The continuing powerlessness of black men affects black women, particularly strong black women. A strong woman knows her strength, has developed it over the years, appreciates it, perhaps even revels in it. Her strength makes her intolerant of weakness. Thus, even though she may love a man, her contempt for weakness will come out. And if her man is black in this society, there will be many opportunities for that weakness to be all too obvious—no matter how successful he is and how strong he tries to be. (p. 78)

In a further discussion of male–female problems, Poussaint (1993) writes, "Since the 1970s, Black people have been made aware of the serious strains in Black male–female relationships by Black female writers who examined issues of racism and sexism from their own racial and gender perspective" (p. 86). The author reports that perceptions by Black women of abusive, disrespectful, and demeaning treatment by Black men are countered by Black men who complain that Black women have condescending and superior attitudes toward them and that they feel devalued. Both Black men and women face difficulties in relating to one another because gender issues are compounded by racism, and "the subordinate roles of Blacks in American society. Sadly, Black men and women themselves harbor racial stereotypes about each other" (Poussaint, 1993, p. 89). Poussaint notes that if these tensions aren't dealt with

> This estrangement threatens our very survival. Not only is the Black family damaged but the unity of the Black community is at stake. Every Black

woman and man has a responsibility to do their share in bringing an end to this internecine warfare. The future of our people, and our children's welfare today, is endangered by our stubbornly refusing to compromise. We need to begin to show more love and respect for one another. We are in a state of crisis and the time to act is now! (p. 89)

To resolve these tensions among Black men and women, Poussaint (1993) indicates the need to respect one another, evaluate and resolve competitive feelings toward one another, eliminate game playing, listen to each other, control angry feelings, and eliminate put-downs and psychological abuse.

Lawson and Sharpe (2000, p. 25) propose similar guidelines for helping Black men following a divorce, but more broadly, with a range of social and emotional problems. The authors provide information for culturally sensitive practice with Black men that:

1) Promotes a culturally competent patient/provider relationships in which clinicians need to be aware of the social marginality, discrimination, and economic inequities that divorced black men face. 2) Develops compassion and awareness for the emotional issues that African American men may not openly show but that are deeply felt feelings of grief over the loss of a relationship. This also suggests screening for symptoms of depression and anger. 3) Respects the ambivalence African American men feel for the helping process and remember the many past and present examples of how badly black men have been treated by the medical and psychiatric communities. 4) Encourages alternative approaches to practice that utilize spirituality, family, support networks, and client strengths. 5) Promotes community education and encourages public concern for the vitality of the Black family and for Black men. 6) Provides services in alternative locations including churches, employment benefit programs, sports arenas, and community health centers. 7) Utilizes self-help groups for the purpose of mutual support and acceptance by other Black men experiencing divorce. 8) Influences social policy changes by training more culturally competent practitioners who are sensitive to the needs and concerns of Black men. 9) Works to encourage legislation that permits flexible property division, child custody, and economic support policies.

THREE CASE EXAMPLES: BLACK MEN AND THEIR FATHERS

CASE 1

I had a wonderful Black student by the name of Arthur Clark. Art is now a close personal friend. We play racquetball together and work out in the gym when I need help keeping in shape, which seems to be all the time. Art is a former football player and in such great shape that he exudes health.

Some years ago, Art took a course from me in crisis intervention. He was testing the waters to further his career, not sure if he wanted to be in education as he currently was or if the larger arenas of life such as public administration, social work, and policy work were more suited to him.

As is my practice whenever I teach a class, I asked for a volunteer to role-play the type of therapy I do. I'm very active in my therapy. Arthur asked to role-play a problem he was having with his father. In Arthur's opinion, his father was an alcoholic. I did what one would normally do. I asked Arthur on what he based this judgment. He said, "My father drinks all day long and I'm afraid that he won't be alive when I need him the most."

"All day long?" I asked.

"Pretty much," Arthur responded.

"How many drinks would that be?" I wondered.

Arthur shook his head. "I don't really know," he said, "I never counted."

"But you're sure that he's an alcoholic," I asked.

Arthur just sat staring at me. No one had ever questioned this view of his father. It just was a fact in his mind. His father was an alcoholic. I asked Arthur to role-play a confrontation with his dad. He was to tell his dad that he worried about his drinking and that he was afraid that his father wouldn't be alive when Arthur needed him most. Mind you, this was all done in front of a class of 25 other students. In responding to the confrontation, Arthur said the following:

"Dad, I worry that you drink too much and that your health will suffer. I want you to be part of my life, to see me when I'm successful in life, to see my kids grow up. I don't want you to die early like so many Black men."

In responding to what Arthur said about his father, I took a chance and said the following in the role of his father:

"Arthur [I used his formal name because I was convinced that his father used it and that it would have more clout in the role play], Arthur where have you gotten this idea that I drink too much? I worked for 40 years. I went to work everyday. I provided for everyone. We had a good life. I'm retired now, Arthur, and I have a nip or two with the boys, with my friends. Does that make me an alcoholic?"

Art's head snapped back, literally. He looked at me for a long time and then he said, "But that's what mom says about you, that you drink too much."

In the role play, I leaned over and touched Arthur on the arm and then I said, "But Arthur, your mom is a very religious woman. Any drink is too much for her, you know that. Why shouldn't I enjoy these retired years and have some fun? And if I take a drink or two, so what? I'm a healthy man, I've worked hard, and I'm not irresponsible. Aren't I entitled to enjoy these years after working so hard? You have your dad alive and well. There aren't many Black sons who can say that. Why not enjoy me instead of criticizing me?"

I looked over at Arthur and tears were forming in his eyes. Like most men who have been given permission to see their fathers as compatriots and friends, he was overwhelmed by the experience. It was liberating not to carry the burden of a father who had somehow failed his son.

When Arthur composed himself, he turned to the class and said that no one had ever given him the opportunity to talk about these things. He thought it wasn't masculine for Black men to discuss problems. Now he knew how wrong that was and that it was clear he wanted to be in social work, if this was what we did to help people. "How many Black boys would benefit from a similar discussion?" he asked the class. And then he answered his own question. "All of them," he said. "All of us."

Arthur was admitted to the Master of Social Work (MSW) Program. He was the winner of many awards and is moving on to getting his doctorate. He hasn't decided where, but because I mentor him, it will be somewhere very good where his career will be as positive and as successful as I know it can be.

Six months after that initial interaction with Arthur, he asked me out for dinner at a nearby Cajun restaurant. He wanted me to meet his father.

The night stands out in my mind. It was such great fun because, much as I had guessed, his father was a man of great joy. A cut-up and a storyteller, charismatic and generous. His father made me think of my own father, who now, passed away, would have been like Arthur's father. I never told this to Arthur but that night was like being with my own father at a point in time when I would have appreciated him all the more for his ability to make an ordinary time so much fun.

Arthur has gone back to Louisiana with his father to meet relatives and to discover his roots. He sees his father often and shares in the ways adult men can share when the curtain has been lifted. Arthur now sees his father as a man with flaws and with goodness, a complex person, too complicated to easily categorize, and it's been freeing for him.

We were having coffee one afternoon after seeing a movie, and Arthur reminded me of the time in class when he was able to work out some issues about his dad. He said the words of an old spiritual to me to describe how he felt. He said to me, "Free at last. Lord all mighty, thank God, I'm free at last."

CASE 2

Another time, a Black technician came to my house to fix an appliance. We got to talking and when he found out that I was a social worker, he shared the following story with me.

My dad left us when I was about ten. I don't remember much about him but my mother said he was a real son of a bitch and that he used to beat up on her and on us a lot because he was into the booze. Funny, but I don't remember any of that. Neither does my sister. For twenty years I had this anger over what he did. I'd listen to my mom, watch her as she got old and alone, think that he was responsible for how poor we were, and just hate the hell out of him for what he did. I mean how to do you just up and leave a family?

So anyway, I get married and about five years into the marriage, damned if I didn't do the same thing. I'm not proud of myself, mind you, but it happens. My wife was just dumping on me all of the time. Nothing I did was good enough. From morning to night all I ever heard was how bad I was. I had my fill of it and, one day, I just took off.

Well, it got me thinking about my dad and I started looking for him. I found him through the V.A. It wasn't easy, but finally, I got his address and phone number. He was living up in Bakersfield, an easy drive. Figured I'd drive up and back in the same day. Thought I'd see him, tell him off, and leave. I ended up staying three days. He was happy to see me. Made me promise to go back to my wife. Said he'd tried going back to my mom a number of times but she wouldn't let him and that he'd written us or called me and my sister, but she stopped the letters. Said he always felt guilty about leaving, but he was just a young man and not very good at talking things through. Mentioned the stuff that my mom was doing to him ... her nagging and her putting him down so's he didn't feel like a man anymore. It sounded pretty familiar. Said he never drank, never abused anyone.

I go back home and confront my mom. She admits to me that he was telling the truth, but that her feelings were hurt so she made up the story. Said he paid child support for a long time. I asked how she could do such a thing, that it had a bad affect on me for a long time. She shrugs her shoulder. Men are all shits, she says. What difference does it make?

Well, it made a difference to me, I said, and I'm gonna get to know him, which is what I did. He's no perfect man, that's for sure. But he's a good man and he's someone I feel proud to call my father. We do a lot of stuff together now. We like the same things, how about that? I see him every week or two. He's almost ready to retire and he may move down here to be closer, or the wife and I may move up there. It depends on where the work is. My dad just did a trust fund for my daughter so she could go to college. Wants me to go too. Says he thinks I'm smart enough and that he's gonna take some courses. Never too old to learn, he says. Goes to show you how wrong you can be when you listen to someone else tell you about your dad. I should have found out for myself a lot sooner. It would have saved me from being so mad all these years. I bet there are a lot of men out there who have the same problem.

I'll bet he's right. In fact, one of my Black colleagues shared a story with me about his father that shows how many men begin to redefine their fathers as they mature in life.

CASE 3

My brother and I were running wild after my old men left us. Why we didn't end up in jail is beyond me. My mother became an alcoholic after he left. Went through men like they were going out of style. Married six times before I left high school. I hated the son of a bitch for what he did to us.

One day I was back from the service visiting my mom. We couldn't find the guy she was living with at the time. We went looking for him and finally found him in the barn where he'd hung himself. There he was, twisting in the wind, dead as hell. My mom just looked at him and said to us, "another son of a bitch bites the dust."

That's what she said to me and my brother. We both looked at her. I think we were thinking the same thing at the same time.

My brother went looking for my dad and found him in some nursing home over in Napa where he'd gone to live after he left my mom. Says my mom was the most difficult woman he'd ever known, that she was drinking before he left, and she was going through men right and left. We couldn't believe him because we thought that he was making it up to make himself look good, but he told us to make a few phone calls to people who knew them when they were still together, and gave us some names, and we called. It was an eye opener. He was telling the truth.

You don't go from hating the guy who left you to loving him, but I feel better about myself now. I thought he left us because he hated me and my brother. It didn't occur to me that it was all about my mom. To me, she was a saint for having kept us together after he left. I could never see her doing anything wrong to anyone. It sounds strange, given the drinking and all the men, but that's the way I felt. I still do, for that matter. I see my dad once in a while. We don't have much to say to each other. I see him out of respect and to remind myself that you need to have a relationship with your dad even if it isn't a good one.

SUMMARY

This chapter on clinical work with Black men suggests the need for cultural awareness and a close check on worker bias. A number of researchers point out that worker bias may lead to misdiagnosis, resulting in much more serious and often stigmatizing ways of viewing Black men and their behavior. A number of social problems experienced by Black men were also noted, including the high rate of incarceration and educational problems, suggesting that treatment is only part of the answer to problems experienced by Black men and that strong social policy changes need to be made to correct historical problems of racism, underemployment, and educational disparities experienced by many Black men.

Clinical Work With Traditional and Newly Immigrated Latino Men

with Mina Garza, MSW

The Latino population in the United States comprises a diverse and heterogeneous group of people with distinct backgrounds. The term *Latino* is used here to represent a group with a shared language and some similar customs and traditions; however, the term *Hispanic* is also used in the literature to describe people from Cuba, Latin America, Mexico, and Puerto Rico. Hernandez (1990) notes that although three disparate groups of Latinos (Cubans, Puerto Ricans and Mexicans) identify very different systems of beliefs related to political orientations, government involvement in their lives, and the extent of discrimination faced by each group in the United States, over 70% feel that all three groups are "very or somewhat similar" (p. 5). It should also be made clear that this chapter is about clinical work with highly traditional or newly immigrated Latinos with very traditional approaches to problems solving when there are social and emotional problems that lead to crisis.

AREAS OF LATINO MALE DIFFICULTY

A University of Arizona (2000) report notes that although the Hispanic population of Arizona was about 20% in 2000, 29% of all arrests for violent crimes (rape, murder, aggravated assault) were Hispanics, whereas

36% of all vehicle crime arrests for drunken driving leading to death and injury were also Hispanics. Another report (University of Arizona, 2000a) indicates that Hispanics comprise 70% of all high school drop-outs in the state of Arizona. Mexican American men have higher rates of alcohol consumption than their non-Hispanic counterparts (Randolph, Stroup-Benham, & Black, 1998, p. 265). According to Howe (1994), Hispanics have lower educational aspirations, despite having college recommended at similar rates as Caucasian students. Latino USA (2002) reports that:

> The dropout rate for Latinos in this country is above 30 percent. That is twice the rate for African Americans and almost four times the rate for Anglo students. Behind the numbers are many stories; poverty interfering with learning, overwhelmed teachers coping with large classes, and schools that promote children to the next grade despite gaps in their knowledge.

Monsivais (1996) provides a reason for high dropout rates and a reduced value for educational attainment:

> Many studies have shown that poor Mexican families see little intrinsic value in acquiring education. Furthermore, a recent Rand study on how immigrants fare in the U.S. education system shows the low academic aspirations of Mexican immigrant children as compared to other immigrant groups. Even more disturbing, the study found that the academic aspirations of subsequent generations of the children of Mexican immigrants, weakened. (p. M2)

MACHISMO

One of the most enduring and often harmful stereotypes of Latino men is the concept of "machismo." Baca Zinn (1980) describes machismo as follows:

> The social science literature views machismo as a compensation for feelings of inadequacy and worthlessness. This interpretation is rooted in the application of psychoanalytic concepts to explain both Mexican and Chi-

cano gender roles. The widely accepted interpretation is that machismo is the male attempt to compensate for feelings of internalized inferiority by exaggerating masculinity. At the same time that machismo is an exaggeration of power, its origin is ironically linked to powerlessness and subordination. (p. 20)

Adding to Baca Zinn's (1980) definition of machismo, Mirande (1979) writes,

The macho male demands complete deference, respect and obedience not only from his wife but from his children as well. In fact, social scientists maintain that this rigid male-dominated family structure has negative consequences for the personality development of Mexican American children. It fails to engender achievement, independence, self-reliance or self worth—values which are highly esteemed in American society. (p. 479)

Pena (1991) conducted an in-depth study on the folklore of Mexican male workers and found that their views of women were heavily influenced by their working class status, particularly because machismo appears to be more pronounced in working-class men than in middle-class men. Pena writes that the principal theme in the machismo folklore is the idea of the "treacherous woman." In the "cancion ranchera" (ranch songs), women are portrayed as heartless women who betray their lovers without remorse. In his conversations with the Mexican men in the fields, Pena found that they believed, "It is a man's inalienable right to exercise control over a woman, to possess her sexually when he wishes ... in effect, to render her defenseless and penetrate her at will" (pp. 35–36).

The concept of machismo has been identified in several studies as a contributing factor to heavy alcohol consumption and its subsequent destructive consequences include domestic violence and child abuse (Neff et al., 1991; Pena, 1991; Shai & Rosenwaithe, 1988). To hold one's liquor and keep up with one's peers is expected of macho males. Pena (1991) again notes that

their code of machismo impelled the men toward cultural behavior that can only be termed destructive. They drank and celebrated with abandon, often with disastrous results, such as bloody fights and vehicular accidents. Almost invariably, alcohol intensified their feelings of machismo and the crudities associated with it. (p. 38)

Chafetz (1974) reinforces Pena's (1991) observations but also cautions us to recognize that machismo is commonly found in all cultures where men are poor:

... more than most Americans, the various Spanish speaking groups in this country (Mexican American, Puerto Rican, Cuban) ... stress, dominance, aggressiveness, physical prowess and other stereotypical masculine traits. Indeed, the masculine sex role for this group is generally described by reference to the highly stereotyped notion of machismo. In fact, a strong emphasis on masculine aggressiveness and dominance may be characteristic of most groups in the lower ranges of the socioeconomic ladder. (Chafetz, 1974, p. 59)

The belief that all Latino men are guided by machismo has made many American clinicians believe that Latino men are too proud to accept help in crisis situations, but Charles Goff (personal communication, July 7, 1994) disagrees:

Mexican men are often described as being very macho which, in the minds of some, translates into being stubborn and unwilling to accept help or advice from others. But we should understand that machismo is a way of providing men who have very little social esteem with self-importance and self- worth. There are bragging rights implied. The best way to approach a Mexican male when help is needed in the family is to focus on his accomplishments, to praise him for his efforts to provide for the family, and to respect him for his hard work in difficult times. You will then get someone who is willing to work hard in treatment in the service of his family.

LATINO MEN AND TREATMENT

Many situations experienced by newly immigrated Latino men or Latino clients living in poverty are created by feelings of being unwelcomed in this country, even when the client has a legal right to be here. This immediate sense of alienation and unfamiliar rules and regulations of American life often place the client in situations that lead to crisis. Unfamiliar child-care laws, expectations that drivers should not drink, and arguments within the family that sometimes become loud and spill onto the streets, may bring the client into immediate contact with the judicial system. Prevention of these unnecessary situations can be made by a process of socialization to the country, a necessary but often neglected function of the social and educational institutions of America. Emphasizing this sense of alienation, Gonzalez (2000) writes that although Latinos are the largest minority group in America

> ... mental health problems of Hispanics living in poverty and undocumented Hispanic immigrants are often exacerbated by socioeconomic stressors, racism, and political oppression. Effective mental health treatment for this segment of the Hispanic population must encompass case advocacy, community outreach, and the mediating of complex social systems. Mental health clinicians who treat poor and/or undocumented Hispanics should be skilled in the implementation of multiple interventive roles such as that of advocate, mediator, broker, and teacher.

Gonzalez suggests that clinicians must assume multiple roles with Latino men because, for the most part, Latino men do not directly seek treatment (Rogler & Malgady, 1987). Velasquez, Arellano, and McNeill (2004) believe that there are several primary reasons for this:

1. The belief that "Psychotherapy is for jotos or maricones (homosexuals), or viejas (old women)" (p. 180)—From an early age, the message given to Latino men is to be strong, tough, and to take it like a man.
2. A further belief that "Psychotherapy is only for people who are mentally ill or locos (crazy)" (p. 180)—Latino men often believe that their problems exist because of other people (their children, spouse, boss, and friends) and only people who have internal problems that originate inside of themselves need help.
3. A common misconception of therapy held by many people that "Psychotherapy is simply chatting with somebody" (p. 180)—

Many Latino men believe that problems that affect one physically (anxiety, depression, headaches, feelings of tension) should be dealt with by seeing a physician who can at least prescribe medication.

4. A sense of futility that "Psychotherapy will simply open up problems that cannot be resolved" (p. 181)—These problems may not only lead to a male feeling vulnerable and inadequate, but the problem may become worse if it's discussed and other people hear about it.

BEFORE SEEING PROFESSIONALS

Traditional Latino men experiencing emotional problems they cannot handle using their typical coping skills may discuss a problem with extended family members or *compadres,* the close friends who baptized their children and who play such an important role in Latino culture. Latino men may also seek help from priests or religious figures in the form of direct advice and suggestions. Elderly people, particularly women, represent wisdom in the Latino culture and they may also be contacted before a professional is seen.

When the problem becomes unsolvable and somatic complaints sometimes result, the client may seek help from the family doctor. Medication to relieve the crisis would be considered an acceptable form of treatment at this stage of coping with the crisis situation. Complaints at the emotional level might be confused in the client's mind with physical difficulties. Problems with anxiety, for example, might be thought to originate in the stomach and the client might first attempt to get medical relief for the stomach ailment.

The family doctor plays a vital role in the treatment of clients in crisis. In many parts of Latin America and Mexico, as well as in the United States, the family doctor may prescribe antidepressive or antianxiety medications but may tell the client that they are for the treatment of a physical ailment. This deception is not considered unethical because it offers the Latino male client some relief and may decrease symptoms. Without counseling, however, the problem may cycle back and forth in severity. In this respect, the Latino male client may have an extremely long duration of the crisis.

TREATMENT SUGGESTIONS WITH LATINO MEN

Congress (1990) notes that the following elements are necessary ingredients of treatment with Latino men: (a) *Confianza*—The development of basic trust of the worker by the client; (b) *Personalismo*—The responsiveness of the client to treatment when the worker personalizes the service and permits latitude in what the client wishes to discuss at the moment; and (c) *Respecto*—The belief that respect is intrinsically a function of all interactions with another person and that it forms a significant part of all crisis work with the Latino client.

Many Latino male clients are fatalistic about life. They have often been socialized to believe in the inevitability of luck, fate, and chance. There is a "dicho," or proverb, that sums up this belief: *Lo Que Dios Mande,* or whatever God wills. This fatalism is partly a result of the historical events that have shaped Latino culture. Change, the client often believes, may take place, but it is usually related to fate rather than anything the worker does in treatment or the attempts at personal change made by the client. To work with fatalism, clinicians need to be positive, emphasizing the client's prior ability to change and the fact that one's luck may always improve.

Latino men experience a considerable imperative to be strong even in the midst of a crisis. The act of discussing feelings or complaining about inequities in life may make Latino men feel weak. One useful technique which reinforces strength is to praise men for their accomplishments, particularly those related to the extended family. Praising strength and accomplishments serve the dual purpose of building trust and provides the client with confidence in the worker as well as in himself.

Latino men often view the family as extensions of themselves. If children do well or do poorly, it reflects on the client. One way to permit Latino men to discuss inner feelings is to pose the following question: "I know that you've experienced much heartache and that you don't feel that your family appreciates you. How would you like your family to treat you differently?" Another useful question is to ask how the client taught his children to handle the issue of respect for a parent because this issue is key to how men view their children, and ultimately, how successful they have been with their children.

There is general respect in Latino culture for highly educated men and women. Placing professional certificates, licenses, and university degrees in public areas and having resumes available which point to the achievements of the worker are important methods of influencing the Latino male client. However, Monsivais (1996), cautions that among many poverty stricken Latinos, there is intrinsic hostility toward professionals and toward their degrees and licenses:

> Whether it is a by-product of a traditional Catholicism that fears reading because, "it poisons the soul," or whether it is rooted in the particular belief that *licenciados* (a professional with a degree) exist only to exploit the people, it is quite common for Mexican families to harbor anti-intellectual attitudes which in turn shape their responses toward education. (p. M2)

THE USE OF *DICHOS* IN TREATMENT

In Latino culture, wise sayings or *dichos* assume considerable importance in guiding the client toward solutions to problems. Zuniga (1992) suggests that *dichos* are actually metaphors which have been traditionally used in treatment. Zuniga (1992) classifies therapeutic metaphors as:

> 1) major stories that address complex clinical problems; 2) anecdotes or short stories focused on specific or limited goals; 3) analogies, similes or brief figurative statements or phrases that underscore specific points; 4) relationship metaphors, which can use one relationship as a metaphor for another; 5) tasks with metaphorical meanings that can be undertaken by clients between sessions; 6) artistic metaphors which can be paintings, drawings, clay models or creations which symbolize something else. (Zuniga, 1992, p. 57)

We have identified several *dichos* which may be commonly used in treatment with Latino male clients. *"Sentir en el alma,"* for example, translates literally as "to feel it in your soul," but the real translation means "to be terribly sorry." *"Con la cuhara se le queman los frijoles"* translates literally as "even the best cook burns the beans," but in reality, it means that everyone makes mistakes. *"Entre azul y buenos noches"* translates directly as "between blue and good night," but its popular meaning is "to be undecided." *"A la buena de Dios"* may translate literally as "as God would have it," but its common meaning is "as luck would have it." *"No hay mal que por bien no venga,"* for example, translates as "there is nothing bad from which good does not come," or "it's a blessing in disguise." Another *dicho* useful in crisis intervention is *"La verdad no mata, pero incomoda,"* which means "the truth doesn't kill, but it can hurt." And yet another *dicho* with relevance for crisis work is *"Al que no ha usado huaraches, las correas le sacan sangre,"* which, loosely translated, means "he who has never worn sandals is easily cut by the straps," or "it's difficult to do things that one is not used to." And finally, as Zuniga (1992) suggests for the client in a deteriorating relationship which might end in termination, the *dicho "Mejor sola que mal acompanada"* might work. Roughly translated, this *dicho* means "it's better to be alone or unmarried than to be in a bad relationship."

FOCUSING ON FEELINGS

Feelings are highly valued in Latino culture. One approach to making feelings part of the therapeutic relationship is to tell the client that you will communicate with them, *"de corazon a corazon,"* or "heart to heart." In Mexico, this concept of a close personal relationship in which true feelings can be communicated has various levels of understanding. It is sometimes associated with the process called *"El Desague de Las Penas,"* or "unburdening oneself." It is what North American therapists call venting.

Velasquez et al. (2004) suggest that men may use Spanish idioms for emotional states. These may include the term *embrujado,* which implies that someone has cast a spell on them. The word *encabronado* indicates extreme anger at someone with potential to harm another person. *Flojo* suggests apathy, lethargy, and fatigue. *Loco de remate* indicates that a man is becoming mentally ill, whereas the term *latoso* suggests that a man is developing a physical or emotional problem that may require care by family members and that he has become a "pain in the neck" as a result.

Considerable credence is given to the significance of dreams in Latino culture. Dreams are considered omens or predictors of the future. Dreams provide answers to problems. The worker should listen carefully to the dreams Latino clients discuss in treatment. They should not, however, ascribe specific meaning or interpretations to a dream but should, instead, ask the client for their own interpretation of a dream. It may also be permissible to ask the client to suggest ways to complete dreams which terminate before a specific message is given. This technique requires the client to finish a dream as if he had control over its ending so that the dream is not a chance occurrence which may imply bad luck over which the client has no control.

CULTURAL ISSUES IN TREATMENT

Altarriba and Bauer (1998) indicate that the following cultural factors must be taken into consideration when working with Latino clients: close family bonds, highly interpersonal relationships, *simparia,* time and language, and acculturation. This can be accomplished, according to the authors, by accessing the client's worldview, which includes the following characteristics: (a) Nature—Hispanics often believe that they have little control over the forces of nature, (b) Time—Most Hispanics prefer to think in the present with the past and the future of minor importance in problem solving and decision making, (c) Behavior—Hispanic immigrants prefer to be openly expressive in their behavior, and (d) Social Relations—Traditional Hispanics believe that an individual may defer to authority on many occasions. The authors conclude by noting the following:

> To engage Hispanic clients in beneficial therapy, it is helpful for the counselor to demonstrate a high level of cultural sensitivity. The counselor should make all attempts to evaluate the client's specific history, including language spoken, family background, and more specifically, the client's cultural identity. It is helpful if counselors have a good understanding of the Spanish language to be able to address culturally related

problems and communicate effectively with non-English-speaking family members. It is imperative that a clear understanding exists of the social and psychological characteristics of the individual subgroups of Hispanic society. Cultural values should form the basis of any treatment program. (Altarriba & Bauer, 1998, p. 396)

CASE EXAMPLE: A LATINO MAN BATTLES A CURSE

This case first appeared in modified form in a volume I wrote on evidence-based practice (Glicken, 2005). It's original purpose was to show the mistakes that can be made when culture isn't factored into diagnosis. In this context, the primary purpose is to show culturally-sensitive work with a Latino man experiencing the symptoms of mental illness.

THE CASE

Jorge Rivera is a 19-year-old Mexican National who came to the United States under the sponsorship of his maternal uncle to attend a California university. Jorge has been in the country a year and was doing well until signs of emotional change became apparent to his loved ones. He was increasingly becoming aloof and secretive, had stopped attending school, and seemed to be a very different person from the happy, motivated young man he had been just a year earlier. Suspecting an emotional or physical problem, Jorge's uncle took him to see his family doctor, an American of Hispanic descent. The doctor was immediately struck by Jorge's aloofness, fearfulness, and social isolation. The doctor performed multiple tests, and, unable to find anything physically wrong with Jorge, urged the uncle to take his nephew to a Hispanic male social worker with whom the doctor had prior positive experiences.

The first interview was conducted in Spanish because it is the language in which Jorge is more proficient, and he could express his inner feelings with more accuracy in Spanish than in English.

Jorge told the therapist that he was hearing voices at night when he tried to sleep and that the voices were telling him to do things that Jorge found repulsive and dangerous. The voices were new to Jorge and he feared that he was going insane. As Jorge began to talk about his fears that he was psychotic and how this would place him in great jeopardy with his family, he said that being *"muy loco"* was what happened to people who were sinful and he would be punished by his family with social isolation and ostracism.

It was clear to the therapist that Jorge was in great distress but pending additional information, the therapist deferred making a diagnosis. Using the *DSM–IV* criteria, however, the therapist saw signs of schizophrenia. He decided to interview the uncle's family to determine the point of onset of his symptoms. Everyone confirmed that Jorge had been very outgoing, showing none of the signs of the mental illness he was now exhibiting. The onset was sudden, within the last three months, and the symptoms had been rapid and were worsening. This didn't sound like the slow onset of mental illness the therapist had seen in other patients, and he was not convinced that he could use this diagnosis with someone so new to the country. He wondered if there were other factors involved.

In the next interview, he asked Jorge to tell him about his life in Mexico and to provide his theory about what was happening to him. It turned out that Jorge had been romantically involved with a young woman who came from a highly affluent family in Mexico. The couple were very much in love but the young woman's parents were strongly opposed to the marriage and had hired a *Bruja* to cast a spell on him so that he would become unattractive to the young woman and she would lose her feelings for Jorge. The *Bruja* (literally a witch, but someone who can cast spells on others) was sending Jorge little totems that represented evil and were scaring him into social isolation and withdrawal. He was convinced the voices he heard were her doing and that as a result of the spells she had cast, he would become insane, lose his beloved, and die a horrible death. He had known others who faced similar fates in Mexico. *Brujas* were evil and they did immense harm, he told the therapist.

The therapist had grown up with stories of witches and spells but wasn't a believer. Nonetheless, he contacted the uncle, told him what had happened, and wondered if he knew of some way to deal with the effects of the *Bruja*. The uncle said that he did and contacted a well-known *Curandero* he knew of in Mexico, paid his way to come to the United States, and had the *Curandero* remove the spell in a ritual that lasted 24 hr. When the ritual was done, the *Curandero* gave Jorge an amulet to wear around his neck to ward off future spells and urged him to break off the relationship with the young woman to cease the *Bruja*'s continued impact on Jorge's mental health. The uncle again intervened, spoke to the young woman's family in Mexico, promised that Jorge would no longer be in contact with the young woman, and urged them to cease any more witchcraft with Jorge. The family agreed, and a brokenhearted but functioning Jorge returned to school, and in time, and with his family's support and an occasional visit to the therapist, is doing well in school, but mourns his lost relationship.

We would like to think that spells, witchcraft, and sorcery do not exist in the modern world, but for many people they do. The therapist spoke to the *Curandero* who told him:

> All of us have demons inside of us. When those demons collide with an outside force, and have no doubt but that Brujas are very powerful outside forces, people often develop the problems we saw in Jorge. You can call this witchcraft which most North Americans don't believe in, but I see the damage Brujas do everyday and myself have been a victim. I went through many of the same problems that Jorge has been having until my dear teacher came and cured me, but everyday I live in fear of the Bruja who cast this spell on me. I don't expect you to believe that, but it's true. In Mexico, these practices date back thousands of years and the Bruja had generations of those before her to give her immense power.

> Whether Jorge believes in Brujas and is susceptible to suggestion or whether their magic really exists isn't for me to prove. My job is to make spells go away as I did with Jorge. I think you would have

called Jorge crazy, put him on strong medicines that would have done him harm, and forgotten about him, believing that he was hopeless. A 24-hour ritual and he is now sad but well again. He'll get over his lost love and he'll be protected for a while from the Bruja if the family pays her off and tells her to leave Jorge alone. But Brujas are cruel and you never know when she'll attack Jorge again just to prove her power over him. Then I'll have to come back to Los Angeles, a place filled with evil, and do this again, only next time I may not be so lucky and Jorge may sink into oblivion. Believe what you'd like. The amulet will help as will the little symbols I've urged Jorge to place around his bed at night when Brujas have the most power, but I offer no guarantee that the Bruja won't come back to haunt Jorge again.

DISCUSSION

In a personal discussion the author had in Mexico with Dr. Pedro Guerrero (July 14, 1994), a University of California at Berkeley-trained cultural anthropologist and codirector of Cemanahuac Educational Community in Cuernavaca, Morelos, Mexico, Dr. Guerrero confirmed the importance of folk cures for a number of problems experienced by Mexicans. He assured me that although the idea of *Brujas* and *Curanderos* is common in Mexico, it has a selective following. However, most Mexicans grow up with stories about the power of witches and black magic. He cautioned against taking that power literally because *Brujas* have been known to take matters into their own hands and told the story of a child molester in a small village whose political influence stymied the police from doing anything. The village hired a *Bruja* known for her expertise in the use of poisons and after observing the man over a period of weeks, observed that he walked barefooted to work every morning and that he used the same route. The *Bruja* sprinkled poison across the path, the man stepped on it, got very ill, and died. Perhaps something similar happened to Jorge but wasn't detected by the laboratory tests run by his physician. In any event, a high degree of cultural awareness saved Jorge from an incorrect, stigmatizing, and probably harmful diagnosis of mental illness, a very good call by the therapist regardless of the cause of Jorge's symptoms.

SUMMARY

This chapter suggests the need to understand the collective nature of Latino life and to respond to Latino men in crisis with social and cultural sensitivity. The chapter also suggests that many Latino clients are placed in crisis situations, not so much because of preexisting pathology, but because they have difficulty navigating the legal and cultural waters of American life. New immigrants face discrimination from North Americans who value their labor but who often do not value Latinos. This may create situations that increase the possibility of crisis. Treatment approaches useful with Latino men focused on the use of *dichos,* culturally-congruent treatment strategies, and the use of ethnically-sensitive practice.

[Some of the material in this chapter was first given in modified form as a paper presented by Mina Garza, MSW, and the author at the *California Conference for Latino Social Workers,* Sacramento, October, 1996, and also appeared in modified form in Glicken (2004, 2005)].

Clinical Work With Asian Men

with Steven M. Ino, PhD

Ino and Glicken (1999, 2002; Glicken, 2004) note that Asian men from traditionally male-dominated Asian families must deal with an internalized belief that they are subordinate, in importance, to family. This collective self, as opposed to the more Western notion of an individualized self, is constantly searching for ways to assimilate self into a social context without losing the prominence of family in all decisions. Ino (1985a, 1985b, 1987, 1991) suggests that, as a result, anglicized Asian men often lead two distinctly different lives. One life is in search of meaning and reinforcement from extended family, whereas the other is in search of meaning and reinforcement from nonfamily members and institutions, such as work and personal life. When the family and the need to assimilate conflict, Asian men often suffer from severe anxiety problems.

When an Asian American male client contacts a mental health professional, the client is probably already emotionally disengaged or estranged from his family and from significant others. Because of feelings of shame or a collective need to protect the family or significant others, the Asian man has often become withdrawn and isolated, increasing his risk for serious emotional problems. If the family is seeking help for the Asian man, then the family has exhausted its strategies for privately and discreetly helping the family member and must now seek outside assistance, and, in the process, risk considerable shame. The emotional danger for the client is that the family may be at a point where it is prepared to "save face" by collectively abandoning the client by removing the client's vital self support and thereby, precipitating a second-order crisis.

Treatment problems arise when the clinician, operating within a strictly European American treatment framework, attempts to implement a cognitive-behavioral-affective intervention strategy that fails to adequately address Asian American men's collective self needs. The clinician must be prepared to consider multiple, overlapping worldviews, self systems, patterns of social life, and therefore, alternate treatment strategies—all of which the client may not be able to consciously explain. When this fails to happen, the Asian American male client may come to believe that treatment is not helpful, may blame himself for not being competent or healthy enough, or may believe that the clinician isn't wise enough, a belief that may cause the client to prematurely terminate treatment.

UNDERSTANDING THE ELEMENTS OF THE COLLECTIVE SELF

For many traditionally male Asian clients, social harmony is the major force governing all meaningful interpersonal relationships (Ho, 1987). Social harmony requires varying degrees of cooperation, adaptation, accommodation, and collaboration by all individuals in the social hierarchy. In the Asian social hierarchy, social roles are based more on family membership and position, gender, age, social class, and social position than on qualification and ability. However, there is a basic belief that age, training, and life experience are associated with wisdom and competency, although deference and respect from an individual in a subordinate role requires that the person in a superior social position look after that individual.

The formal idea of family in Asian society extends family identity and membership backwards in time through all of the ancestors in the male family line, continuing on in the present time, and then on to those future descendants who have yet to appear (Lee, 1996). One's sense of family is not time-bound or limited to only those important kin who are living. Although the father is the head of the nuclear family household and is responsible for the family's economic and physical well-being, he still shows deference and loyalty to his father and older brothers as well as to his mother and older sisters. Elders in the father's extended family are also respected. The mother becomes included in the extended family of her husband and is the "emotional hub" of her nuclear family of creation, responsible for nurturing her husband and their children. Although wielding considerable emotional power and often acting as the relational and communication link between father and children, she, nevertheless, has little public power and authority and defers to her husband, his mother, and the elders in the husband's extended family.

Self-restraint and stoicism, inhibiting disruptive emotional expression, conscientious work to fulfill one's responsibilities, heightened social sensitivity and other-directedness, all contribute to maintaining social harmony. However, a person's breech of social obligation or duty can potentially damage the social harmony of the family, group, or larger community. Significant others will condemn their loss of confidence in that individual's ability to fulfill obligations to the family or group through the mechanism of shaming that person.

From an Asian perspective, the prescribed forms of interpersonal interaction are intended to preserve dynamic social harmony by minimizing direct conflict and social discordance. Communication is highly contextual and tends to flow downward from superior to subordinate, often in the form of directives. Both verbal and written communications are indirect, in the passive tense, and at times may appear convoluted. Much of the communication is nonverbal, where the conduct of the superior and not the content of the message is most meaningful. These principles of Asian communication styles serve to maintain social harmony in any interpersonal interaction.

The Asian socialization process develops highly differentiated adult individuals with mature levels of deep emotional interdependency and strong feelings of role responsibility and obligation. But within the context of Asian social reality, physical distress may appropriately exemplify psychosocial distress (Root, 1993). For instance, a gastrointestinal disorder can be viewed as a normal expression of psychological stress over an intense interpersonal conflict and is not necessarily seen as a "symptom" or indicator of the client's inability to cope with psychosocial conflict. To alleviate the physical symptom may be an appropriate treatment for a relational conflict over which one has no control.

THE ASIAN CLIENT AND TREATMENT

As a group, Asians tend to seek help from mental health professionals only when all other more familiar and usual coping strategies, interpersonal resources, and safer avenues of help, have been exhausted. Despite the underutilization of existing services, many Asian mental health professionals believe that there is a significant unmet need for appropriate mental health care (e.g., Furuto, Biswas, Chung, Murase, & Ross-Sheriff, 1992; Gaw, 1993; Sue & Morishima, 1982; Uba, 1994). In a study of nonpatient Southeast Asian Americans, Gong-Guy (1987) estimated that 14.4% of the sample needed inpatient mental health services and 53.75% could benefit from outpatient care, in comparison to corresponding 3% and 12% rates in the general population.

Several reasons explain the discrepancy between the perceived need and the limited use of services: (a) the Asian conception of mental health–mental illness and their management, (b) the strong Asian stigma and shame attached to seeking "out-of-the-family" assistance for mental illness, (c) the inappropriateness of European American mental health care approaches for Asians, (d) shortages of culturally-sensitive mental health professionals, and (e) socioeconomic barriers (Sue & Morishima, 1982; Uba, 1994).

Asians initially seek mental health services only after they are in serious emotional crisis. They will have first exhausted their usual and then their atypical coping strategies and will have sufficiently "overridden" their guilt at breaching family privacy and "loss of face" by seeking help from outside the family. The Asian man who is experiencing the emotional "disequilibrium" of a crisis situation may be very responsive to outside assistance (Golan, 1978; Roberts, 1990). However, the same client is also very vulnerable to family and community influences, leaving the client concerned about the possibility of worrisome miscommunication and misinterpretation of the need for mental health services by the client's family, friends, and the Asian community.

The high level of stigma associated with intractable emotional problems and mental disturbance has its origin in the strong Asian belief that an individual can endure hardship and overcome personal problems through individual perseverance, hard work, stoicism, and the avoidance of disturbing thoughts and feelings. If the client is unable to benefit from these beliefs, then he is felt to have a weak character, be biologically defective, or is the unfortunate victim of bad luck, a curse, vengeful spirits, or fate.

The Asian man experiencing unmanageable emotional pain may assume, from a mainstream Euro-Anglo American cultural viewpoint, a very passive-dependent interpersonal stance as he seeks a wise and benevolent worker to act as an authority figure who can advise and assist him in alleviating his pain. If the client has confidence in the worker's wisdom and respects the worker's authority, timely intervention can provide vital emotional support and guidance, leading to more adaptive coping patterns, which encourage the client to make corrective life changes.

UNIQUE TREATMENT CONSIDERATIONS

From the beginning of treatment, the Asian male client should have considerable say in selecting the worker. Maximizing the therapist–client "fit" can strengthen client motivation and facilitate the relationship. However, it is the responsibility of the worker to sensitively inquire about this because the client may not wish to insult or embarrass anyone by making such a request. There may also be a natural preference by the client to work with an Asian worker who has a similar ethnic and sociocultural background. Leong (1986) notes the tendency for Asian clients to "... describe their therapists as more credible and competent if they are Asian" (p. 198).

Generally, working with an older, professionally trained and credentialed male or female worker can engender an implicit and immediate trust in the clinician. In some cases, however, the client may be very threatened by an Asian therapist who also shares a similar background with the client. There is great fear of "gossip" in which the client's family or community finds out about the client's need for treatment. In this case, the client may feel more comfortable with a biculturally-aware Asian worker who is "removed" from the client's family and community by virtue of coming from a different ethnic background. On the other hand, both first-generation and highly acculturated Asians may wish to work with a mainstream White worker, believing that they are the best-trained and most competent to help. Whatever the worker's background, he or she must be prepared to be a sociocultural translator or "culture broker," negotiating between and among multiple social worlds (the therapeutic relationship and the Asian American client's life), as the worker helps the client understand the nature of his emotional problem.

The client's feelings about the effectiveness of the initial encounter with the worker will determine whether there will be further meetings. A substantial amount of material must be covered in the first session as the worker attempts to establish rapport, clarify the problem, evaluate the client, and develop a treatment plan. This treatment effort must balance the Asian client's natural reluctance to self-disclose intimate life details to the therapist-as-stranger. Because time and interpersonal activity have a different culturally-dictated meaning and pace to the Asian client, the worker must be more flexible in allowing sufficient time—both in terms of session length, frequency, and number of sessions—to accomplish a successful intervention. First and foremost, the worker must be able to ensure that the Asian male client feels respected and is able to maintain personal dignity.

If possible, the initial session should last as long as necessary for the client to feel a completion in the disclosure of relevant life issues and the basic establishment of a trusting relationship. This may take 30 minutes or 3 hours. The client may be adamant that this is to be a one-session meeting, which means that the worker must be prepared to provide, in concise form, the entire sequence of interventions in that single session (Ewing, 1990). If it appears that the client is willing to return for an additional session, it is the worker's responsibility to outline an understandable schedule of further sessions and to describe clear and reasonable goals to be accomplished, asking, of course, for feedback and clarification from the client to determine if the proposed plan is acceptable.

Collective Self Issues

A fundamental task for the worker is the need to accurately assess the quality and degree of the client's collective identification. One simple "collective self" assessment question might be to ask the following: "When you think about yourself, or when you are asked to identify yourself, do you seem to resonate more to your family name or to your first name?" In traditional Asian social situations, personal introductions are made by giving one's family name first and then one's given name. Asian social etiquette implicitly acknowledges and values one's family identity or "collective self" over one's individual identity (Ino, 1985b, 1991).

The worker should not expect the Asian male client to be able to readily explain the central problem that brought him into treatment. Fear of losing face, mistrust because of experiences with racism and discrimination, or suspiciousness of the therapist and mental health services, can make the client reluctant to self-disclose personal and family information. When asked, the client may initially focus on physical symptoms or somatic complaints. Consequently, physical complaints must be seen as valid problems to be treated in a competent and respectful way. Suggesting that the physical symptoms have an emotional base may initially alienate the client and can create unmanageable conflict.

On the other hand, the client may begin talking so globally about life history or the family situation that it appears only tangential to a clear depiction of the immediate problem. For example, when asked, "What brings you here today?" or "How can I be of help to you?" the client may respond by going into great detail about how he was born in Cambodia, how he and part of his family escaped Cambodia back in 1979, and how they gradually made their way to a refugee camp in Thailand and eventually on to America, England, Australia, or Canada. This need to situate the perceived problem in the larger context of the person's entire life history is the client's way of explaining to the worker why he or she has come for help and to provide the relevant information necessary to understand the client's perception of the origins of the problem. Sometimes, the client may begin by seeking help for a "minor" or less pertinent problem as a way of testing "the therapeutic situation" and the trustworthiness of the worker. If the clinical experience is deemed helpful, the client may then proceed to disclose the true reason for coming.

Ino (1985a, 1985b, 1987) suggests that there are five primary reasons why Asian men may come for treatment: bicultural identity development, significant non-Asian relationships, significant loss, expulsion from one's family, and dysfunctional families of origin.

FIVE PRIMARY REASONS ASIAN MEN SEEK TREATMENT

Bicultural Identity Development

For second- and later-generation Asian Americans, the multicultural socialization process may result in a mix of self identities that are, at times, conflictual and contradictory. For example, an immigrant Asian American may possess a basic sense of collective self and yet practice very acculturated and assimilated attitudes and behaviors and even claim conscious "allegiance" to the mainstream American way of life. At best, bicultural Asian American self development can result in resolvable internal psychic confusion and an affective commitment to some form of multicultural self. At worst, it may develop into critical intrapsychic disorganization and instability of self. The strength and durability of the client's "individual self" depends on how psychosocially sound the other significant family members are and the internal consistency of family interrelationships.

Significant European American–Asian American Relationship

Asian Americans having an essential collective self will naturally seek collective as opposed to individualistic relationship involvement with those who become a part of their significant social world. However, the individual may not always be conscious of these needs and he or she may be unaware of who can best fulfill them. Consequently, he or she may become socially involved with others in an apparently assimilated and acculturated fashion. Serious interpersonal conflicts can arise when a couple having very different self dynamics and accompanying interpersonal needs unwittingly attempt to realize a shared, deep, fulfilling, and intimate bond. The following case example describes treatment with an Asian man and his non-Asian wife.

CASE EXAMPLE: JAMES AND LISA

James is a 41-year-old Sansei (third-generation Japanese American) who has been married for about two years to Lisa, a 35-year-old Anglo American. Lisa is very unhappy with the marriage and frustrated that they have not been able to effectively communicate with each other about her unhappiness. Whenever she tries to initiate a conversation about the marriage, James avoids discussing their problems, saying only that their marriage is good and that they just have to work harder at it. He has consistently rejected her earlier requests that they talk to a counselor. James feels very embarrassed about sharing their marital problems with a stranger. Although Lisa's family is aware of their marital problems and tries to be supportive, James does not want to disclose their marital problems to his family. As Lisa has become more adamant about separating and as James has become more desperate to save the marriage, he has finally agreed to join Lisa for five treatment sessions.

When they came in for treatment, Lisa was friendly, self-assured, worried, and verbally expressive. James, on the other hand, looked tired, disheveled, tense, constricted, depressed, and seemed to be on the verge of tears. Separately, both denied any serious physical risk to either of them, although Lisa continued to worry about James. Both acknowledged that they still cared very deeply for each other, despite the serious marital stress, and that there was more disappointment than animosity in their feelings about the marriage. The short-term goal of the marital counseling, agreed on by the couple, was to help James better deal with the stress of their marital problems and to do some preliminary exploration to help identify the reasons for their conflicts.

In the course of the five sessions, James began to feel more emotionally stable. He was getting considerable support from his older brother and his wife as well as from two close friends. Major sociocultural differences were uncovered which neither James nor Lisa thought were present. Although James identified himself as "all American" and highly assimilated into mainstream America, his core "self" was collective rather than individualistic, in origin. His own Nisei parents, who seemed as "American as apple pie" and only spoke English at home, had nevertheless raised James and his older siblings in a more traditional Japanese way. Although James had mostly non-Asian friends throughout his life, he developed a "thick" layering of individualistic "self" which he actualized in his social relationships, but which concealed a core collective "self" base. As he settled into a secure married life, he began to relax his defenses, allowing his collective needs to emerge and seek fulfillment. James had a very traditional view of marriage and was critical of Lisa for not understanding, although he had failed to explain the traditions of his culture sufficiently for Lisa to recognize that James expected Lisa to defer to him and place his needs above hers. There were many other unspoken expectations of Lisa that James had not explained but felt Lisa should understand and respect just because she was his wife.

By the end of the five sessions, both Lisa and James realized that they had entered into a much more complex marriage than imagined. Both agreed that they needed to talk further with a marriage counselor and accepted a referral to another therapist who was culturally-sensitive to both Asian and European American ways of being. James left treatment feeling much more in touch with the traditions of his culture and felt ready to enter into a dialogue with Lisa to explain and process those traditions. Lisa left treatment recognizing their cultural differences and agreeing to learn much more about the traditions that had shaped James, but uncertain that she could meet all of James's

needs. Both were impressed with the process which they described as not only positive, but which James said

> Helped me understand not only the problems my cultural heri-
> tage created in our marriage, but many of the positives in those tra-
> ditions which I have a deep appreciation for. It also confirmed my
> feelings for Lisa and helped me realize the hard work she had done
> to maintain our marriage. What I thought would be an embarrass-
> ing experience turned out to be very touching and I'm grateful to
> Lisa for not giving up on me.

Significant Loss

For the Asian American man who has an important established relationship with someone, the loss of that person, either through death or
the dissolution of the relationship, has profound implications for the
integrity of the individual's collective self. The process of mourning
and grieving the loss of that individual and the subsequent emotional
reconstitution entails a major psychosocial reconstruction of the collective self. When there is a major loss through death, all Asian cultures
have their distinct rituals and practices to help with the healing process
of "re"—collective self—integration. This reaffirms the collective self
integrity of all parties and helps them continue on in life. In the extreme case, a crippling loss may so severely disrupt the person's collective self integrity and desire to live, that he or she cannot imagine living
without the lost other. Such an individual, who is unable to experience
emotional collective self support from others, may be at serious suicidal risk.

Family Expulsion

In Asian tradition, the son never truly leaves his family of origin. The
family he establishes becomes incorporated into the continuous family
line as the next generation. Generally speaking, the daughter leaves her
family of origin only when she marries, relocates to her husband's family

of origin, and establishes a new collective self, incorporating his significant family members. Her emotional bond with her own father and mother is "transferred" to her husband and his mother. If the son or daughter is "disinherited" or cast out from the family for some perceived travesty by the family before the right developmental time, this can cause a serious emotional collective self fragmentation and a deep sense of self loss.

Dysfunctional Asian American Family

A dysfunctional, traditional Asian American family is one where the significant adult family members are incapable of managing their role responsibilities and obligations and cannot provide a sufficient level of care and appropriate childrearing to promote the development of a healthy collective self. Occasionally, this includes promoting a confusing, contradictory self experience without any inherent coherence and psychosocial integrity, or imposing family roles and responsibilities on its member that are self-destructive. When this takes place, a family-level therapeutic intervention is ideally called for.

SUMMARY

This chapter on work with Asian American men suggests that strong family ties create what Ino (1987) calls a collective self, which is very strongly identified with family. Work with Asian men requires an understanding of Asian traditions and the importance of family life. Five types of problems were identified that might bring Asian men into therapy, and a case example of a relationship between an Asian husband and a non-Asian wife were included in the chapter.

   Note: [We acknowledge the initial publication of some of this material in *The Smith College Studies in Social Work,* June\July 1999, originally titled: "Treating Asian American Clients in Crisis: A Collectivist Approach," and "Understanding and Treating the Ethnically Asian Client: A Collectivist Approach" in the *Journal of Health and Social Policy*

(2002), Vol. 14 (with Steven Ino, first author on both articles), and thank the editors for permission to reprint some of the material in this chapter. The material also appeared in modified form in Glicken (2004), [again with Steven Ino as the first author.]

PART V

Aging and Substance Abuse

Clinical Work With
Male Substance Abusers

Substance abuse is a very serious health and mental health problem in America today. Substance Abuse and Mental Health Service Administration (SAMSHA), an office of the U.S. Department of Health and Human Services (HHS) (2000b), estimates that 14.5 million Americans age twelve and older are classified with dependence on or abuse of either alcohol or illicit drugs. This amounts to 6.5% of the total population. Of this number, 1.9 million Americans were classified with dependence on or abuse of both alcohol and illicit drugs (0.9% of the population). An estimated 2.4 million Americans were dependent on or abused illicit drugs but not alcohol (1.1% of the total population), whereas an estimated 10.2 million Americans were dependent on or abused alcohol but not illicit drugs (4.6% of the population). *Alcohol Alert,* a publication of the National Institute of Alcohol Abuse and Alcoholism (2000), reports that more than 700,000 Americans receive alcoholism treatment, alone, on any given day. Using HHS data, Kann (2001), writes,

> Alcohol and other drug use are among our nation's most pervasive health and social concerns, contributing to leading causes of death such as motor vehicle crashes, other injuries, homicide, suicide, cancer, and HIV infection and AIDS (U.S. Department of Health and Human Services, 2000). In addition, alcohol and other drug use contribute to social problems such as crime, lost workplace productivity, and lower educational achievement. Alcohol and other drug use among youth are com-

mon and contribute to health and social problems during adolescence, and are predictive of substance-related problems in adulthood. (p. 725)

Men are twice (21%) as likely as women (10%) to be heavier drinkers as measured by consumption of two or more drinks a day on average (National Council on Alcoholism and Drug Dependence, 1998). Nearly 95% of all D.W.I. cases involve men, and male alcohol-related cirrhosis of the liver is fully two and a half times the rate for that of women (Gupta, 2003). Peele (1989) indicates that studies support the notion of alcoholism as a problem mainly affecting men and suggests that when D.W.I. referrals for alcohol abuse and consumption levels are compared, that women have a third to a tenth of the drinking problems of men. When they do have a problem, women seek help sooner and more often than men.

Epperly and Moore (2000) contend that men are at much greater risk of alcohol abuse than women, with the highest rates of alcoholism occurring in men between 25 and 39 years of age. However, age is not a deterrent for risk factors in men. Fourteen percent of men over 65 are alcohol dependent as compared to 1.5% of women in the same age group, with male suicides for men over 65, six times the rate of the general population, often with alcohol and depression as coexisting conditions, according to Reuben, Yoshikawa, and Besdine (1996).

Drinking by young men is a frequent problem with binge drinking on college campuses creating a much more prevalent and damaging problem than many people realize. Hingson et al. (2002) found that alcohol consumption is linked to at least 1,400 student deaths and 500,000 unintentional injuries annually. Alcohol consumption by college students is associated with drinking and driving, diminished academic performance, and medical and legal problems. Nondrinking students and community residents also experience the consequences of alcohol consumption through increased rates of crime, traffic accidents, rapes, assaults, and property damage. More than 600,000 students are assaulted by other students who have been drinking, and 70,000 sexual assaults are related to alcohol consumption by men on college campuses (Hingson et al., 2002).

In explaining the high rates of alcoholism among male college students, Johnston, O'Malley, and Bachman (2001) report that many young men enter college with preexisting drinking problems. In a study by the authors, 30% of male twelfth graders reported heavy "episodic drinking" in high school, over 50% had been drunk, and almost 75% reported that that they had been drinking in the year preceding college.

DIAGNOSTIC MARKERS OF SUBSTANCE ABUSE

The *DSM–IV* uses the following diagnostic markers to determine whether substance use is abusive—A dysfunctional use of substances causing impairment or distress within a twelve-month period as determined by one of the following: (a) frequent use of substances that interfere with functioning and the fulfillment of responsibilities at home, work, school, and so forth; (b) use of substances that impair functioning in dangerous situations such as driving or use of machines; (c) use of substances that may lead to arrest for unlawful behaviors; and (d) substance use that seriously interferes with relations, marriage, childrearing and other interpersonal responsibilities (American Psychiatric Association, 1994). Substance abuse may lead to slurred speech, lack of coordination, unsteady gait, memory loss, fatigue and depression, feelings of euphoria, and lack of social inhibitions (APA, 1994).

Short Tests

Miller (2001) reports that two simple questions asked of substance abusers have an 80% chance of diagnosing substance abuse: "In the past year, have you ever drunk or used drugs more than you meant to?" and, "Have you felt you wanted or needed to cut down on your drinking or drug abuse in the past year?" Miller reports that this simple approach has been found to be an effective diagnostic tool in three controlled studies using random samples and laboratory tests for alcohol and drugs in the bloodstream following interviews.

Stewart and Richards (2000) and Bisson, Nadeau, and Demers (1999) suggest that four questions from the CAGE Questionnaire are predictive of alcohol abuse. CAGE stands for Cut, Annoyed, Guilty, and Eye-Opener (see the questions that follow). Because many people deny their alcoholism, asking questions in an open, direct, and nonjudgmental way may elicit the best results. The four questions are as follows:

> 1) **Cut:** Have you ever felt you should cut down on your drinking? 2) **Annoyed:** Have people annoyed you by criticizing your drinking? 3) **Guilty:** Have you ever felt guilty about your drinking? 4) **Eye-Opener:** Have you ever had a drink first thing in the morning (Eye-opener) to steady your nerves or get rid of a hangover? (Bisson et al., 1999, p. 717)

Stewart and Richards (2000) note that, "A patient who answers yes to two or more of these questions probably abuses alcohol; a patient who answers yes to one question should be screened further" (p. 56). Not everyone is as certain that the CAGE instrument, developed in the late 1970s to distinguish heavy from moderate drinkers, is an effective diagnostic tool. Bisson et al. (1999) write the following:

> If the CAGE had any utility as an instrument informing on the prevalence or incidence of heavy drinking within the population, it would have discriminated between heavy and non-heavy drinkers. Our results show that this is not the case. (p. 720)

The authors think the instrument is less than accurate because many people have a new awareness of alcoholism and have tried to do something to limit their alcohol use. Furthermore, the instrument asks about last year's alcohol consumption and because the participant may have changed his or her alcohol-related behavior, the answers may be misleading. Alcohol consumption has also decreased somewhat nationally. Consequently, a direct series of questions answered truthfully may fail to distinguish those who drink heavily from those who drink moderately because the responses of both groups may tend to be the same. This finding supports the notion that short questions may not be accurate in diagnosing substance abuse and that diagnosis requires an in-depth social, emotional, and medical history in which the guidelines of the *DSM–IV* provide direction for the types of historical and medical issues for which one might look. Perhaps this lack of an in-depth history is why Backer and Walton-Moss (2001) found that fully 20% to 25% of all patients with alcohol-related problems were treated medically for the symptoms of alcoholism rather than for the condition itself, and that a diagnosis of alcohol abuse was never made in almost one-fourth of all alcoholics seen for medical treatment.

Psychosocial Histories

Another problem when a complete psychosocial history is lacking is that services are often withheld from elderly patients with substance abuse problems. Pennington, Butler, and Eagger (2000) report that older patients referred to a psychiatric service with a diagnosis of alcohol abuse failed to receive the clinical assessment recommended by the American Geriatrics Society. Rather than being treated for alcoholism as a primary problem, most elderly clients abusing alcohol (four out of five, most of whom are men) were treated for depression or associated medical problems. The authors believe that the reason elderly patients are not adequately screened for alcohol abuse is that, "Some health professionals harbor a misguided belief that older people should not be advised to give up established habits or they may be embarrassed to ask older patients personal questions about alcohol use" (Butler & Eagger, 2000, p. 183), although those behaviors may be self-injurious and possibly dangerous to others.

Writing about female alcohol abuse, Backer and Walton-Moss (2001) note the following gender differences:

> Unlike men, women commonly seek help for alcoholism from primary care clinicians. Further, the development and progression of alcoholism is different in women than in men. Women with alcohol problems have higher rates of dual diagnoses, childhood sexual abuse, panic and phobia disorders, eating disorders, posttraumatic stress disorder, and victimization. Early diagnosis, brief interventions, and referral are critical to the treatment of alcoholism in women. (p. 13)

The authors point out the following differences in the diagnostic markers for male and female alcoholics: Because women metabolize alcohol differently than men, they tend to show signs of becoming intoxicated at a later age than men (26.5 vs. 22.7), experience their first signs of a recognition of alcohol abuse later (27.5 vs. 25), and have diminished control over their drinking later in life (29.8 vs. 27.2). The mortality rate for female alcoholics is 50% to 100% higher than it is for men. Liver damage occurs in women in a shorter period of time and with lower amounts of intake of alcohol. Backer and Walton-Moss (2001) also report that, "Female alcoholics have a higher mortality rate from alcoholism than men as a result of suicide, alcohol-related accidents, circulatory disorders, and cirrhosis of the liver" (p. 15). Use of alcohol by women in adolescence is almost equal to that of male adolescents. The authors report that although men use alcohol to socialize, women use it to cope with negative moods and are likely to use alcohol in response to specific stressors in their lives.

Kuperman et al. (2001) report several risk factors for male adolescent alcoholism that include home problems, personal behavioral problems, and early use of alcohol. Home problems are considered problems with parental use and acceptance of alcohol and drugs, problems with family bonding and family conflict, ease in obtaining alcohol, a high level of peer use of alcohol, and positive peer attitudes toward alcohol and drug use. Personal behavioral problems include rebellious behavior against parents, gaining peer acceptance by drinking and other risky behaviors meant to impress peers, and self-treatment through the use of alcohol and drugs for mental health or academic problems. Grant and Dawson (1997) report that early use of alcohol is a very strong predictor of lifelong alcoholism. They note that 40% of young adults ages 18 to 29, who began drinking before the age of 15, were considered to be alcohol-dependent as compared to roughly 10% who began drinking after the age of 19. Although Kuperman et al. (2001) suggest that these three domains are predictive of alcoholism, they also note that no one domain, by itself, can predict a diagnosis of alcoholism. In their study, all three domains were evident in adolescents who did not develop alcohol and drug problems and are idiosyncratic of a society in which many adolescents are rebellious and partake in risky behaviors. Nonetheless, the wise clinician will be aware that early and frequent use of alcohol has a fairly high probability of leading to prolonged alcohol use and will consider it as a screening and treatment issue.

Related Medical Problems

Stewart and Richards (2000) suggest that a number of male medical problems have their origins in substance abuse and may be indications of heavy alcohol and drug use. Many accident-related head injuries and spinal separations may be caused by substance abuse. Because heavy drinkers often fail to eat, they may have nutritional deficiencies that result in psychotic-appearing symptoms including abnormal eye movements, disorganization, and forgetfulness. Stomach disorders, liver damage, and severe heartburn may have their origins in heavy drinking because alcohol destroys the stomach's mucosal lining. Fifteen percent of all heavy drinkers develop cirrhosis of the liver and many develop pancreatitis. Weight loss, pneumonia, muscle loss because of malnutrition, and oral cancer have all been associated with heavy drinking. The authors note that substance abusers are poor candidates for surgery. Anesthesia and pain medication can delay alcohol withdrawal for up to five days postoperatively:

> Withdrawal symptoms can cause agitation and uncooperativeness and can mask signs and symptoms of other postoperative complications. Patients who abuse alcohol are at a higher risk for postoperative complications such as excessive bleeding, infection, heart failure, and pneumonia. (Stewart & Richards, 2000, p. 58)

Stewart and Richards (2000, p. 59) provide the following blood alcohol levels as measures of the impact of alcohol in screening for abuse:

- 0.05% (equivalent to one or two drinks in an average-sized person)— impaired judgment, reduced alertness, loss of inhibitions, euphoria.
- 0.10%—slower reaction times, decreased caution in risk taking behavior, impaired fine-motor control. Legal evidence of intoxication in most states starts at 0.10%.
- 0.15%—significant and consistent losses in reaction times.
- 0.20%—function of entire motor area of brain measurably depressed, causing staggering. The individual may be easily angered or emotional.

- 0.25%—severe sensory and motor impairment.
- 0.30%—confusion, stupor.
- 0.35%—surgical anesthesia.
- 0.40%—respiratory depression, lethal in about half of the population.
- 0.50%—death from respiratory depression.

THE EFFECTIVENESS OF TREATING MALE SUBSTANCE ABUSERS

Short-Term Treatment

Herman (2000) believes that individual psychotherapy can be helpful in treating male substance abusers and suggests five situations where therapy is indicated: (a) as an appropriate introduction to treatment; (b) as a way of helping mildly or moderately dependent drug abusers; (c) when there are clear signs of emotional problems such as severe depression because these problems will interfere with the substance abuse treatment; (d) when clients progressing in twelve-step programs begin to experience emerging feelings of guilt, shame, and grief; and (e) when a client's disturbed interpersonal functioning continues after a long period of sustained abstinence, therapy might help prevent a relapse.

One of the most frequently discussed treatment approaches to addiction in the literature is brief counseling following an accident requiring an emergency room contact. Bien, Miller, and Tonigan (1993) reviewed 32 studies of brief interventions with alcohol abusers and found that, on the average, brief counseling reduced alcohol use by 30%. In a study of brief intervention with alcohol abusers, Chang, Wilkins-Haug, Berman, and Goetz (1999) found that both the treatment and control groups significantly reduced their alcohol use. The difference between the two groups in the reduction of their alcohol abuse was minimal. In a study of 175 Mexican Americans who were abusing alcohol, Burge et al. (1997) report that treated and untreated groups improved significantly over time, raising questions about the efficacy of treatment versus natural recovery. In an evaluation of a larger report by *Consumer Reports* on the effectiveness of psychotherapy, Seligman (1995) notes that, "Alcoholics Anonymous (AA) did especially well, ... significantly bettering mental health professionals [in the treatment of alcohol and drug related problems]" (p. 10).

Bien et al. (1993) found that two or three ten- to fifteen-minute counseling sessions are often as effective as more extensive interventions with older alcohol abusers. The sessions include motivation-for-change strategies, education, assessment of the severity of the problem, direct feedback, contracting and goal setting, behavioral modification techniques, and the use of written materials such as self-help manuals. Brief interventions have been shown to be effective in reducing alcohol consumption, binge drinking, and the frequency of excessive drinking in problem drinkers, according to Fleming, Barry, Manwell, Johnson, and London (1997). Completion rates using brief interventions are better for elder-specific alcohol programs than for mixed-age programs (Atkinson, 1995), and late-onset alcoholics are also more likely to complete treatment and have somewhat better outcomes using brief interventions (Liberto & Oslin, 1995).

Miller and Sanchez (1994) summarize the key components of brief intervention using the acronym FRAMES: feedback, responsibility, advice, menu of strategies, empathy, and self-efficacy:

1 Feedback—This includes the patient's risk for alcohol problems, his or her reasons for drinking, the role of alcohol in the patients' life, and the consequences of drinking.

2. Responsibility—Includes strategies to help patients understand the need to remain healthy, independent, and financially secure. This is particularly important when working with older clients and clients with health problems and disabilities.

3. Advice—Includes direct feedback and suggestions to clients to help them cope with their drinking problems and other life situations that may contribute to alcohol abuse.

4. Menu—List of strategies to reduce drinking and to cope with such high-risk male situations as loneliness, boredom, family problems, and lack of social opportunities.

5. Empathy—Bien et al. (1993) strongly emphasize the need for a warm, empathic and understanding style of treatment. Miller and Rollnick (1991) found that an empathetic counseling style produced

a 77% reduction in patient drinking as compared with a 55% reduction when a confrontational approach was used.

6. Self-efficacy—Strategies to help clients rely on their inner resources to make a change in their drinking behavior. Inner resources may include positive points of view about themselves, helping others, staying busy, and good problem-solving coping skills.

Some additional aspects of brief interventions suggested by Menninger (2002) are as follows: drinking agreements in the form of agreed-on drinking limits that are signed by the patient and the practitioner, ongoing follow-up and support, and appropriate timing of the intervention to the patient's readiness to change. Completion rates for elder-specific alcohol treatment programs are modestly better than for mixed-age programs (Atkinson, 1995). Late-onset alcoholics are also more likely to complete treatment and have somewhat better outcomes (Liberto & Oslin, 1995). Alcoholics Anonymous (AA) may be helpful, particularly AA groups oriented toward the elderly.

Babor and Higgins-Biddle (2000) discuss the use of brief interventions, a set of treatment approaches used with people involved in "risky drinking," but who are not classified as alcohol dependent. Brief interventions are usually limited to three to five sessions of counseling and education. The intent of brief interventions is to prevent the onset of more serious alcohol-related problems. According to Babor and Higgins-Biddle

> Most programs are instructional and motivational, designed to address the specific behavior of drinking with information, feedback, health education, skill-building, and practical advice, rather than with psychotherapy or other specialized treatment techniques. (p. 676)

Higgins-Biddle, Babor, Mullahy, Daniels, and Mcree (1997) analyzed fourteen random studies of brief interventions that included more than 20,000 risky drinkers. They report a net reduction in drinking of 21% for men and 8% for women. To improve the effectiveness of short-term interventions, Babor and Higgins-Biddle (2000) encourage the use of early identification of problem drinking, life-health monitoring by health and mental health professionals, and risk counseling that includes screening and brief intervention to inform and motivate potential alcohol abusers of the risk of serious alcohol dependence and to help change their alcohol use.

Fleming and Manwell (1998) report that people with alcohol-related problems often receive counseling from primary care physicians or nursing staff in five or fewer standard office visits. The counseling consists of rational information about the negative impact of alcohol use as well as practical advice regarding ways of reducing alcohol dependence and the availability of community resources. Gentilello, Donovan, Dunn, and Rivara (1995) report that 25% to 40% (mostly men) of the trauma patients seen in emergency rooms may be alcohol dependent. The authors found that a single motivational interview, at or near the time of discharge, reduced drinking levels and readmission for trauma during six months of follow-up. Monti et al. (1999) conducted a similar study with 18- to 19-year-olds admitted to an emergency room with alcohol-related injuries. After six months, all participants had decreased their alcohol consumption, however, "the group receiving brief intervention had a significantly lower incidence of drinking and driving, traffic violations, alcohol-related injuries, and alcohol-related problems" (Monti et al., 1999, p. 3).

Lu and McGuire (2002) studied the effectiveness of out-patient treatment with substance abusing clients and came to the following conclusions: (a) the more severe the drug use problem before treatment was initiated, the less likely clients were to discontinue drug use during treatment when compared to other users; (b) clients reporting no substance abuse three months before admission were more likely to maintain abstinence than those who reported abstinence only in the past one month; (c) heroin users were very unlikely to sustain abstinence during treatment, whereas marijuana users were less likely to sustain abstinence during treatment than alcohol users; (d) clients with "psychiatric problems" were more likely to use drugs during treatment than clients without psychiatric problems; (e) clients with legal problems related to their substance abuse had reduced chances of improving during the treatment; (f) clients who had multiple prior treatments for substance abuse were less likely to remain abstinent during and after treatment; (g) more educated clients were more likely to sustain abstinence after treatment; and (h) clients treated in urban agencies were less likely to maintain abstinence than those treated in rural agencies.

Longer-Term Treatments

Walitzer, Dermen, and Connors (1999) report that treatment attrition is such a pervasive problem in programs offering long-term treatment services that it affects our ability to determine treatment effectiveness. Bakeland and Lundwall (1975) report dropout rates for inpatient treatment programs of 28% and that 52% and 75% of the outpatient alcoholic patients in their study dropped out of treatment before their fourth session. Leigh, Osborne, and Cleland (1984) indicate that of 172 alcoholism outpatients studied, 15% failed to attend their initial appointment, 28% attended only a session or two, and 19% attended only three to five times. In studying 117 alcoholism clinic admissions, Rees (1986) found that 35% of the clients failed to return after their initial visit and that another 18% terminated treatment within 30 days.

To reduce the amount of attrition in alcohol treatment programs, Walitzer, Dermen, and Connors (1999) randomly assigned 126 clients entering an alcohol treatment program to one of three groups to prepare them for the treatment program: a role induction session, a motivational interview session, or a no-preparatory session control group. They found that clients assigned to the motivational interview "attended more treatment sessions and had fewer heavy drinking days during and 12 months after treatment relative to control group" (p. 1161). Clients assigned to the motivational interview also were abstinent more days during treatment and in the first three months following treatment than the control group, but the difference, unfortunately, did not last for the remaining nine months of follow-up. Clients assigned to the role induction group did no better than the control group in any of the variables studied.

In describing the motivational interview, Walitzer, Dermen, and Connors (1999) indicate that it consists of the following:

(a) Eliciting self-motivational statements; (b) reflective, empathic listening; (c) inquiring about the client's feelings, ideas, concerns, and plans;

(d) affirming the client in a way that acknowledges the client's serious consideration of and steps toward change; (e) deflecting resistance in a manner that takes into account the link between therapist behavior and client resistance; (f) reframing client statements as appropriate; and (g) summarizing. (p. 136)

Kirchner, Booth, Owen, Lancaster, and Smith (2000) considered the factors related to entry into alcohol treatment programs following a diagnosis of alcoholism. They found that many male patients who might benefit from treatment were not referred by their medical providers because of a belief that treatment wasn't effective, although a number of

well-designed and methodologically sound studies have repeatedly shown that treatment for alcohol related disorders can be effective not only for reducing the consumption of alcohol but also for improving the patient's overall level of functioning. (p. 339)

The authors also report that improved detection of alcoholism, the first step in the provision of services, is often negatively influenced by a number of factors that include younger age, non-White ethnicity, the severity of the alcohol use, lower socioeconomic status, and male gender. Drug and alcohol use to self-medicate for psychiatric disorders is also a key predictor of detection as are alcohol-related medical problems such as liver disorders, high blood pressure, and adult onset diabetes. Herman (2000) reports that the reasons substance abusers enter treatment are usually external in nature and include legal problems with drug use (e.g., license suspension because of drunk driving), marital problems, work-related problems, medical complications caused by drug and alcohol abuse, problems with depression and anxiety that lead to self-medicating with alcohol and drugs, and referral by mental health professionals (a major reason women enter treatment programs, but not men).

Treatment Strategies

Herman (2000) believes that the primary strategy in the treatment of substance abuse is to initially achieve abstinence. Once abstinence is achieved, the substance abuser can begin to address relationship problems that might interfere with social and emotional functioning. Herman (2000) also believes that the key to treatment is to match the client with the type of treatment most likely to help. He suggests that the following phases exist in the treatment of substance abuse:

Phase 1: Abstinence.

Phase 2: Teaching the client coping skills to help prevent a relapse through cognitive-behavioral techniques that help clients manage stressful situations likely to trigger substance abuse. These may include recognizing cues that lead to substance abuse, managing external cues, avoiding peers who are likely to continue to abuse substances and encourage the client to do the same, and alternative behaviors that help the client avoid drug use.

Phase 3: Because the underlying problems that contribute to substance abuse are often deeply internalized feeling of low self-worth, depression, and self-loathing, therapy should help the client deal with internalized pathologies that are likely to lead to relapse. The therapies that seem most effective in doing this are cognitive-behavioral therapies, the strengths approach, and affective therapies, including Gestalt therapy. Herman (2000) suggests the use of psychodynamic therapy but research evidence on the effectiveness of this form of treatment is not overly promising.

In a review of 30 years of research, the National Institute on Drug Abuse (1999) reports that the following are necessary elements of effective treatment of substance abuse:

1) Treatment involves matching the patient to the correct treatment modality; 2) treatment is readily accessible; 3) treatment attends to the ancillary needs of patient; 4) treatment is based on a comprehensive and regularly updated treatment plan; 5) treatment involves the patient remaining in treatment for an adequate period of time; 6) treatment assures the patient of receiving a sufficient amount of counseling; 7) treatment includes adjunctive pharmacotherapy, if necessary; 8) treatment is provided for coexisting mental disorders, if present; 9) treatment is provided beyond detoxification; 10) treatment accommodates patients that are mandated into treatment; 11) the treatment staff mon-

itors the patient's drug use regularly; 12) an assessment is made for human immunodeficiency virus/acquired immune deficiency syndrome
(HIV/AIDS) and other infectious diseases; 13) multiple treatment episodes are provided for, if necessary. (Lennox & Mansfield, 2001, p. 169)

Other factors found to provide best evidence of treatment effectiveness
are suggested by Dahlgren and Willander (1989) who compared women-
only and mixed-gender treatment groups. Clients in the women-only
group remained in treatment longer, had higher completion rates, and
improved biopsychosocial rates compared with women who were in
mixed-gender programs. Burtscheidt, Wolwer, and Schwartz (2002)
studied the treatment effects of long-term treatment by comparing non-
specific supportive therapy with two different forms of behavioral therapy (coping skills training and cognitive behavioral therapy). One
hundred and twenty patients were randomly assigned to each of the three
therapy approaches and were seen in treatment for 26 weeks with a follow-up period of 2 years. Patients receiving behavioral therapy showed
consistently higher abstinence rates. Differences in treatment effectiveness between the two behavioral therapies could not be established. The
study also established that cognitively-impaired and severely personality-
disordered clients had less benefit from any of the therapies than clients
not fitting into these two categories of dysfunction. The authors conclude
that behavioral treatment had the best long-term effects and met high client acceptance, but more needs to be done to develop effective behavioral
therapies for clients who abuse substances.

Natural Recovery

Granfield and Cloud (1996) estimate that as many as 90% of all problem
drinkers never enter treatment and that many suspend problematic use
of alcohol without any form of treatment (Hingson, Scotch, Day, &
Culbert, 1980; Roizen, Cahalan, Lambert, Wiebel, & Shanks, 1978; Stall
& Biernacki, 1989). Sobell, Sobell, Toneatto, and Leo (1993) report that
82% of the alcoholics they studied who terminated their addiction did
so by using natural recovery methods that excluded the use of a professional. In another example of the use of natural recovery techniques,

Granfield and Cloud found that most ex-smokers discontinued their tobacco use without treatment (Peele, 1989), although many addicted substance abusers "mature-out" of a variety of addictions, including heavy drinking and narcotics use (Snow, 1973; Winick, 1962). Biernacki (1986) reports that addicts who naturally stop their addictions use a range of strategies which include breaking off relationships with drug users, removing themselves from drug-using environments (Stall & Biernacki, 1986), building new structures in their lives (Peele, 1989), and using friends and family to provide support for discontinuing their substance abuse (Biernacki, 1986). Trice and Roman (1970) suggest that self-help groups with substance abusing clients are particularly helpful because they tend to reduce personal responsibility with its related guilt and help build and maintain a support network that assists in continuing the changed behavior.

Granfield and Cloud (1996) studied middle-class alcoholics who used natural recovery alone without professional help or self-help groups. Many of the participants in their study felt that the "ideological" base of self-help programs were inconsistent with their own philosophies of life. For example, many felt that some self-help groups for substance abusers were overly religious whereas other self-help groups believed in alcoholism as a lifetime struggle consistent with a belief in the disease model. The participants in the study by Granfield and Cloud (1996) also felt that some self-help groups encouraged dependence and that associating with other alcoholics would probably make recovery more difficult. In summarizing their findings, Granfield and Cloud (1996) report that:

> Many [research subjects] expressed strong opposition to the suggestion that they were powerless over their addictions. Such an ideology, they explained, not only was counterproductive but was also extremely demeaning. These respondents saw themselves as efficacious people who often prided themselves on their past accomplishments. They viewed themselves as being individualists and strong-willed. One respondent, for instance, explained that "such programs encourage powerlessness" and that she would rather "trust her own instincts than the instincts of others." (p. 51)

To further underscore the significance of natural healing, Waldorf, Reinarman, and Murphy (1991) found that many addicted people with supportive elements in their lives (a job, family, and other close emotional supports) were able to "walk away" from their very heavy use of cocaine. The authors suggest that the "social context" of a drug user's life may positively influence their ability to discontinue drug use. Granfield and Cloud (1996) note that many of the respondents in their sample had a great deal to lose if they continued their substance abuse.

> The respondents in our sample had relatively stable lives: they had jobs, supportive families, high school and college credentials, and other social supports that gave them reasons to alter their drug-taking behavior. Having much to lose gave our respondents incentives to transform their lives. However, when there is little to lose from heavy alcohol or drug use, there may be little to gain by quitting. (p. 55)

Humphreys (1998) studied the effectiveness of self-help groups with substance abusers by comparing two groups: one receiving inpatient care for substance abuse, and the other attending self-help groups for substance abuse. At the conclusion of the study, the average participant assigned to a self-help group (AA) had used $8,840 in alcohol-related health care resources as compared to $10,040 for the inpatient treatment participants. In a follow-up study, Humphreys compared outpatient services to self-help groups for the treatment of substance abuse. The clients in the self-help group had decreased alcohol consumption by 70% over three years and consumed 45% less health care services (about $1,800 less per person). Humphreys argues that

> From a cost-conscious point of view, self-help groups should be the first option evaluated when an addicted individual makes initial contact with professional services (e.g., in a primary care appointment or a clinical assessment at a substance abuse agency or employee assistance program). (p. 16)

CASE EXAMPLE: A BRIEF INTERVENTION
AFTER AN ALCOHOL-RELATED CAR ACCIDENT

This case first appeared in a volume I wrote on evidence-based practice (Glicken, 2005). The reader may want to consult that volume for a discussion of evidence-based practice as a model for work with men.

THE CASE

Jim Larson is a seventeen-year-old high school student who was taken to the emergency room after his car spun out of control and hit an embankment. Three passengers in the car were slightly injured. Jim and his friends had been drinking "Ever Clear," a 180% proof alcoholic beverage they purchased through an older friend. All four friends were highly intoxicated and had walked a block and a half from a party they were attending to their car wearing T-shirts in 40-degree below-zero weather. Jim sustained minor injuries. After he became sober enough to recognize the seriousness of the accident and that his blood alcohol level was in excess of .25%, three times the allowed drinking and driving level of .08%, he became antagonistic and withdrawn. His parents rushed to the hospital and were very concerned about Jim's behavior. His drinking was unknown to them, although Jim had begun drinking at age ten and had been regularly becoming intoxicated at weekend parties by age thirteen. Jim thought he was doing social drinking and felt that he was no different than his other friends. The accident, however, seemed to be a wake-up call to do something about his risky drinking.

A social worker and nurse met with Jim and his parents three times over the course of a two-day stay in the hospital. They gave out information about the health impact of drinking and did a screening test to determine Jim's level of abusive drinking. They concluded that Jim was at high risk of becoming an alcoholic because his drinking impaired his judgment, affected his grades, and was thought to be responsible for high blood sugar readings consistent with early onset diabetes and moderately high blood pressure. A psychosocial history taken by the social worker revealed that Jim had begun experimenting with alcohol at age ten and was using it at home and with friends from age thirteen on. He was drinking more than a quart of alcohol a week, some of it very high in alcohol content. Jim's driver's license was revoked by the court, and, on the basis of the report made by the emergency room personnel, Jim was sent for mandatory alcohol counseling.

Jim is a reluctant client. He discounts his drinking problem claiming that he drinks no more than his friends and that were it not for the accident, he would not be in counseling because he was not having any serious problems in his life. That isn't altogether true, however. With an IQ of over 130, Jim's grades are mostly in the "D" range. He misses classes on a regular basis and often misses class in the mornings because of hangovers. His parents are having marital and financial problems and fail to supervise Jim closely. Furthermore, Jim has been fantasizing about harming his friends whom he thinks have been disloyal to him for reasons he can't validate. "Just a feeling, ya know?" he told the therapist. Was the accident really an accident? "Sure," Jim says, "what else?" His therapist isn't so certain. He has hints of Jim's antagonism toward other students and has heard Jim talk about dreams in which Jim harms others. Jim spends a great deal of time on the Internet and has assumed various identities, many of them harboring antisocial and violent intentions. The therapist believes that Jim is a walking time bomb of emotional distress and that his alcoholism, although robust, is just one way of self-medicating himself for feelings of isolation, low self-esteem, and rejection by parents and classmates.

After months of treatment during which time Jim would often sit in silence and stare at the therapist, he has begun to talk about his feelings and admits that he has continued drinking heavily. He also drives, although his license has been suspended. He is full of self-hate and thinks that he is doomed to die soon. He feels powerful when he drinks, he told the therapist, and loves the peaceful feeling that comes over him as he gets drunk. Like his parents, he romanticizes his drinking and can hardly wait to have his first drink. Sometimes he drinks when he wakes up and often drinks rather than eat. He is aware that this cycle of drinking to feel better about himself can only lead to serious life problems, but doesn't think he is capable of stopping.

Jim's therapist asked Jim to help him do an Internet search to find the best approach to help Jim with his drinking problem. It seemed like a silly request to Jim because the therapist was supposed to be the expert, but Jim was intrigued and did as he was asked. When he next met with the therapist, Jim had printed out a number of articles suggesting ways of coping with adolescent alcoholism that seemed reasonable to him and to the therapist. From the work of Kuperman et al. (2001), they agreed that Jim had a number of problems that should be dealt with at home, with friends, and with his alcohol abuse. They decided that a cognitive-behavioral approach would work best coupled with homework assignments and cognitive restructuring as additional aspects of the treatment. Jim was intrigued with an article he found on the strengths approach and showed the therapist an article by Moxley and Olivia (2001) that they both found quite useful. Another article on self-help groups by Humphreys (1998) convinced them that a self-help group for adolescent alcohol abusers might be helpful. Finally, Jim brought up the issue of working with his parents and it was decided that the family would be seen together to identify some of the problems they were having and to develop better communication with Jim.

Jim has been in treatment for over a year. He is applying himself in school and has begun thinking about college. His drinking has modified itself somewhat. Although he still drinks too much at times, he won't drive when he is drinking or engage in risky behavior. He feels much less angry and has developed new friendships with peers who don't drink or use drugs. The changes seem very substantial, but it's much too early to know if the alcoholism is likely to display itself when he deals with additional life stressors. Jim is unsure and says that

> Yeah, it's all helping me but my head isn't always on straight and sometimes I do dumb stuff. I'm more aware of it now but I still do it. I'm getting along with my folks a lot better and my new friends are real friends, not drinking buddies. I don't know. I looked at some studies on the Internet and it looks like I have a pretty good chance

of becoming an alcoholic. I like booze. It makes me feel good. That's not a good sign, is it? And I'm still pretty mad about a lot of things. I spend a lot of time on the Internet in chat rooms and it's pretty bizarre, sometimes, the things I say. But yeah, I know I'm better. I just hope it keeps up.

Jim's therapist added the following:

Jim has a good handle on himself. I wouldn't argue with anything he said. He has lots of potential but he also has enough problems to make me unwilling to predict the future. What I will say is that he works hard, is cooperative, and seems to be trying to work on some long standing issues with his family and his perception of himself. I think that addictions are transitory and you never know when his desire to drink will overwhelm his desire not to. The self-help group he's in keeps close tabs on his drinking, and his new friends are a help. I'd caution anyone who works with adolescents not to expect too much from treatment. I do want to applaud the professionals he worked with in the hospital. Even though the treatment was brief, it made a lasting impact on Jim to hear that he was considered an alcoholic and it did bring him into treatment. That's exactly what you hope for in serious alcoholics who are in denial.

SUMMARY

In this chapter on working with male substance abusers, research findings are reported that suggest disagreement about the effectiveness of certain types of treatment, particularly very brief treatment with high-risk abusers. Promising research on natural recovery and self-help groups suggests that treatment effectiveness may be positive with these two types of treatment. A case example is provided that shows the use of short-term intervention followed by longer-term treatment with a young male substance abuser initially seen in an emergency room following an accident.

Chapter 17

Working With Older Adult Male Clients

Some of the material found in this chapter was first presented in Glicken (2004, 2005). The reader may want to consult those sources for additional information about aging, terminal illness, and bereavement.

Large numbers of anxious and depressed older adult males often go undiagnosed and untreated because underlying symptoms of anxiety and depression are thought to be physical in nature and professionals frequently believe that older men are even less motivated for therapy than their younger male counterparts. This often leaves many older men trying to cope with serious emotional problems without adequate help. The numbers of older men dealing with anxiety and depression is considerable and growing as the number of older men increases in America. Health problems, loss of loved ones, financial insecurities, lack of a support group, a growing sense of isolation, and a lack of worth are common problems among older men that often lead to serious symptoms of anxiety and depression, problems that often coexist. This is particularly true among traditional older men who have lost status at work or have retired only to find that they have little in the day to keep them occupied. Many of these men have never developed hobbies, support groups, taken care of their health, or saved enough money to live the good lives they envisioned as a reward for years of hard work. And sadly, many have alienated children who neither want to see them nor, when they develop serious health and emotional problems, to help them. Work no longer occupies their time and if it does, many older men are on the downside of careers that long ago stopped giving them the support and positive regard for which all workers long. This combination of isolation, loss of status, and loneliness often makes aging very difficult for men.

ANXIETY IN OLDER MALE ADULTS

The prevalence of anxiety disorders has usually been thought to decrease with age, but recent findings suggest that generalized anxiety is actually a more common problem among the elderly than depression. A study reported by Beekman et al. (1998) found anxiety to affect 7.3% of an elderly population. However, Smith, Sherrill, and Celenda (1995) found that elderly women have almost three times the rates of anxiety, panic disorder, and obsessive compulsive disorder than elderly men, a rate that may be influenced more by older men not seeing their physicians and admitting anxiety problems than by gender differences. Lang and Stein (2001) estimate that the total number of older Americans suffering from anxiety could be in excess of ten percent. Since many anxious elderly people, particularly men, do not meet the criteria for anxiety found in a number of research studies, the prevalence of anxiety-related problems in the elderly could be as high as eighteen percent and constitutes the most common psychiatric symptom for older adults (Lang & Stein, 2001). Anxiety and depression among older adults frequently coexist with typical physical manifestations, including chest pains, heart palpitations, night sweats, shortness of breath, essential hypertension, headaches, and generalized pain. Because physicians often fail to diagnose underlying symptoms of anxiety and depression in older men, the emotional component of the symptoms are frequently not dealt with. Definitions and descriptions of anxiety used to diagnosis younger patients often fail to capture the unique stressors that older men deal with, or the fragile nature of life for older adults as they attempt to cope with limited finances, failing health, the death of loved ones, concerns about their own mortality, and a sense of uselessness and hopelessness because their roles as adults have been dramatically altered with age and retirement.

Because anxiety in older men may have a physical base or may realistically be connected to concerns about health, Kogan, Edelstein, and McKee (2000) provide some guidelines for distinguishing an anxiety disorder with an emotional cause in older men from anxiety related to physical problems. A physical cause is more likely if the onset of anxiety comes suddenly, the symptoms fluctuate in strength and duration, and if fatigue has been present before the symptoms of anxiety were felt. The authors identify the following medical problems as reasons for symptoms of anxiety that exist in much higher frequency among men: (a) medical problems that include endocrine, cardiovascular, pulmonary, or neurological disorders; and (b) the impact of certain medications, most notably, stimulants, beta-blockers, certain tranquilizers, and, of course, alcohol. An emotional cause of anxiety is more likely if the symptoms have lasted two or more years with little change in severity and if the person has other emotional symptoms. However, anxiety may cycle on and off, or a lower level of generalized anxiety may be present that causes the elderly client a great deal of discomfort. Obsessive concerns about financial issues and health are common and realistic worries that trouble older men. The concerns may be situational, or they may be constant but not serious enough to lead to a diagnosis of anxiety; nonetheless, they cause the client unhappiness and may actually lead to physical problems, including high blood pressure, cardiovascular problems, sleep disorders, and an increased use of alcohol and over-the-counter medications to lessen symptoms of anxiety.

TREATING ANXIETY IN AN OLDER MALE POPULATION

Beck and Stanley (1997) and Stanley and Novy (2000) report positive results with anxious older men using cognitive- behavioral therapy and relaxation training. Benefits for older clients experiencing anxiety appear as positive as they are with younger clients. Smith et al. (1995) found that older adults respond well to psychotherapy for anxiety, "especially if it supports their religious beliefs and encourages life review that helps to resolve both hidden and obvious conflicts associated with specific events in the patient's life history" (p. 6). The authors recommend medications only after all options have been considered. Most anxiety problems are treated with benzodiazepines and have only a "marginal efficacy for chronic anxiety and are especially bad for older adults because the body accumulates the drug and may produce excess sedation, diminished sexual desire, worsening of dementing illness, and a reduction in the general level of energy" (Smith et al., 1995, p. 6). The authors also warn that Prozac may actually cause anxiety as a side effect and recommend pinpointing the cause of the anxiety problem before considering the use of medications.

Although the benefits of cognitive-behavioral approaches seem positive, Lang and Stein (2001) recommend that treatment of anxiety in older male adults should be tailored to the individual needs and cognitive abilities of the client. Many older male clients resent advice given by professionals younger than they are. They may find relaxation approaches inappropriate or childish. Systematic desensitization may be seen as unrelated to their situation or to the origins of their anxiety. And they may view changes in the way they are told to perceive life events as dangerous to their survival because long-held beliefs and behaviors have often served them well in the past. Being asked to view a situation with clarity and rationality may suggest to the older male client that workers believe they are lying about an event. Older men may discount psychological explanations for their anxiety and prefer to think that it has a physical origin. All of these cautionary suggestions should be taken into account when working with anxious older men or one runs the risk of having psychological treatments dismissed completely.

A suggestion to get better acceptance of any intervention is to give male clients reading materials to help them understand the origins of their anxiety and the approach most likely to help relieve their symptoms. Testimonials from other men might be helpful, or suggestions made by other professionals they trust could also help the client accept treatment. Keep in mind that older men may be suffering, but they also fear that accepting new ways of approaching life may actually increase their level of anxiety. However, as Lang and Stein (2001) report, there are harmful side effects to the long-term use of many antianxiety medications. Although some of the cognitive-behavioral approaches used in the treatment of anxiety may not always fit an older male adult's frame of reference, it's wise to let them know about medical treatments and the potential for harm as one way to acknowledge that medications have risks that should be considered, just as there are associated risks in doing nothing.

DEPRESSION IN OLDER MALE ADULTS

Although symptoms of depression are consistent across age groups, Wallis (2000) suggests that older men may express depression through such physical complaints as insomnia, eating disorders, and digestive problems. They may also show signs of lethargy, have less incentive to do activities they did before they became depressed, and experience symptoms of depression while denying that they are depressed. Mild and transient depression brought on by situational events usually resolve themselves in time, but moderate depression may interfere with daily life activities and can result in social withdrawal and isolation. The *DSM–IV* (American Psychiatric Association, 1994) does not distinguish depression in older adults from depression in a younger population, and the subtle as well as the overt signs of depression in the elderly are not discussed, and neither are differences in symptoms by gender. This lack of differentiation of depression makes diagnosis more problematic and is one explanation why depression is often not treated when elderly clients have coexisting medical problems. Whether the medical problem results in the depression or the depression contributes to the medical problem is difficult to determine and remains an area requiring more study. Clearly, however, older men have intrusive health and mental health issues that may cause depressed feelings and lead to changes in functioning.

Casey (1994) reports a study that found rates of suicide among adults 65 and older almost double that of the general population, with men having a much higher rate of suicide attempts and completion than women. The completion rate for suicide among older men is 1 in 4 as compared to 1 in 100 for the general population, suggesting that older men are much more likely to see suicide as a final solution rather than a cry for help. Older men who commit suicide often suffer from major depression, alcoholism, severe medical problems, and social isolation (Casey, 1994). Mills and Henretta (2001) indicate that more than 2 million of the 34 million older Americans suffer from some form of depression, yet late-life depression is often undiagnosed or underdiagnosed.

When studying the impact of natural disasters on elderly adults demonstrating predisaster indication of depression, Tyler and Hoyt (2000) found that elderly adults with high levels of social support had lower levels of depression before and after a natural disaster. Throughout this book, it has been noted that men are less likely to have social support networks than women. One could certainly assume that men are therefore less able to cope with traumatic events than women. In research on successful aging, Vaillant and Mukamal (2001) believe that predictors of longer and healthier lives can be made before the age of 50 by using the following indicators: parental social class, family cohesion, major depression, ancestral longevity, childhood temperament, and physical health at age 50. Seven variables suggesting personal control over physical and emotional health having a negative effect on length of life and overall health, include alcohol abuse, smoking, marital instability, lack of exercise, obesity, unsuccessful coping mechanisms, and lower levels of education. The authors believe that we have greater control over our health following retirement than had been previously recognized in the literature. Because men have poorer generalized health at 50, particularly when smoking, drinking, unsuccessful coping mechanisms, and overall health are considered, one can expect men to have much more difficulty with aging than women.

TREATING DEPRESSION IN AN OLDER MALE POPULATION

Cochran and Rabinowitz (2003) believe that although men are often thought to be "immune" from depressive disorders

> there is mounting evidence that many men suffer from various manifestations of depression. These manifestations are often associated with alcohol and drug abuse, interpersonal conflict, and externalizing or acting-out behavior patterns. (p. 139)

The authors believe that therapists must be sensitive to the ways in which men express depression and to the social and cultural issues that affect them. Among these issues are gender role stereotypes and work and personal problems, which often cause men to feel powerless and defeated. The authors go on to note that, "undiagnosed and untreated depression in men may be one reason why many more men than women commit suicide" (Cochran & Rabinowitz, 2003, p. 132).

Gallagher-Thompson, Hanley-Peterson, and Thompson (1990) followed older clients for two years after completion of treatment and found that 52% of the clients receiving cognitive treatment, 58% of the clients receiving behavioral treatment, and 70% of the clients receiving brief dynamic treatment, had no return of depressed symptoms two years following treatment. The authors report that these rates of improvement are consistent with a younger population of depressed clients. However, Huffman (1999) reports high rates of recurrence of depression in older adults following treatment. In participants over 70 who received psychotherapy and a placebo as an antidepressant, the recurrence rate for depression was 63% within a three-year period of time. For participants 60 to 69, the recurrence rate was 65%. Participants treated with just an antidepressant and scheduled office visits to check on progress did least well with a 90% recurrence rate for both age groups (Huffman, 1999).

Lenze et al. (2002) studied the effectiveness of interpersonal treatment in conjunction with antidepressives with elderly depressed clients. Not surprisingly, given the lack of awareness of late onset depression in elderly clients, they report the following: "To our knowledge, this is the first report concerning social functioning in a controlled randomized study of elderly patients receiving maintenance treatment for late-life depression" (p. 467). The authors found improved social adjustment attributable to combined interpersonal psychotherapy and maintenance medication. Although improvements in social functioning could not be related directly to therapy, maintenance of the gains made in social functioning seemed directly related to therapy. The most significant gains reported by the authors were in the areas of interpersonal conflict role transitions and abnormal grief.

Kennedy and Tannenbaum (2000) suggest compelling evidence that older patients experience a variety of emotional problems, including depression, anxiety, caregiver burden, and extended bereavement. The authors believe that many older clients can benefit from psychotherapeutic interventions and suggest that adjustments for clinical practice should include consideration of "sensory and cognitive" problems, the need for closer collaboration with the client's family and other care providers, and a belief by the clinician, shared with the elderly client and his or her family, that treatment will result in improved functioning and symptom reduction to offset stereotypes that elderly clients with emotional problems are untreatable or unlikely to improve. The authors suggest that work with elderly clients also requires skill with a variety of approaches, including work with couples, families, and groups. They also report that the use of pharmotherapy may produce very positive results with late-onset social and emotional problems experienced by older clients.

O'Connor (2001) notes that clients usually get better after their first episode of depression but that the relapse rate is 50%. Clients with three episodes of depression are 90% more likely to have additional episodes. O'Connor suggests that we need to accept depression as a chronic disease and that therapists must be prepared to "give hope, to reduce shame, to be mentor, coach, cheerleader, idealized object, playmate, and nurturer. In doing so, inevitably, we must challenge many of our assumptions about the use of the self in psychotherapy" (p. 508). O'Connor goes on to say:

... When patients are trying their best but their environment is not rewarding them, one obvious alternative source of reinforcement that we have near at hand is the therapist him/herself. Most depressed patients acutely desire the therapist's approval, and it is an effective therapist who gives it warmly and genuinely.... We know that we shape patients' behavior by showing interest and approval or showing boredom or condemnation. And we know that we can do this very subtly ... a smile, a nod, an indication that you recognize the patient has accomplished something difficult, an indication that you share the patient's valuation of what he/she has accomplished, an emotional mirroring of the patient's pride—these can have powerful impact on the depressed patient. (p. 522)

In discussing prolonged grieving in older clients, Kennedy and Tannenbaum (2000) suggest that older men who have suffered a loss should be "encouraged to reestablish life's routine and social rhythm, maintaining regular sleep, exercise, and meals, attending church, synagogue or senior center, and participating in volunteer organizations and family affairs" (p. 405). The authors also suggest that older men should be encouraged to confront painful memories of the lost loved one in the midst of a support group. "The ultimate goal of Bereavement Therapy," the authors write, "is to assist the patient in processing the past relationship and current loss in order to bear the future separation and maximize existing, positive relationships" (p. 405).

Although this appears to be sound advice, coping with aging can be particularly difficult for men who not only lose physical strength and find it difficult to reach out to others as they experience prolonged grief, but are also unlikely to seek treatment because they don't think it will help them. The depression of the famous author Primo Levi is instructive here (Glicken, 2004). Levi was the author of *The Periodic Table* (1995b), *If Not Now, When?* (1995a), and other books about the human spirit and the Holocaust experience. In his youth, he was imprisoned for a year at the notorious Auschwitz Concentration Camp during World War II, a subject he wrote about with great humanity and sensitivity. Many think his books about the concentration camp experience are among the best examples of man's ability to deal with incredible trauma. In his mid-60s and at the height of his recognition as a writer, Levi suffered a severe depression. He was ill with prostate problems, was finding writing increasingly difficult, and was entering a severe and unrelenting late-onset depression.

Writing about Levi's depression, the biographer Carole Angier (2002) says, "The real pit of his depression had begun. It was so bad that he had lost interest in everything and didn't want to see anyone" (p. 706). She also reports a letter written to a friend in which he said, "I am going through the worst time of my life since Auschwitz, maybe the worst time in my life because I am older and less resilient. My wife is exhausted. Forgive me for this outburst" (p. 708). And later, he called his doctor and said, "I can't go on" (p. 731). Moments after talking to his doctor, he walked outside the apartment where he had lived all of his life, stood at the railing of the staircase, perhaps paused for a moment, and then jumped five stories to his death.

Did Levi commit suicide because of his experiences in Auschwitz? Angier writes, "... Primo Levi held up a light for us ... And if he had laid down that light himself [because of his suicide], was he saying that he no longer believed in [the light], that he no longer believed in us?" (p. 726). Or was his suicide the culmination of a writer's inability to write, a serious illness, and an increasing age-related depression that many older men experience because they are unable to do many of the things they did so well before? Certainly the traumas of the concentration camps contribute to feelings of depression in many Holocaust survivors. But this experience of a famous author taking his life, someone with many social contacts and a rich personal life, should give us pause when we think about the lives of older men who no longer work, have perhaps lost a mate, live alone, are alienated from their children and extended families, are beginning to have serious physical problems, and experience a deterioration in their ability to do many activities they did so well just a few years earlier. Angier (2002) believes that Levi's decision to commit suicide was a private decision. She writes the following:

> Auschwitz caused him guilt and shame, and torment about human evil; but he contained these in decades of writing and talking, and with the knowledge that he had done everything he could to right them. What we suffer from most in the end is our own private condition. It was his own private condition that killed Primo Levi. (p. xx)

To further suggest that Levi's suicide may have taken place for reasons unrelated to his experiences at Auschwitz, Waern, Runeson, Allebeck, and Beskau (2002) believe that elderly people commit suicide for reasons because of depression, failing health, aloneness, changing cognitive abilities, family deterioration, death of loved ones, and for a variety of other complex reasons. However, according to Waern et al., the primary reason for elder suicide is a severe late-life depression that is unresponsive to treatment. This certainly describes Primo Levi who, in addition to receiving psychotherapy, was also placed on antidepressive medications. In studies of Holocaust survivors such as Primo Levi; Baron, Eisman, Scuello, Veyzer, and Liberman (1996) suggest that survivors who were aware of their ethnic identities and cultural heritage were less vulnerable to emotional traumas. Newman (1979) found that religious beliefs were beneficial to survivors and that religious beliefs provided many survivors with feelings of personal control over the experience that helped give meaning to the concentration camp experience. However, Tech (2003) says that women were more likely to survive the Holocaust experience than men because men defined themselves on the basis of their level of achievement and status whereas women, having virtually none of either at that time in history, were focused on the positive experiences they had as cooperative and helping partners to other inmates. She notes that the Holocaust experience didn't allow Jewish men to do what traditional society expected of them, something that often left them demoralized or depressed and more subject to feelings of hopelessness.

Angier (2002) describes Primo Levi as a highly assimilated Jew who wrote little about the Jewish experience in the death camps but wrote, more precisely, about the human experience. She believes that he told us very little about himself in his books and was often aloof from people, even people he knew well, a condition with which many older men can identify. She writes, "He very rarely betrays his feelings, and almost never has negative feelings—this is the first and most important thing everyone notices in his great books about the Shoah [The Holocaust]" (p. xv). Angier also says that Levi was a deeply conflicted man and that the "torments" of his experiences with the Holocaust, which he tried to cope with by living a highly rational life (he was also a well-known chemist), began to fail him. As a traditional man, Levi dealt with failing health and the inability to work, with great self-blame, which ultimately resulted in depression and suicide. This same self-blame plagues many traditional men throughout their lives.

How interesting that a highly educated and successful man would have the same self-destructive tendencies as less educated and less successful men when his capacity to work and live a healthy life began to fail him. Neither therapy nor medication helped Levi as it so often doesn't help other older men who find that with aging comes inactivity, isolation, and a great sense of failure.

CASE EXAMPLE:
TREATING DEPRESSION IN AN OLDER MALE ADULT

Jake Kissman is a 77-year-old widower whose wife, Leni, passed away a year ago. Jake is emotionally adrift and feels lost without Leni's companionship and guidance. He has a troubled relationship with two adult children who live across the country and has been unable to turn to them for solace and support. Like many men, Jake has no real support group or close friends. Leni's social circle became his, but after her death, her friends left Jake to fend for himself. Jake is a difficult man who is prone to being critical and insensitive. He tends to say whatever enters his mind at the moment no matter how hurtful it may be and then is surprised when people take it badly. "It's only words," he says. "What harm do words do? It's not like smacking somebody." Before he retired, Jake was a successful salesman and can be charming and witty, but, sooner or later, the disregard for others comes through and he ends up offending people.

Jake's depression shows itself in fatigue, feelings of hopelessness, irritability, and outbursts of anger. He doesn't believe in doctors and never sees them. "Look what the 'Momzers' (bastards) did to poor Leni? A healthy woman in her prime and she needed a surgery like I do. They killed her, those butchers." Jake has taken to pounding on the walls of his apartment whenever noise from neighbors upsets him. Complaints from surrounding neighbors have resulted in the threat of an eviction. Jake can't manage a move by himself and someone from his synagogue contacted a professional in the community who agreed to visit Jake at his apartment. Jake is happy that he has company, but angry that anyone thought he needed help. "Tell the bastards to stop making so much noise and I'll be fine. The one next door with the dog, shoot her. The one on the other side who bangs the cabinets, do the same. Why aren't *they* being kicked out?"

The therapist listens to Jake in a supportive way. He never disagrees with him, offers advice, or contradicts him. Jake is still grieving for his wife, and her loss has left him without usable coping skills to deal with the pressures of single life. He's angry and depressed. To find out more about Jake's symptoms, the therapist has gone to the literature on anger, depression, and grief. Although he recognizes that Jake is a difficult client in any event, the data he collected helped him develop a strategy for working with Jake. The therapist has decided to use a strengths approach (Glicken, 2004; Saleebey, 1992; Weick, Rapp, Sullivan, & Kisthardt, 1989) with Jake. The strengths approach focuses on what clients have done well in their lives and uses those strengths in areas of life that are more problematic. The approach comes from studies on resilience, self-healing, and on successful work with abused and traumatized children and adults. Jake has many positive attributes that most people have ignored. He was a warm and caring companion to Leni during her illness. He is secretly very generous and gives what he has without wanting people to know where his gifts come from. He helps his children financially and has done a number of acts of kindness for neighbors and friends but in ways that always make the recipients feel ambivalent about his help. Jake is a difficult and complex man and no one has taken the time to try and understand him. The therapist takes a good deal of time and listens closely.

Jake feels that he's been a failure at life. He feels unloved and unappreciated. He thinks the possibility of an eviction is a good example of how people do him in when he is least able to cope with stress. So the therapist listens and never disagrees with Jake. Gradually, Jake has begun discussing his life and the sadness he feels without his wife, who was his ballast and mate. Using a strengths approach, the therapist always focuses on what Jake does well and his generosity while Jake uses their time to beat himself up with self-deprecating statements. The therapist listens, smiles, points out Jake's excellent qualities, and waits for Jake to start internalizing what the therapist has said about him. Gradually, it's begun to work. Jake told the therapist to go help someone who needed it when Jake's anger at the therapist became overwhelming. Jake immediately apologized. "Here you're helping me and I criticize. Why do I do that?" he asked the therapist. There are many moments when Jake corrects himself or seems to fight an impulse to say something mean-spirited or hurtful to the therapist, who recently told him, "Jake, you catch more flies with honey than you do with vinegar." To which Jake replied, "So who needs to catch flies, for crying out loud? Oh, I'm sorry. Yeah, I see what you mean. It's not about flies, it's about getting along with people."

Gradually, Jake has put aside his anger and has begun talking to people in the charming and pleasant manner of which he is so capable. The neighbors who complained about him now see him as a "doll." Jake's depression is beginning to lift and he's begun dating again, although he says he can never love anyone like his wife, "but a man gets lonely so what are you supposed to do, sit home and watch soap operas all day? Not me." The therapist continues to see Jake and they often sit and quietly talk. This is what Jake said in summarizing his therapy experience:

> I was a big deal once. I could sell an Eskimo an air conditioner in winter. I could charm the socks off people. But my big mouth, it always got in the way. I always said something that made people mad. Maybe it's because my dad was so mean to all of us, I got this chip on my shoulder. Leni was wonderful. She could put up with me and make me laugh. When she died, I was left with my big mouth and a lot of disappointments. You want to have friends, you want your kids to love you. I got neither, but I'm not such an "alte cocker" [old fart] that I don't learn. And I've learned a lot from you. I've learned you can teach an old dog new tricks and that's something. So I thank you and I apologize for some things I said. It's hard to get rid of the chip on the shoulder and sometimes it tips you over, that big chip, and it makes you fall down. You're a good person. I wish you well in life.

DISCUSSION

Most of the treatment literature on work with older depressed adults suggests the use of a cognitive approach. Jake's therapist felt that the oppositional nature of Jake's personality would reject a cognitive approach. Instead, a positive and affirming approach was used that focused on Jake's strengths because, "Most depressed patients acutely desire the therapist's approval, and it is an effective therapist who gives it warmly and genuinely" (O'Connor, 2001, p. 522). Although much of the research suggests the positive benefits of cognitive therapy, the therapist found the following description to be at odds with what might best help Jake. Rush and Giles (1982) indicate that cognitive treatment attempts to change irrational thinking through three steps: (a) identifying irrational self-sentences, ideas, and thoughts; (b) developing rational thoughts, ideas, and perceptions; and (c) practicing these more rational ideas to improve self-worth, and ultimately, to reduce depression. Although this approach might work with other older clients, the therapist believed that Jake would take offense and reject both the therapy and the therapist, finding them preachy, critical, and completely off the mark.

The therapist decided instead to let Jake talk, although he made comments, asked questions to clarify, and made connections that Jake found interesting and oddly satisfying. "No one ever said that to me before," Jake would say, shaking his head and smiling. "You learn something new everyday, don't you." The therapist would always bring Jake back to the positive achievements of his life which initially Jake would toss away with comments like, "That was then when I paid taxes, this is now when I ain't gotta penny to my name." Soon, however, Jake could reflect on his positive achievements and begin to use those experiences to deal with his current problems. In discussing the conflict with one of his neighbors, Jake said the following:

> Maybe I should bring flowers to the old hag. Naw, I can't bring flowers, but she's no hag. I've seen worse. What about flowers? Yeah, flowers. Down at Vons I can buy a nice bunch for a buck. So it costs a little to be nice. Beats getting tossed out on my keester.

Or he would tie something he had done when he was working to his current situation. "I had something like this happen once. A customer complained to my boss, so I go over and ask her to tell me what she's mad about so I can fix it, and she does, and it gets fixed. Sometimes you gotta eat a little crow." As Jake made connections, and as he began to trust the therapist, this process of self-directed change reinforced his sense of accomplishment and led to a decrease in his depression. It also led to a good deal of soul searching about how he had to make changes in his life now that his wife was gone. "So maybe I should stop feeling sorry for myself and take better care. What do you think?"

SUMMARY

This chapter discusses anxiety and depression in older male adults. Both problems exist in large numbers among older men and frequently coexist. Because older male adults are often not thought to be amenable to therapy, underlying symptoms of anxiety and depression may be missed, ignored, or avoided, with medication or other nontherapy approaches used instead. Research suggests that older men are as positively affected by treatment as younger clients, but are more susceptible to suicide and other serious problems resulting from untreated symptoms.

PART VI

The Future:
Improving the Lives of Men

Chapter *18*

Changing the Way We Respond to Men

This chapter discusses the ways in which the crisis among men might be dealt with through a combination of social programs and innovative approaches to treatment. Foremost in the discussion is the need to recognize that the health, educational, and mental health problems men experience are serious and need our considerable attention. Gender conflicts which suggest that a men's agenda might harm the progress made by women need to be put aside and in its place, hard work must to be done to help men get beyond the current crisis.

WHAT NEEDS TO BE DONE

Recognizing the Crisis

In discussing the crisis of male educational underperformance, O'Neill (2000) writes,

> We have created a monster which is very difficult to escape from. There is nobody who is going to stand on a platform and start talking about the problems that face young boys, especially if it means criticizing the kind of education policies that got us into this position in the first place. (p. 54)

O'Neill (2000) believes that those policies have worked against the best interests of boys by creating an educational system where the primary focus is on the achievement and learning styles of girls, creating an atmosphere where boys think no one cares about them.

One way this lack of attention to boys shows itself is in the way boys are portrayed in young adult fiction. In a review of young adult novels from 1940 to 1997, Bereska (2003) found that the depiction of masculinity had remained static and suggests that although social change is depicted in novels for young adults in accurate ways, the way masculinity is described remains unchanged: "This means that a significant portion of the discourse surrounding masculinity has remained unchanged for more than 50 years, despite other social changes having occurred" (Bereska, 2003, p. 161).

Bereska (2003) argues that most of the research on gender and the culture of adolescents in the 1980s and 1990s has focused on girls and asks the following: "But what about boys? What do their popular cultural products tell them about how to understand the world and themselves?" (p. 161).

In answering that question, Forbes (2003) suggests that boys are experiencing a severe crisis which hampers their development and can be harmful to others. Forbes blames this crisis on a restrictive male norm that

> ... pressures male youths to prove their masculinity through stoic inexpressiveness and control, avoidance of qualities considered to be feminine, homophobia, competition, domination, and aggression. Influential and highly visible institutions, such as the government and the media, tend to favor male values such as aggression as a means to solve problems. Equally problematic is that male youths often grow up without adequate emotional and conceptual tools that enable them to distance themselves from the norm and become conscious of their own development. Recent incidents of school violence are examples of the destructive effects of boys caught up in the norm. Schools contribute to gender formation and the making of masculinities but do so in an unreflective, inchoate way. (p. 146)

Recognition of the Positive Aspects of Male Socialization and Behavior

In response to male bashing and the many attacks on men as perpetrators and abusers, Morrow and Dickerson (1994) ask why men are so angry these days. In providing one answer to that question, they note that,

"Federal, state and local governments spend hundreds of millions of dollars protecting women workers from sexual harassment, while millions of men are still left substantially unprotected from premature death by industrial hazard" (p. 56). They go on to suggest that the real reason men are angry isn't the danger they face in the workplace with its potential for premature death, but that they feel so unappreciated.

Farrell (2004) believes that although we encourage men to be heroic, the behavior that develops is the exact behavior we criticize repeatedly in traditional men. Heroic behavior, Farrell writes, requires men to

> repress feelings, not express feelings. The more a man values himself the less he wants to die. To teach a man to value himself by dying—to give him promotions to risk death, to tell him he's powerful, he's a hero, he's loved, he's a "real man"—is to "bribe" a man to value himself more by valuing himself less. Thus volunteer firefighters are virtually 100% males; all the Drug Enforcement Agency officials who have died in "The War on Drugs" are male; men died in the Gulf War at a ratio of 27 to 1, and, overall, 93% of people killed in the workplace are males.

> We think of a hero as someone who has power. In fact, a servant and slave possess the psychology of disposability, not the psychology of power. Many men have learned to define power as "feeling obligated to earn money that someone else spends while he dies sooner." Real power is best defined as "control over one's life."

The Need for Practice Research on What Works Best With Men

Before a revolution in therapy for men can take place, a well-funded, empirical set of research studies is needed to determine the following:

1. How can we get men to voluntarily attend and stay in treatment?
2. What types of therapeutic alliances and therapy approaches work best with a range of male clients by the type of social and emotional problems experienced and by race, ethnic, educational, and socio-economic variables?
3. Does the level of masculinity or traditional maleness suggest the need for a very different type of treatment than we have at present?

4. Are there institutional ways of helping men go for health and mental health services that might include use of the popular culture, ad campaigns, and perhaps monetary rewards for seeking help when needed?

The need for a more knowledge-guided therapy for men is also noted by Peebles (2000), who writes,

> In North America, policymakers have been taking an interest in the scientific evidence underlying the practice of clinical psychology. Demands for accountability have been mounting from both government agencies and managed care companies. (Barlow, 1996; Parloff & Elkin, 1992) (p. 660)

When therapy was offered in private or nonprofit settings, its effectiveness was of little concern to policymakers. With the advent of large, public sector expenditures for therapeutic services, "the public gained a right and a responsibility to determine who is entitled to receive services, what conditions warrant treatment, and what treatments will be authorized" (Parloff, 1979) (Peebles, 2000, p. 559). This need for accountability, in light of the large cost for therapeutic services, has been growing, and mental health providers are "scrambling," in Peebles's words, to prove the need and worth of our services to policymakers and to a skeptical public, particularly services provided to such underserved populations as men and minority clients who have infrequent contacts with therapists and when they do, the contacts are often brief and unhelpful.

New Approaches to Treatment

Clearly, much more needs to be done to develop approaches to therapy that work well with men. The negative data on the lack of use of treatment and a sense that when men do go for help, it isn't a positive or helpful experience is reinforced by Forbes (2003) who writes,

> Traditional counseling, especially school counseling, has not adequately addressed the mental health needs of all *male* youths ... A model that transcends traditional counseling elements and encompasses

emergent ones can point toward a fuller meaning of *development* for everyone. (p. 142)

In discussing the response men get when they seek help for a variety of problems, but particularly when they are being abused by wives, lovers, or coworkers, Migliaccio (2001) writes that men in his study who attempted to seek out assistance

> felt they were met with prejudice and demoralizing reactions from institutions that could have aided them with their situations. Regardless of the intentions of the people of these institutions, it is the perceptions of the men in this study that such displays can emasculate them. (p. 215)

In further noting the way institutions treat men who are abused by others, and in giving a strong reason why men don't often choose to voluntarily seek help, Migliaccio (2001) concludes,

> Those men that chose to face public ridicule claimed they were denied help and were "unmasked" by public, legal, and social institutions as well as private citizens. In essence, while struggling to understand a situation that contradicted gender expectations, many chose to see the abused husband as less than a man. When individuals do not fit into the prescribed notion of what is expected, they are sanctioned, which may include being marginalized. In this instance, an individual can no longer be considered a man; he is displaying a feminine face. As Goffman (1979) states, "females are equivalent to subordinate males" (p. 5). When a man assumes such a face it is accompanied by certain attributes, which are also gendered. Such characterizations can " 'desex' the man, making him appear as not fully a man" (Kimmel, 1994, p. 127). (p. 215)

In discussing the general ineffectiveness of therapy, Wampold et al. (1997) write,

> We would cherish the day that a treatment is developed that is dramatically more effective than the ones we use today. But until that day comes, the existing data suggest that whatever differences in treatment efficacy exist, they appear to be very small, at best. (p. 230)

Developing effective male models of treatment could have substantial impact on the effectiveness of therapy with all client groups.

320 CHAPTER 18

Social Programs for Men

A number of programs have been used to treat young men involved with or at risk of involvement in violence, crime, drugs, early school dropout, and joblessness, with some success (Rae-Grant, McConville, Fleck, & Stephen, 1999). Among those programs are school-based conflict resolution training programs; gun-free zones around schools; evening curfews; weekend and evening recreational programs; summer camps; job and training programs for youths at risk; and community policing (Ash, Kellermann, Fuqua-Whitley, & Johnson, 1996). Caplan et al. (1992) studied programs treating the early onset of substance use in teenagers. The outcomes of these programs resulted in better problem-solving skills, better control of impulsive behavior, and reduced alcohol use. Hansen and Graham (1991) found that fewer adolescents used alcohol and had better awareness of the risks of alcohol after drug and alcohol intervention. Borduin (1999) reports that multifocused diversion programs providing services to repeat youth offenders before they enter the court system have shown positive results. Greenwood, Model, Rydell, and Chiesa (1996) indicate that programs focusing on prevention of crime in youthful offenders were more cost-effective in lowering serious crime than mandatory sentences for adult repeat offenders.

For children with multiple risk markers to develop violent or antisocial behavior, many programs target specific aspects of the child's family life. Olds, Henderson, Tatelbaum, and Chamberlin (1988) provide an example of how an early infancy project for economically disadvantaged mothers with poor prenatal health, self-damaging behaviors, and poor family management skills, can improve maternal diet, reduce smoking during pregnancy, result in fewer premature deliveries, increase the birth weight of babies, and result in significantly less child abuse. Johnson (1990) reports that providing social, economic, and health-related services to preschool children and their families with multiple risk markers improved academic success, reduced behavioral problems in at-risk children, improved parenting skills, decreased family management problems, and lowered the subsequent arrest rates for children in families provided services. However, Johnson (1990) cautions that some of these positive outcomes are only effective for several years after follow-up. Johnson (1990) suggests the reasons for the lack of long-term effectiveness may be the result of diminished services to at-risk families, poor school experiences for children, and the often troubled lives of the families served. Weikart, Schweinhart, and Larner (1986) found similar results. Zigler, Tausig, and Black (1992) believe that pre-school services to at-risk families coupled with programs such as Head Start may actually help prevent antisocial behavior in young children.

Rae-Grant, McConville, and Fleck (1999) suggest that in elementary grade school boys, "interpersonal cognitive problem-solving programs gave rise to better problem-solving skills and fewer behavior problems in children with economic deprivation, poor impulse control, and early behavioral problems" (p. 338). Hawkins et al. (1992) report that a social development program in Seattle for similarly at-risk grade school children demonstrated positive results. Preschool and elementary school programs may be one proactive approach to preventing future delinquent and violent behavior.

Another way to help boys and young men is through conflict resolution curricula. These approaches teach boys to use alternatives to violence when resolving interpersonal conflict. They may include programs that teach conflict resolution strategies, actual conflict resolution teams headed up by students who patrol the school grounds and can provide conflict resolution as a way of reducing tension before the conflict is reported to the school authorities, and programs to teach children ways of avoiding situations where violence might occur. Films, role plays, and simulations may be used and parents might become involved to extend conflict resolution to problems in the home. Topics covered in conflict resolution curricula include anger management; learning to identify and express feelings about others; discussing issues related to racial, ethnic, and gender differences; and learning to cope with stress.

Another way boys can be helped to cope with aggression is assertiveness training, which teaches boys that one can be assertive without being aggressive. Studer (1996) explains the difference between aggression and assertiveness:

> Aggression is an action that enhances the aggressor while it minimizes and violates the rights of others. The intent of the aggressive behavior is to

humiliate and dominate. This behavior is in contrast to passive behaviors that are self-denying and inhibiting, as a person's own rights are disregarded and he or she gives in to demands of others. Instead, Baer defined assertiveness as "win–win" behavior in which an individual can stand up for his or her own rights in such a way that the rights of others are not disregarded. (p. 188)

Huey and Rank (1984) found assertiveness training to be very helpful with disruptive, low achieving boys who were referred for counseling because of their aggressive, acting out behavior. The authors noted that after being given eight hours of assertiveness training, these children were less aggressive but were more assertive in the classroom. Mathias (1992) reports that the "DeBug" System, a training program to teach children assertiveness, showed overwhelmingly positive results in the classroom and substantially reduced aggressive behavior.

Other Programs to Help Men

There are many additional ways to help men including the following: (a) learning to work cooperatively through projects where boys are rewarded for their individuality as well as their ability to work together. These cooperative skills can begin to be learned early in life and should be reinforced throughout the life cycle; (b) programs to teach young boys to deal with aggression while retaining the ability to be assertive; (c) reducing the amount of abandonment by fathers through helpful social programs. When fathers are absent, using male mentors in place of absent or uninvolved fathers; (d) an educational system that focuses on the way boys learn and allows boys to develop at their own pace without applying generalized ideas of where learning should be at a specific point in time; (e) national service to help socialize young men, make up for educational loss, and help young men to work cooperatively with others; (f) identifying and training indigenous helpers who are part of the workforce but are particularly helpful to co-workers because they provide empathic listening, good advice, and are considered trustworthy and helpful by co-workers; and (g) finally, let's admit that boys and men need to be seen as a special class just as girls and women have driven our national agenda for the past 30 years. As Bereska (2003) writes,

> Many contemporary efforts at gender change have been directed at the girls' world, for example, in the behavior of parents and teachers aimed at increasing girls' self-esteem, encouraging them to try traditionally male educational programs or careers, and teaching them that their lives are complete without boyfriends. In the 1960s, feminism encouraged women to become independent, find their own interests, develop their own careers, and claim their power. However, in contrast males have only been expected to change in terms of accommodating those changes in women's lives. We have also expected males to tolerate and accept the entrance of women into the **boys'** world. And yet, there is evidence to suggest that this expectation for men to change merely in accommodation to changes in women's lives has not worked. (p. 170)

Resolving the Gender Wars

This is a chapter from a book I wrote (Glicken, 2004) based on conversations with men and women in a very informal setting over several years. I think the people included in the volume have a good deal to say about resolving the gender wars I see between men and women, a war that has no winners and often ends with the children in America as the worst losers of all.

COFFEEHOUSE WISDOM

Most mornings I go to a local café in Southern California for coffee. It's a sort of ritual for me. Sometimes I write checks for bills I owe or read the dismal news in the paper. Other times I try and organize my day or grade the accumulated papers I must read as a professor of social work at a California university.

The local men often walk by my table and nod in recognition. Sometimes they stop and talk to me about my articles in the local papers about men. These men are the workingmen of America; the plumbers and construction workers, the common laborers and retired railroad workers, the illegal immigrants from Mexico. Their trucks and beat up old cars line the parking lot outside of the restaurant.

I have come to value my conversations with these men. Many of them have done badly by women and children, and readily admit it. Some of them are extraordinary people who have done better than most of us. And there are always the men who sit and talk about women and you want to get up and ream them out. They sound like abusers. Worse, they sound like children in adult bodies.

I've learned a lot from listening and talking to these men in the morning. Academics often hear pretty unrealistic versions of life, but these men talk like real people; people with flaws, human beings we all know in our daily lives.

When the wives and children of these men talk to me, you get a different picture of their behavior. They talk about abuse and neglect, about put downs and absences, and sometimes, about abandonment. They describe how the insensitive behavior of their men affects the very people who are trying so hard to love their husbands, boy friends, and fathers.

Sometimes I get a chance to sit with the men and women and listen to them talk about the gender wars they have fought. The men often sit with their mouths open and ask, "Was I that bad?" Everybody nods their heads. The men have mellowed so it isn't easy for them to imagine that they've acted so badly in the past.

Sometimes the men hang around, after the women leave, to assure me that they weren't so bad, but there's an emptiness to their denial that rings hollow. Many times they walk away shaking their head, angry at me for making them hear so much bad stuff about behavior they'd rather forget; mean, nasty, hurtful behavior that has been like a knife in the hearts of the women and children trying so hard to understand them.

The men who interrupt me as I try and drink my coffee are ordinary men. They're men who have had troubles in their lives, men who drink too much, from time to time, and men who can be mean and petty. They're the men who regret their past and have done a thing or two that leave them with the night sweats when they wake up from bad dreams. Normal men who have made mistakes. Decent guys who cared for the baby at night and provided for families when it was nearly impossible.

Sensitive men? Probably not. Romantic men? I doubt it. Men who sweep women off their feet with the power and brilliance of their lovemaking? It doesn't seem very likely. Just regular "Joes" who need the guidance and the sweet and tender loving of a woman. Men who are better when a woman is in their life. Men who can hardly navigate the complexities of life and who depend on women in ways that are sometimes childlike.

Men like Roger, a plumber, who joins the early morning construction gang at my coffee shop. He sees me sitting in the back reading the paper and comes over to sit with me. Today he complains about his wife. She's too fat, he says. He's lost interest in her. I look over at Roger, who is perhaps 60 or 70 pounds overweight, and I ask if he's looked in the mirror lately. Does he know that his obesity is as off-putting to his wife as hers is to him? He mumbles something derogatory about my mother, but I see him everyday and he looks somehow, thinner. When I see him weeks later with his wife, they look nice together. Warm, maybe even tender in the way older men and women can be with each another.

He doesn't thank me for my advice or say how much his life has improved because of my simple suggestions. All he does is bring his wife over, an attractive woman in her forties, while I drink my coffee and try and read the paper. He beams at me. See how great my wife looks, his smile says? See what a hunk I must be to attract such a great looking lady? It is thanks enough and I smile at their happiness.

Another guy, Richard, one of the few Black men who sit in the café, complains to me about the way his wife spends his money. "She's a shopping junky," he says. "Ain't no way anyone can spend so much money."

He brings her in one morning, a nice, soft-spoken young woman. She talks to me about how difficult it is for a Black family to make ends meet, but Richard is a good husband and father and they make the money go a little further. Richard wants to buy me breakfast. He feels like dancing in the café. His wife has touched a part of his heart with love seeds.

How strange men must seem to women. How they talk so badly about the women in their lives but depend on them for everything. And how badly men do in giving women credit for so much that women do to make their lives easier. And yet women are there to help in the small and large ways that men almost never regard as important or admit make a difference.

How absolutely contradictory male behavior must seem to most women. How men prance, and strut, and brag without end when inside they often feel as inadequate as anyone can feel and still manage to get up in the morning and put their clothes on. And yet to listen to them, men seem on top of the world, kings of the hill, beyond pain.

Were it only so. If men were so secure, they wouldn't do the often terrible things they do to wives, girlfriends, co-workers and children. They wouldn't abuse and abandon their loved ones, or fly into jealous rages, or harass women in the workplace. If men were the winners in this war between the genders, they wouldn't fall apart in mid-life, or suffer the indignity of bodies, which fail them and leave them old and emotionally wrecked well before God meant for such a thing to happen.

Just as I talk to the men when I have coffee in the mornings, I have come to cherish the time I spend talking to the women who come in for a quick cup of coffee before their impossibly long and complicated days begin. They are the working women of America, the unglamorous women who get up at 5 A.M. and care for their families before driving an hour or more to thankless jobs. I have come to think of these women as very special people. They have been the prisoners in the war among the sexes. Although they are often war weary trying to keep families and marriages together, they still have an optimism about the flawed men they often meet, fall in love with, and marry.

They are the women like Betty Sue who asks me what to do when a man loses interest in sex. As I begin to talk to her, some of the women in the coffee shop join us.

"He's a good man," she says, "and we used to have a great love life. I'm sure something is really wrong."

One of the women sitting at the table says, "Why not just say to him something like, 'Honey, it sure used to be nice how we'd spend our time in bed. It would sure be nice to have that again.' Why not give it a try?" Betty Sue looks over at me and I nod in support.

The next day she comes back with a big smile on her face. All of the ladies at the table rib her until she says, "He thought I wasn't interested anymore. He thought maybe I was with another man, and it was making him crazy."

"How could he think something like that?" someone asks, and one of the ladies says, "Because, he's a man. That's the way men think."

Another time, Denise, a woman perhaps in her late thirties is going through the early stages of knowing that her marriage is all but over. "I don't understand it, doc," she says to me. "We were such good friends. We really liked being together. But now, he just always seems like he's in another world. When we talk, it's always about the house or the car, it's never about how unhappy we are together."

It's very early in the morning but Denise has been up for hours and her bloodshot eyes suggest that she's been crying in the car on the way to the coffee shop. "It's tough," I tell her, "when a man shuts off. Have you asked him if something is wrong at work or in his personal life?"

She shakes her head. "He always tells me when something is wrong," she says. "He's not one to keep things inside."

We sit in silence for a while and watch the regulars walk in, many of them still sleepy from nights too short to make up for the hours of driving and the hard work ahead of them. I look at Denise and gently touch her hand. "Maybe there's something wrong, Denise, that's so troubling to your husband that he can't discuss it with you. Men often find it hard to talk about really personal problems. Try asking him tonight and stay with it. Don't let him slough you off or avoid talking."

Denise looks at me with a look I've seen all too often. The moment comes in a relationship when you've tried everything and you've unconsciously begun to give up. It's the moment of being psychologically divorced. Denise looks up and nods her head, her shoulders slumped. "O.K. doc," she says, "I'll try for you, but I don't think it's gonna work."

A week goes by and Denise hasn't come in for coffee. I'm all too ready to blame myself for bad advice, but one morning she comes in with her husband. They find their way over to my booth and after introductions and handshakes, Denise and her husband, Ed, sit for a while and drink their coffee while we make small talk. Finally, Denise tells me what's happened in the past week with Ed looking on, a serious look on his face.

"I didn't want to do it, doc, but I knew you'd be hurt if I came to you for advice and didn't use it. So I waited until Ed was sitting in his chair after dinner and I made the kids go outside so we could talk. I said to Ed how he seems to be unhappy all the time and that I don't think we're gonna make it. And he says back to me that he's fine and that it's my imagination. But I won't let it go, doc, and I kept at it until he finally says to me that he thinks he might lose his job and he doesn't think I'll stay with him if he doesn't have a job."

I look over at Ed and he's nodding quietly as Denise tells the story. We pause for a moment to drink our coffee and then Denise continues.

"Where did he get that crazy idea? I asked him and he says, 'from you, Denise, from you.' I argued with him about that but he reminded me of the many times I've said, sarcastically, that I'd never take care of a man. And it's true. I've said it a lot but I didn't mean *my* man. But of course, that's the way he took it. We talked most of the week about the situation and we got it straightened up. We didn't think we could because there were so many other things that were going wrong, but we did and it's so much better now I can't even believe it was possible. I thought that Ed was like most men and that he couldn't talk about the really tough stuff. He fooled me, though. Once I reached out a little, he could talk just fine."

I've had hundreds of conversations like this with the men and women of the coffee shop. Not all of them end as dramatically or as well, but I think that men and women are much better together with a little gentle guidance, some good information, and some timely help. I also think this gender war we keep fighting needs to be resolved. Too many good people get hurt. What better war for us to fight and win in the helping professions.

I think men and women hunger for better times. No one wants to be in a constant war between the sexes. When relationships between men and women improve, we all gain. Love is everything it's cracked up to be and nothing in this world beats the wonder of two people in love.

SUMMARY

This chapter notes that continued male problems including high rates of violence, health problems, and low educational achievement require a much greater effort on the part of policymakers and therapists. Few men voluntarily use therapy and new approaches to therapy are required to encourage men to change troubled behavior, suggesting the need for more research on treatment with men and a willingness by therapists to experiment with new ideas about the best way to help men in treatment.

Female Therapists and Academics Respond

I sent the manuscript of this volume to six women I know who are either therapists or academics in the helping professions. I consider all of the women to be supportive of men's problems and I feel confident that they all read the manuscript objectively. I'm reporting their feedback here and although I did some editing for length and the removal of duplicate ideas, I tried not to change the essence of the feedback. You will note more feedback than respondents.

RESPONSES FROM FEMALE THERAPISTS

Response 1

Without question, men are doing badly, but the reasons need to be explored a bit further than the author takes them. The author suggests that the national agenda has changed from men to women and that the agenda is to blame for men doing badly. How can that be? During a time of increased opportunity for all groups in America, men have done badly, not because of women, but because those who do best get rewarded. If the unequal playing field had been taken away from women much earlier, the shift from an all men's agenda to a people's agenda would have taken place sooner. Certainly we should be concerned about male problems and try and correct them. That goes without saying, but to suggest that male bashing is the cause of male problems, or that a lack of respect causes men to go into decline is to deny that men have been doing badly for a very long time. Health data and data on drinking and violence would support the notion that men were in decline well before the feminist movement began in America.

The author is correct in pointing out that men need specialized help and that institutional disregard for any group in difficulty is a sign of trouble. Ignoring male problems is bad for society and particularly bad for family life. However, women have a long way to go as well. After 30 years of feminism, women still make appreciably less money than men in the workplace and expect less than men when it comes to both initial and life time salaries (Heckert, Droste, Adams, et al., 2002). This is a particularly serious problem for women raising families alone without, as the author points out, very much help from their ex-husbands. That men live several years less than women paints an erroneous picture of women's health. Women suffer more depression and anxiety over the life span. They're also more prone to PTSD because of family violence and sexual assault including child molestation. The reason they use therapists more than men is that their lives are full of stress.

Response 2

I laughed when I read chapter 4 on male bashing. After all, men have been saying terrible things about women for as long as anyone can remember. I'm not a fan of gender bashing but men have done a pretty good job of stereotyping women as flaky, obsessed with material objects, using men for their own gain, needing to be told who's boss, liking sex to be forced on them, dumb, and I could go on. The point is that most women I know have heard just about every demeaning thing imaginable said to their faces by men. Go to any bar or men's locker room in America and if you don't hear men bashing women or painting unflattering pictures of them, it's my turn to buy.

The fact is that men have practiced a form of very serious and harmful gender bias against women for a very long time ... in the jokes they tell, in their abandonment of women and children, in their physical and sexual abuse of women and children, and in the institutional bias against women that has kept us out of high end corporate and political positions, yet we've persevered. The author believes that the playing field isn't level anymore and that the national agenda is now focused on women. For how many thousands of years has it been focused on men? Does he mean to imply that after just 30 years of concern about women and our needs and aspirations, that men can't take it anymore and are giving up? If that's the case, men really are the weaker sex, not women.

Response 3

The author argues that men need a new type of therapy just as women argued that they also needed a new type of therapy. I don't think women had any objection to the techniques of therapy other than to feel that many therapists had values and beliefs about women that negatively affected us. Our concern with therapy wasn't as fundamental as the author's concerns about therapy for men. He argues for a new approach to therapy that takes into consideration male ambivalence about introspection. How can we do therapy when clients resist a primary element of treatment? He even admits that when therapy is expressed in terms that men can accept, they still resist coming for treatment. It seems to me that therapy is just not a process that most men find helpful because they resist change. You have to want to change your behavior for therapy to work. I don't know what that new type of help would be but it doesn't sound like anything I'm familiar with.

Let's be realistic. You have to want to change your behavior as a first step in treatment. You have to admit that what you're doing isn't working, and you have to have some acceptance of your involvement in the problem. It doesn't sound as if men have a desire to admit that what they're doing is harmful to themselves or others, or to become part of a process that involves introspection and change. Perhaps what this leaves is self-help groups or some involvement is spirituality and religious based practices, but it isn't therapy as I or anyone else I know defines therapy.

While I think the author does a good job of describing the problems men have, I'm not certain his solutions, at least his therapy-based solutions are very practical. What I think might be more realistic are programs to help men deal with the loss of fathers in their lives through abandonment and the heavy burden on single mothers to raise children with limited financial, educational, and social resources. I agree that more effort needs to be made in the schools to work with young male children and to provide helping approaches that take into consideration the way boys learn. We could also do a much better job of offering guidance to children after school while parents work. And perhaps most importantly, we can provide help to all parents in their struggle to survive financially. Canada's system of financial help to all parents is something America might learn from. Taking financial burdens away from parents would go a long way to help parents do a better job with their children.

Response 4

The author talks a great deal about male socialization as if it's something unchangeable and set in stone, but the reality is that many boys grow up with very good models of behavior that permit them to be sensitive to others, unwilling to participate in violence, and excited and challenged by education. They also have very positive attitudes toward women and to their responsibilities as parents. I think much would be gained from finding out more about boys with good values, the type of parenting they've received, and how they develop so well in the midst of others who develop less well. I suspect a good deal of what makes these boys so healthy has to do with a positive family environment. I'm sure the author would agree, since he speaks so much about the strengths perspective, that more is to be gained by studying healthy behavior than dysfunctional behavior. Would he also agree that there are large numbers of boys and young and older men who do very well in life and that the dismal problems he describes are more limited to a subset of men rather than to all men? Seen this way, the troubled lives of *some* men would be a better title than the implication that all men have difficulties in their lives.

Response 5

The author mentions in passing the Harvard Study where high functioning men at Harvard were studied years later to see how their lives
had gone and that many of these young men had very privileged backgrounds yet had done badly in their personal lives while doing very well
in careers that bored them and for which they often felt ill suited. I don't
think this says anything about men in particular since one would find
the same thing about young women from privileged backgrounds. The
mistake made is to assume that men are so other-oriented that they
choose careers and relationships to please parents without any thought
to their own happiness. This rings true for women as well. Which brings
up the point I'd like to make. If you forget gender and just consider men
and women in America, I think you'll find a very heavy overlay of depression, anxiety, a sense of failure and a longing for a more fulfilling
life. There is something about life in America that produces a terrible
sense of isolation, loneliness and failure.

Men are fond of saying that women do better than men since they
have more friends, but all too many women I know recognize that the
people they describe as friends are people men would describe only as
superficial acquaintances. I think women talk a good game about their
happiness but if that were the case, why do women have such high rates
of depression, anxiety, and symptoms of PTSD across the life span? The
emphasis on men or women ignores the fact that we're an unhappy people with increasing problems of relating to one another, and that many
of us live lonely and desperate lives. All too many women are moving
into middle age without any hope of marriage or having children because the conflicts between the genders set up relationship problems
that all but negate healthy and happy bonding. I know a number of
women in their late 30's and early 40's who have a ton of female friends
and think that life is going to depend on these and other friends rather
than a relationship leading to marriage or a long term commitment.
Maybe this is a good way to realistically handle a growing problem but I
don't think it leads to happiness or fulfillment for many women.

I've been hearing more and more about Japan where men and women
have given up on marriage and the birth rate is falling so dramatically

that the population will begin declining by 2006. Imagine a society that can't maintain itself and stagnates and that's the feeling I get about America. I think the truer question we need to study is why increasing numbers of men and women are unable to have committed relationships that lead to family life and what this will do to us as a nation.

Response 6

The male mystique the author seems to allude to just doesn't wash with what most therapists see in male clients. I don't think men are resistant to therapy or that their socialization negates a willingness to work on personal problems in therapy. I have a number of men in treatment, some of them very traditional in their world view, and some of them very modern and hip. I can't really generalize about the work they do in therapy since it doesn't seem a whole lot different than the work my female clients do. Some are motivated for change and others aren't. Some work well with me and some don't. What I do find is that men seem to be very driven to resolve the problem as quickly as they can. They take advice and direction very well once they feel you're OK and that what you're doing with them is going to help. More than my female clients, perhaps, they want to work the problem out as fast as possible and get on with their lives. They don't want to meander along as some women do, developing the relationship and using therapy more as support and a social event. This doesn't mean that men get better faster than women; it's just a difference in style.

Many of the men I work with have been deeply wounded by women or feel as if they've acted badly, but they remain optimistic. I can't say the same for women, many of whom have given up on relationships and are very angry at men. Again, I don't find the end result very different but it's an observation I find interesting. Men seem more willing to forgive both past partners and themselves while many women find it hard to give up their anger at men or their feelings of naiveté at having been taken advantage of in past relationships. These are observations that some therapists I know are in agreement with but I wouldn't generalize them to all therapists. I think we all have different styles and that style attracts a certain client population. I also think the way we present our goals sets up a certain type of working relationship. What I've found helpful is to focus on what the male client wants to do to get better and not make light of it. Once men feel you're on their side, they have a way of being open to other points of view and suggestions. I find women mainly interested in the process and men mainly interested in the results, but after that, both genders work hard, resolve their problems in good time, and do a lot better in their lives. I'm optimistic about men and therapy and I think we'd be much better off looking at therapists who work successfully with men and learning from them than to continually suggest that therapy isn't something men use well.

Response 7

I found a good deal of the material interesting, particularly the data on health problems and the discussion of male socialization. My problem is that focusing on male health problems and their reasons sets up a gender competition. Yes, prostate cancer is a terrible thing but is it as disfiguring or serious as breast cancer? Most men do well when prostate cancer is diagnosed early enough but can we say the same thing about breast cancer? I just find the gender competition hides the fact that we have a very uneven health care system in America. If we had universal health care, I think everyone's health would benefit.

The other problem with a gender competition is that it begins to blame the victim. If a woman has a health problem it's because she doesn't adhere to proper exercise or diet, but how many women are so overburdened with family and work responsibilities that just getting through the day is amazing, let alone living it in a healthy way. The same can be said for men. Life in America is stressful, medical care is expensive, and to deal with the multiple stressors in life, few men or women have the time or discipline to take good care of themselves. I'm convinced it's one of the reasons we have an obesity epidemic in America. And I think the upshot is going to be that people who don't take care of themselves will be denied health care or will have to pay higher premiums. I think that's a regressive way to go because it will punish the poor, the working poor, single mothers, and others of us with terribly stressful lives.

Response 8

What I found interesting were the numerous negative statements made by clients. They didn't seem gender specific at all but had to do with the competence of the therapist. There was nothing the good therapists did with male clients that also wouldn't work with female clients. The bad therapists would have been bad with any client. I think the reality is that a lot of therapists have a great deal of work to do on their professional competency. Bad therapists seem evident in this book to a greater degree than I think is the reality when all therapists are considered. Perhaps the author was trying to find clients who epitomized negative experiences. Anyway I hope that's the case. Perhaps there is an argument to be made for specializing in work with certain client groups. I know that some therapists are highly effective with borderline personality disorders, for example, a problem many therapists would prefer not to treat or at least feel less than competent to treat. Perhaps just as we have therapists who specialize in women's issues we can encourage the development of therapists with expertise in working with men's issues. I see a strong argument for women therapists to work with men. I've known a number of male therapists who tell me they prefer doing their own therapy with women therapists. The reason they give is usually that female therapists provide them with a different point of view than male therapists and it's usually a point of view that helps them see a problem in a unique way.

Response 9

For most women who have been on the receiving end of bad behavior by men, there's something troubling about portraying men in a sympathetic way. Men rape, beat spouses and girlfriends, sexually harass and physically intimidate women. How sympathetic is that? While I appreciate the helpful way the author approaches much of the material, the chapter on male bashing seemed gratuitous and unnecessary. I know men think the playing field at work isn't level but the fact is that women make a whole lot less money than men and have a much harder time of it at work than men. There's still an old boy network that makes the lace curtain the author describes pretty meaningless. Men still run the show and if some woman breaks out and does well, it isn't very long before men come gunning for her or the rumor mill makes her life impossible. I don't know why men are doing so badly but it isn't because of women and that's the sense I get from the chapter on male bashing and sexual harassment; women take advantage of men and use prevailing laws to move up the ladder occupationally while being as sexist and harassing as men. I just find that a little preposterous.

Response 10

I would have been far less sympathetic to this book were it not for the fact that I have 2 sons under the age of 12. What I see in the video games, films, and TV programs they watch reinforces much of what the author says in his book. Young males are surrounded by images of violence with a great deal of emphasis placed on them to be stoic, impervious to pain, and to act like grown men. I see many challenges for leadership in the boys my sons have as friends and much too much dangerous competition. What goes on at school is appalling with frequent fights and a sense that boys who achieve academically are nerds. My sons only do well enough in school to get by when they're both extremely bright and capable children with a great many sophisticated interests. At school, however, the pressure is such that to do really well suggests either feminine qualities or a nerdiness that precipitates ridicule and can be isolating.

My husband understands it all better than I do and tells me that boys change as they age and that highly achieving boys learn to discount social pressures and ridicule, but it all seems self-destructive and dangerous to me. I'm bothered by the attitude toward women I see in my sons and their friends. It's not directed at me as much as it suggests a public attitude they're supposed to have to be accepted by other boys. I've already heard my sons mention female body parts in terribly condescending ways. Again, my husband says that this posing is natural for boys and that secretly, they're scared to death of girls. But you have to believe that some boys are influenced by sexist notions of women and that potential abusers and rapists get reinforcement for future behavior from this macho way of viewing women.

I'm sure the author is right in describing compensatory masculinity and risk taking to prove that boys have all the right stuff to be men. Both my sons have broken legs or arms in activities which, besides being dangerous, are outrageously stupid, all for the sake of proving themselves to other boys. And my sons are terrific kids. I can't even imagine what boys do who come from troubled families.

Finally, the workplace problems faced by men are all too real. My husband, a really wonderful guy, tells me stories from his corporate job that make me fearful that someday he'll lose his job for some small mistake or indiscretion. It isn't funny when you're in your late 30's and already you worry about saying something that somebody will take wrong, or that a woman wanting to get promoted will accuse your husband of sexual harassment knowing full well that a woman's side of a story always wins out over a man's. So I was very positively impressed with the book. I wish there were more like it instead of the fluff you read in the book stores about people from other planets or co-dependence. No doubt not all women who read this book will feel as positively as I do but then they may not have sons and they may not see what pressures boys go through to be men, pressures that often have very troubling consequences.

Response 11

I wonder why the author didn't discuss gay men. It seems to me that the ability to accept one's sexual preference is complicated by traditional views of masculinity that hold gay men to be outside of the acceptable boundaries of male behavior. I think there is a great deal of homophobia, not only among traditional men but among most straight men. The issue of coming out of the closet is an enormously complicated one for many gay men, particularly when it comes to letting male friends, fathers, and brothers know they're gay. And homophobia translates into bad behavior in the workplace, in the community, and certainly among family members. And more than just talking about gay men, I wish the author had discussed the traditional view of male behavior with women in more detail, and I'm not just talking about abusive behavior. I think men often see women as inferior and have difficulty dealing with women who may be smarter and more able than they are. My friends in administrative positions complain about gender bias all the time, among men and women, and how they are held to a higher standard than male administrators. This comes from stereotypic beliefs about the competency of women that are almost always male driven. It seems to me that the same male bias against gays goes hand in hand with bias against women and the origins, I believe, are in traditional male notions of masculinity which just have to change.

I don't see how the author can argue for a new therapy that works with traditional men without also accepting the need for traditional men to change their behavior related to gender stereotyping. In my view, there are really unhealthy aspects of male socialization that just have to be changed and a respectful approach to treatment might help, but the bottom line is that men need to change their attitudes about gays, lesbians, women and anyone who deviates even slightly from traditional notions of gender behavior.

AUTHOR'S COMMENTS

I've categorized the major criticisms into several parts with comments.

Male Bashing

I understand that women feel a good deal of provocation to bash men and that many women have considerable reason to be angry. Still, bashing is just unacceptable. What good can come of it? When bashing occurs, it always generates a dysfunctional response. As Poussaint (1993) argues in the reaction of Black men to male bashing by Black women:

> Unfortunately, some Black men tend to direct their destructive rage against Black women, employing violence, rape, battery and sexual ha-

rassment. Extremist rap musicians have even advocated sexual abuse and murder of "the bitches." And Black men, unlike most Black women, engage in self-destructive behaviors—their involvement in crime and drugs has resulted in too many ending up in jail, unemployable or dead! (p. 88)

Men Aren't Able to Use Therapy

I'm surprised that my call for a new approach to therapy was so widely criticized when the same thing has been said about women and people of color. After all, therapy is a helping process. If it doesn't work well with a certain group, we shouldn't blame that group, but we should use the criticism to develop new helping approaches. I don't see that this has been done and I wonder if the reason has less to do with the inability of men to use therapy as much as the unwillingness of therapists to change their approaches to helping, approaches which have been roundly criticized in the literature. O'Donnell (1997) says that the current practice of therapy is a process that makes the same mistakes, with growing confidence, over a long number of years. Issacs and Fitzgerald (1999) call current practice "vehemence-based practice," where clinicians substitute volumes of clinical experience for evidence, which is "an effective technique for brow beating your more timorous colleagues and for convincing relatives of your ability" (p. 1).

Flaherty (2001) believes that there is a "murky mythology" behind certain treatment approaches that causes them to persist and that

> Unfounded beliefs of uncertain provenance may be passed down as a kind of clinical lore from professors to students. Clinical shibboleths can remain unexamined for decades because they stem from respected authorities, such as time-honored text-books, renowned experts, or well-publicized but flawed studies in major journals. (p. 1)

Flaherty (2001) goes on to note that even when sound countervailing information becomes available, clinicians still hold onto myths. And more onerous, Flaherty points out that we may perpetuate myths, "by indulging the mistaken beliefs of patients or by making stereotypical assumptions about patients based on age, ethnicity, or gender" (p. 1), concerns in the mental health field that still plague us.

In a review of the effectiveness of psychotherapy over a 40-year period, Bergin (1971) writes,

> It now seems apparent that psychotherapy has had an average effect that
> is modestly positive. The averaged group data on which this conclusion is
> based obscures the existence of a multiplicity of processes occurring in
> therapy, some of which are now known to be unproductive or actually
> harmful. (p. 263)

In a more recent evaluation of the effectiveness of psychotherapy,
Kopta, Lueger, Saunders, and Howard (1999) report the following:

> The traditional view that the different psychotherapies—similar to medi-
> cation treatments—contain unique active ingredients resulting in spe-
> cific effects, has not been validated [and that] the aforementioned
> situations are evidence of a profession in turmoil. (p. 22)

Kopta and colleagues (1999) go on to say that "The field is currently experiencing apparent turmoil in three areas: (a) theory development for
psychotherapeutic effectiveness, (b) research designs, and (c) treatment
techniques" (p. 1). Kopta and colleagues note that researchers have failed
repeatedly to find best evidence that different therapies are effective in
different situations with different groups of clients.

If We Change the Agenda to Men It Will Hurt Women

I've heard this argument many times and I find it troubling. It feels
self-serving and hostile and I suspect that an exclusively female agenda
would also argue, although quietly, that racial and ethnic groups
should also be put on the back burner because their needs might make
the needs of women secondary. Men have been going through difficult
times for a long while. We need to resolve male problems if we are to
continue having normal family life and marriage. Poussaint (1993) argues for a cooperative relationship between men and women where
their mutual problems can be satisfactorily resolved without a sense
that one gender is giving up something for the purpose of helping the

other gender. Some of the ways we can develop cooperative relations include the following:

- Recognizing sexist behaviors and eliminating gender stereotypes.
- Eliminating competition between genders and avoiding destructive game playing.
- The genders need to listen better to one another and to be more empathic.
- We need to fund and study couples whose relationships work particularly well.
- Much effort should be spent for treating one another well, which means eliminating put-downs and name calling.

Including Material About Gay Men and Homophobia

It's true that I didn't write about gay and bisexual men. This wasn't so much an omission as a sense that gay and bisexual men often have the same problems as other men and that those problems are covered in the book. But I also have to say that the opinions of gay and bisexual men on appropriate treatment approaches are more likely to be accurate and helpful when made by those men. Enough straight men have said ridiculous things about gay and bisexual men for me not to want to repeat past mistakes. Although I did discuss homophobia in a number of chapters, not enough can ever be said about the harm caused by rigidly traditional male attitudes toward anyone whose sexuality even hints of homosexuality. A good example of that harm is described by Bidsrup (2000):

There are the obvious murders inspired by hatred. In the U.S., they number in the dozens every year. Abroad, the numbers run to the hundreds to thousands, no one knows the precise number for sure, as in many countries, the deaths of homosexuals are not considered worth recording as a separate category.

But there are other ways in which homophobia kills. There are countless suicides every year by gay men and lesbians, particularly youth, which mental health professionals tell us are not the direct result of the victim's homosexuality, but is actually the result of how the homosexual is treated by society. When one lives with rejection day after day, and society discounts one's value constantly, it is difficult to maintain perspective and realize that the problem is *others'* perceptions, not one's own, which is why suicide is several times as common among gay men as it is among straight men.

Perhaps the highest price is paid by youth. The young person just emerging into adulthood who has begun to realize that he is different, and the difference is not approved of, finds acceptance of self particularly difficult. This is especially true when others perceive the young person as different, and persecute him as a result, with little effort made by authority figures to stop the torment. This is why gay youth commit suicide at a rate of about seven times that of straight youth. Yet it is surprising how often homophobes actually try to prevent intervention by teachers in the schools!

Traditional Men Are More Likely to Have Physical and Emotional Problems

The concept of traditional men is in many ways an abstraction. The more rigidly traditional the attitudes, in theory, the more unlikely men are to use helping services. That doesn't mean traditional men are unhealthy in their views of life or that their behavior is necessarily dysfunctional. It just means that they hold to notions of masculinity that are historically traditional in our culture. I think this desire for a make-over from traditional to sensitive man is troubling. You take what you have and you work with it, and what many traditional men have is a desire for a healthy, respectful family life. They often want to be productive at work and to contribute to the world. The way to help them when the need arises is to develop strategies that make sense to them. Offering the advice of other men and women is one way to help. Strategically-placed helping professionals in the workplace and positive messages in films and TV programs about the importance of taking care of one's self and using helping professionals when needed, all have an impact on men. And let's face it, more and more men are moving away from notions of rigidly, traditional, masculine values. Fewer people are getting divorced. Family violence and spousal abuse rates have dropped in the past few years. Change is taking place and out of it, so is the notion of rigidly, traditional masculinity.

I recently spoke to a doctor who treats very poor immigrant farm workers in the Coachella Valley near Palm Springs, CA. She told me that more and more men who have emotional problems are coming to her with an understanding of their behavior and a desire to change it. A local mental health clinic serving Hispanic men and women is overflowing with male clients receiving counseling. People have become educated through the information they receive in the media on mental health, even very poor traditional people, and the rigid masculinity we associate with dysfunction is changing. The mental health clinic uses much of what we've discussed in the developmental model and is highly cooperative and respectful, with very short-term, educationally-oriented treatment. You know that male client satisfaction is great because men are referring other men to the clinic.

Women Are Doing Better Than Men Because They Are Better

This is one of those arguments that makes me wonder about how far we will go with gender politics. Women are doing well but you can't deny that many years of affirmative action and attempts to make education more accessible to women have helped them. I'm asking that the same be done for men. In my field of social work, where men constitute less than ten percent of the student population, and men of color are almost nonexistent, affirmative action and equal opportunity statements about programs still stress that women are encouraged to apply. I haven't seen similar statements about men although they're so underrepresented in the field. That women are doing well is cause for joy. That men aren't doing well certainly isn't cause for women to say they were better than men all along. Those statements are just an extension of male bashing and sexual politics. We get them in many different ways. Women tell us they're more conciliatory and cooperative as managers and that they run organizations in highly collegial styles because that's the way women are. But many of us have worked with women managers who are as dictatorial, autocratic, and mean spirited as many male administrators. Gender stereotyping is getting us into deep trouble in this society because it paints outrageous and stereotypic pictures of men and women which interfere with our relationships with one another. Let's stop bragging about which gender is better and get on with the job of equity between the genders and the needed help to maintain equity when necessary. As Migliaccio (2001) writes in discussing the way men have become marginalized in our society

> Being marginalized in Western society involves denial of access to resources, inability to assume a dominant identity, and the perception by others as a deviant. Being marginalized constitutes being defined as "other" by the dominant group, which designates an individual to a lower status in the social hierarchy. It is a determinant of power that maintains the inequality of the system. (p. 205)

FEEDBACK, CRITICISM, AND THANKS

I know that many of you, men and women, have strong opinions about the material in this book on men. Because this is an initial book and there will hopefully be more editions or more books on men in the future, please send me your comments. Feedback, criticisms, and opinions are very much welcomed, and do give me permission to use them in future work. You can contact me at mglicken@msn.com

Thank you for reading my book on men. Men are not doing well these days. Poor men and minority men are doing least well. I hope this book helps in your practice with men and that you feel a bit more aware of how men think about change, the approaches that may work best with a particular type of man and a particular problem, and that the difficult male client who seems so resistant to change will now be seen as someone who has a great deal of gender influences that make change difficult. Don't give up!

References

Chapter 1

Allen, J. (2003, June 23). Are men obsolete? *U.S. News & World Report, 134*(22), 33.

Balcom, D. A. (1998, April 30). Absent fathers: Effects on abandoned sons. *Journal of Men's Studies, 6*(3), 283–302.

Conlin, M. (2003, May 26). The new gender gap. *Business Week*, 74–81.

Courtenay, W. (1998). College men's health: An overview and a call to action. *Journal of American College Health, 46*(6), 279–290.

D'Antonio, M. (1994, December 5). The fragile sex. *L.A. Times*, p. 16.

Dead-Beat Dads. (1993, March 12). *L.A. Times*, Metro Section, Part B, p. 6. Author.

DiIulio, J. J., Jr. (1996a, February 28). *Fill churches, not jails: Youth crime and super predators: Statement before the United States Senate Subcommittee on Youth Violence*. Retrieved May 17, 2003, from http://www/brook.edu/pa/hot/diiulio.htm

DiIulio, J. J., Jr. (1996b, July 13). Stop crime where it starts. *The New York Times*. Retrieved May 17, 2003, from http://www.brook.edu/pa/hot/arttoppics/diiulio.htm

Dunn, J. (1994, April 10). The fear of violence. *L.A. Times*, pp. 26–29.

Ellum, F. (1994, December 5). Found in the fragile sex, by M. D'Antonio. *L.A. Times*, p. 26.

Families and Work Institute. (1995). *Women: The new providers* (Whirlpool Foundation Study, Part One).

Farrell, W. (1992). Farrell addresses the future of the men's movement. *Transitions, 12*(1), pp. 1–12.

Freudenberger, H. (1987, December). Today's troubled man: Afraid of commitment, they flee it through hard work and play. *Psychology Today*. Retrieved November 26, 2004, from www.findarticles.com/p/articles/min_m1175/is_n12-v21/ai_6145395/pg2

Furstenberg, F. F., Jr., Nord, C. W., Peterson, J. L., & Zill, N. (1983). The life course of children of divorce: Marital disruption and parental contact. *American Sociological Review, 48,* 656–668.

Herzog, E., & Sudia, C. (1971). Boys in fatherless families. DHEW (Pub. No. [OCD] 72–33). Washington, DC: U.S. Government Printing Office.

Krugman, S. (1995). Male development and the transformation of shame. In R. Levant & W. Pollack (Eds.), *A new psychology of men* (chap. 4, pp. 83–97). New York: Basic Books.

Levant, R. F. (1997, February 28). The masculinity crisis. *Journal of Men's Studies, 5*(3), pp. 221–231.

Marin, P. (1991, July 8). The prejudice against men. *The Nation, 253*(2), 85–91.

O'Neill, T. (2000, December 4). Boys' problems don't matter. *Newsmagazine, 27*(15), 54–56.

Osofsky, H. J., & Osofsky, J. D. (2001). Violent and aggressive behaviors in youth: A mental health and prevention perspective. *Psychiatry, 64*(4), 285–295.

Roach, R. (2001, May 10). Where are the Black men on campus? *Black Issues in Higher Education.* Retrieved September 13, 2004, from http://www.findarticles.com/cf_0/m0DXK/6_18/75561775/print.jhtml

Schenk, R., & Everingham, J. (Eds.). (1995). *Men healing shame: An anthology.* New York: Springer.

Slater, E. (June 23, 2003). Democratic candidates skewer Bush in appeal to Black voters. *Los Angels Times,* p. A13.

Steinmetz, S. K., & Lucca, J. S. (1988). Husband battering. In V. B. Van Hasselt, R. L. Morrison, R. L. Bellack, & N. Hesen (Eds.), *Handbook of Family Violence.* New York: Plenum.

Svoboda, S. (2002, January 31). Why boys don't talk and why we care: A mother's guide to connection. *Everyman: A Men's Journal, 52,* 67–82.

U.S. Census Department. (1998). United States Census Department report. Washington, DC: Author.

U.S. Office of Child Support Enforcement. (2003, April 29). Child Support Enforcement (CSE) FY 2002 Preliminary Data Report. U.S. Department of Health and Human Services. Administration for Children and Families. Retrieved May 2, 2004, from http://www.acf.dhhs.gov/programs/cse/pubs/2003/reports/prelim_datareport/

Wolfgang, M. E., Figlio, R. M., & Selling, T. (1972). *Delinquency in a birth cohort.* Chicago: University of Chicago Press.

Chapter 2

Bereska, T. M. (2003). The changing boys' world in the 20th century: Reality and fiction. *Journal of Men's Studies, 11*(2), 157–183.

Brannon, R. C. (1976). No "sissy stuff": The stigma of anything vaguely feminine. In S. Sailid & R. Brannon (Eds.), *The forty-nine percent majority* (pp. 57–87). Reading, MA: Addison-Wesley.

Brooks, G. R. (1998). *A new psychotherapy for traditional men.* San Francisco: Jossey-Bass.

Cowley, G. (2003, June 16). Why we strive for status. *Newsweek*, pp. 67–70.

Fabes, R. A., Eisenberg, N., Karbon, M., Troyer, D., & Switzer, G. (1994). The relation of children's emotion regulation to their vicarious emotional responses and comforting behaviors. *Child Development, 65*, 1678–1693.

Farrell, W. (1992). Farrell addresses the future of the men's movement. *Transitions, 12*(1), 1–12.

Fivush, R. (1989). Exploring sex differences in the emotional content of mother–child conversations about the past. *Sex Roles, 20*, 675–691.

Gilligan, C. (1982). *In a different voice.* Cambridge, MA: Harvard University Press.

Hopkins, W. D., & Bard, K. A. (1993). Hemispheric specialisation in infant chimpanzees (Pan troglodytes): Evidence for a relation with gender and arousal. *Developmental Psychobiology, 26*, 219–235.

Keller, A. K., & West, M. (1995). Attachment organisation and vulnerability to loss, separation, and abuse in disturbed adolescents. In S. Goldberg, R. Muir, & J. Kerr (Eds.), *Attachment theory: Social, developmental and clinical perspectives* (p. 327). Hillsdale, NJ: Analytic Press.

Kohlberg, L. (1987). *Child psychology and childhood education: A cognitive developmental view.* London: Long Group United Kingdom.

Kraemer, S. (2000). The fragile male. *British Medical Journal, 321*, 1609–1612

Levinson, D. J., Darrow, C. N., Klein, E. B., Levinson, M. H., & McKee, B. (1978). *The seasons of a man's life.* New York: Ballantine.

Mahalik, J. R., Locke, B. D., Theodore, H., Cournoyer, R. J., & Lloyd, B. F. (2001). A cross-national and cross-sectional comparison of men's gender role conflict and its relationship to social intimacy and self-esteem. *Sex Roles: A Journal of Research.* Retrieved May 21, 2004, from http://www.findarticles.com/cf_0/PI/search.jhtml?key=men%27s+health&page=3&magR=all+magazines

Mead, M. (1935). *Sex and temperament in three primitive societies.* New York: William Morrow and Co.

Murray, L., Kempton, C., Woolgar, M., & Hooper, R. (1993). Depressed mothers' speech to their infants and its relation to infant gender and cognitive development. *Journal of Child Psychiatry; 34*, 1083–1101

O'Neil, J. M. (1981). Patterns of gender role conflict in: Sexism and fear of femininity in men's lives. *Personnel and Guidance Journal, 60.*

O'Neil, J. M., & Egan, J. (1992). Men's gender role transitions over the life span: Transformations and fears of femininity. *Journal of Mental Health Counseling, 14*, 305–324.

Parker, J. D. A., Keightley, M. L., Smith, C. T., & Taylor, G. (1999). Interhemispheric transfer deficit in alexithymia: An experimental study. *Psychosomatic Medicine, 61*, 464–468.

Pitman, F. S. (1993). *Man enough: Fathers, sons, and the search for masculinity.* New York: Putnam.

Pleck, J. H. (1980). Men's power with women, other men, and society: A men's movement analysis. In E. Pleck & J. H. Pleck (Eds.), *The American man* (pp. 417–433). Englewood Cliffs, NJ: Prentice Hall.

Pleck, J. H. (1987). The contemporary man. In M. Scher, H. Stevens, G. Goud, & G. A. Eichenfeld (Eds.), *Handbook of counseling & psychotherapy with men* (pp. 16–27). Newbury Park, CA: Sage.

Pleck, J. H. (1995). The gender role strain paradigm: An update. In R. F. Levant & W. S. Pollack (Eds.), *A new psychology of men* (pp. 11–32). New York: Basic Books.

Pollack, W. (1990). Men's development and psychotherapy. *Psychotherapy, 27.*

Pollack, W. (1998). *Real boys: Rescuing our sons from the myths of boyhood.* New York: Random House.

Robertson, J., & Fitzgerald, L. (1992, April). *Journal of Counseling Psychology, 39*(2), 240–246.

Rout, U. (1999). Gender differences in stress, satisfaction and mental well-being among general practitioners in England. *Psychological Health Medicine, 4*, 345–354.

Sackett, G. P. (1972). Exploratory behavior of rhesus monkeys as a function of rearing experiences and sex. *Developmental Psychology, 6*, 260–270.

Sargent, J. (1999). Review of William Pollack, PhD. Random House, New York, 1998, 450 pages. *Everyman: A Men's Journal, 36*, 45.

Scher, M. (1979). On counseling men. *Personnel and Guidance Journal,* 252–254.

Scher, M. (1990). Effect of gender role incongruencies on men's experiences as clients in psychotherapy. *Psychotherapy, 27*, 322–326.

Spielberg, W. E. (1990). Why men need to be heroic. *Journal of Men's Studies, 2*, 173–178.

Van Wormer, K. (1999). The strengths perspective: A paradigm for correctional counseling. *Federal Probation, 63*, 51–58.

Wade, J. C., & Brittan-Powell, C. (2000, September). Male reference group identity dependence: Support for construct validity. *Sex Roles: A Journal of Research,* *12*(5), 45–63. Retrieved June 17, 2004, from http://www.findarticles.com/cf_0/m2294/2000_Sept/71118810/p1/article.jhtml?term=men+%2B+Counseling

Wilson, J. Q. (1993). On gender. *Public Interest,* 3–27.

Worell, J. (1981). Life-span sex roles: Development, continuity, and change. In R. M. Lerner & N. A. Busch-Rossnagel (Eds.), *Individuals as producers of their development: A life-span perspective* (pp. 37–71). New York: Academic.

Yacovene, D. (1990). Abolitionists and the "language of fraternal love." In M. C. Carnes & C. Griffen (Eds.), *Meanings for manhood: Constructions of masculinity in Victorian America* (pp. 85–95). Chicago: University of Chicago Press.

Zaslow, M. J., & Hayes, C. D. (1986). Sex differences in children's response to psychosocial stress: Toward a cross-context analysis. In M. E. Lamb, A. L. Brown, & B. Rogoff (Eds.), *Advances in Developmental Psychology* (Vol. 4, pp. 285–337). Hillsdale, NJ: Lawrence Erlbaum Associates.

Chapter 3

Aaron, F., Hughes, J., Buehler, J., Mittelmark, M., Jacobs, D., & Grimm, R. (1985). Do Type A men drink more frequently than Type B men? Findings in the Multiple Risk Factor Intervention Trial (MRFIT). *Journal of Behavioral Medicine,* *8*, 227–235.

Anderson, R., Kochanek, K., & Murphy, S. (1997). *Report of final mortality statistics* (Monthly Vital Statistics Rep. No. 45). Hyattsville, MD: National Center for Health Statistics.

Cochran, S. V., & Rabinowitz, F. E. (2003, April). Gender-sensitive recommendations for assessment and treatment of depression in men. *Professional Psychology: Research and Practice,* *34*, 132–140.

Courtenay, W. H. (1996). *Health mentor: Health risk assessment for men.* Berkeley, CA: Author.

Courtenay, W. H. (2000). Behavioral factors associated with disease, injury, and death among men: Evidence and Implications for prevention. *Journal of Men's Studies,* *9*, 81–104.

Epperly, T. D., & Moore, K. E. (2000, July 1). Health issues in men: Part II. Common psychosocial disorders. *American Family Physician.* Retrieved January 25, 2005, from http://www.findarticles.com/cf_0/m3225/1_62/65864000/print.jhtml

Gupta, S. (2003, May 12). Why men die young. *Time,* *161*(19), 84.

Harrison, J., Chin, J., & Ficarrotto, T. (1988). Warning: Masculinity may be dangerous to your health. In M. S. Kimmel & M. A. Messner (Eds.), *Men's lives* (pp. 271–285). New York: MacMillan.

Heifner, C. (1997). The male experience of depression. *Perspectives in Psychiatric Care, 33,* 10–18.

Huyck, M. H. (1993). Middle age. *Academic American Encyclopedia, 13,* 390–391.

Karlberg, L., Unden, A.-L., Elofsson, S., & Krakau, I. (1998, Fall). Is there a connection between car accidents, near accidents, and Type A drivers? *Behavioral Medicine, 16*(5), 207–219. Retrieved May 14, 2003, from http://www.findarticles.com/cf_0/m0GDQ/3_24/53478953/p1/article.jhtml

Kogan, M. J. (2000). The pressure men feel to live up to the macho image is literally making them sick. *Monitor on Psychology, 31,* 48–49.

Kraemer, S. (2000). The fragile male. *British Medical Journal, 321,* 1609–1612

Kruger, A. (1994). The mid-life transition: Crisis or chimera? *Psychological Reports, 75,* 1299–1305.

Levinson, D. (1979). *The seasons of a man's life.* New York: Ballantine.

MacDoniels, J. (1997, December 1). *Mid-life crisis: Recent research.* Retrieved January 25, 2005, from http://www.hope.edu/academic/psychology/335/webrep2/crisis.html

Men's health at a glance: A fact sheet for pharmacists. (1998, July 20). *Drug Store News.* Retrieved January 25, 2001, from http://www.findarticles.com/cf_0/m3374/n11_v20/20969541/p1/article.jhtml? term=men+%2B+health

Misener, T. R., & Fuller, S. G. (1995). Testicular versus breast and colorectal cancer screen: Early detection practices of primary care physicians. *Cancer Practice, 3,* 310–316.

Moore, T. (1995). *Type A personality: A collection of traits consisting of competitiveness, urgency, high achievement, and irritability.* From *Gale Encyclopedia of Psychology,* January 1, 1995, by Timothy Moore. Retrieved July 15, 2003, from http://www.findarticles.com/cf0/g2699/0006/269900648/p1/article.jhtml?term=Type+A+Personality

National Center for Chronic Disease Prevention and Health. (2001). *Suicide facts and statistics.* Retrieved May 17, 2004, from http://www.nimh.nih.gov/suicideprevention/suifact.cfm

National Center for Chronic Disease Prevention and Health. (2003). *Prostate cancer: The public health perspective.* Retrieved May 17, 2004, from http://www.cdc.gov/cancer/prostate/prostate.htm#public Promotion

National Institute for Occupational Safety and Health. (1993). *Fatal injuries to workers in the United States, 1980–1989: A decade of surveillance* (DHHS [NIOSH] No. 93–108). Cincinnati, OH: Author.

Reuben, D. B., Yoshikawa, T. T., & Besdine, R. W. (Eds.). (1996). *Geriatrics review syllabus; a core curriculum in geriatric medicine* (3rd ed., pp. 207–210). New York: American Geriatric Society.

Saunders, C. S. (2000, June 15). Where are all the men? *Patient Care*. Retrieved May 15, 2003, from http://www.findarticles.com/cf_0/m3233/11_34/63602907/print.jhtm

Seligman, D. (2004, June 7). Why the rich live longer. *Forbes, 173*, 113–114.

Shek, D. T. L. (1996). Mid-life crisis in Chinese men and women. *Journal of Psychology, 130*, 109–119.

Chapter 4

Abernathy, M. (2003, January 9). *Popmatters.com: An Internet Journal*. Retrieved April 17, 2003, from http://popmatters.com/tv/features/030109-male-bashing.shtml

Alkon, A. (2003, September 17–23). All you need to know about men. *The Boise Weekly, 16*(5), 17.

Association for Advanced Training in the Behavioral Sciences. (1991). Preparation course for the psychology licensure examination (Vol. 4). Westlake Village, CA: Author.

Cary, S. (1998, October 8). The big bash (men bashing). *Men's Fitness, 3*(10), 14–17. Retrieved September 12, 2004, from http://www.findarticles.com/cf_0/m1608/n10_v14/21148337/print.jhtml

Farrell, W. (1999). *Women can't hear what men don't*. New York: J. P. Tarcher.

Grant-Bowman, C. (1994, April 4). *USA Today, 14*(26), 15A.

Heckard, I. D. (1998). Male bashing: Is it trash talk or harmless humor? *Christianity Today International: Today's Christian Woman, 20*(1), 46.

Kaufman, G. (1999, September 10). The portrayal of men's family roles in television commercials. *Sex Roles: A Journal of Research, 30*(9), 36–43. Retrieved May 17, 2004, from http://www.findarticles.com/cf_0/m2294/1999_Sept/58469479/p1/article.jhtml?term=psychotherapy+%2B

Kelly, K. R, & Hall, A. S. (1992). Toward a developmental model of counseling men. *Journal of Mental Health Counseling, 16*(4), 257–273.

Kelly, K. R., & Hall, A. S. (1994). Affirming the assumptions of the developmental model for counseling men. *Journal of Mental Health Counseling, 16*, 475–483.

Lamb, M. E., Frodi, A. M., Hwang, C.-P., & Frodi, M. (1982). Varying degrees of paternal involvement in infant care: Attitudinal and behavioral correlates. In M. E.

Lamb (Ed.), *Non-traditional families: Parenting and child development* (pp. 117–137). Hillsdale, NJ: Lawrence Erlbaum Associates.

Lehrman, K. (1994, April 14). Has sexual correctness gone too far? *USA Today, 14*(26), 15A.

Leo, J. (1994, April 18). DE-escalating the gender war. *U.S. News & World Report, 116*(15), 24.

Morrison, P. (1994, October 4). Woman who killed abusive mate may be set free. *Los Angeles Times,* p. A3.

Morrow, L. (1994, February 14). *Time, 143*(7), 52–60.

Stillman, D. (1994, February 27). Has feminism missed the point? *Los Angeles Times, 107,* p. 32.

Nathanson, P., & Young, K. (2001). *Spreading misandry: The teaching of contempt for men in popular culture.* Toronto, Canada: McGill-Queen's University Press.

Wetzstein, C. (2000, January 10). Has man-bashing become the hallmark of greeting cards? *Insight on the News, 1.* Retrieved September 11, 2004, from http://www.findarticles.com/cf_0/m1571/2_16/58617319/print.jhtml

Young, C. (2000, March). The man question [Review of the book *Stiffed: The betrayal of the American male*]. Retrieved August 12, 2003, from http://www.findarticles.com/cf_0/m1568/10_31/59580158/print.jhtml

Chapter 5

Alcohol Alert. (2003). *National Institute of Alcohol Abuse and Alcoholism, 49.*

American Psychiatric Association. (1994). *Diagnostic and statistical manual of mental disorders* (4th ed.). Washington, DC: Author.

Bisson, J., Nadeau, L., & Demers, A. (1999). The validity of the CAGE scale to screen heavy drinking and drinking problems in a general population. *Addiction, 94,* 715–723.

Cloud, J. (2003). How we get labeled. *Time, 161*(3), 102–106.

Davis, R. T., Blashfield, R. K., & McElroy, R. A. (1993). Weighting criteria in the diagnosis of a personality disorder: A demonstration. *Journal of Abnormal Psychology, 102,* 319–322.

DeGrandpre, R. (1999). *Ritalin nation: Rapid-fire culture and the transformation of human consciousness.* New York: Norton.

Dwyer, K. P., Osher, D., & Warger, W. (1998). *Early warning, timely response: A guide to safe schools.* Washington, DC: U.S. Department of Education. (ERIC Document Reproduction Service No. ED 418 372)

Evidence-Based Medicine Working Group. (1992). Evidence-based medicine: A new approach to teaching the practice of medicine. *Journal of the American Medical Association, 268,* 2420–2425.

Franklin, A. J. (1992). Therapy with African American men. *Families in Society: The Journal of Contemporary Human Services, 26*(7), 350–355.

Gambrill, E. (2000, October). *Evidence based practice.* A handout to the dean and directors of schools of social work meeting, Huntington, Beach, CA.

Glicken, M. D. (2004a). *Using the strengths perspective in social work practice: A positive approach for the helping professions.* Boston: Allyn & Bacon/Longman.

Glicken, M. D. (2004b). *Violent young children.* Boston: Allyn & Bacon/Longman.

Glicken, M. D. (2005). *Improving the effectiveness of the helping professions: An evidence-based approach to practice.* Thousand Oaks, CA: Sage.

Havercamp, B. (1993). Confirmatory bias in hypothesis testing for client-identified and counselor self-generated hypotheses. *Journal of Consulting Psychology, 40,* 305–315.

Lynam, D. (1996). Early identification of chronic offenders: Who is the fledgling psychopath? *Psychological Bulletin, 120,* 209–234.

Markowitz, F. E. (1998). The effects of stigma on the psychological well-being and life satisfaction of persons with mental illness. *Journal of Health & Social Behavior, 39*(4), 335–347.

McLaughlin, J. E. (2002). Reducing diagnostic bias. *Journal of Mental Health Counseling, 24,* 256–270.

Moffitt, T. E. (1994). Adolescence-limited and life-course persistent antisocial behavior: A developmental taxonomy. *Psychological Review, 100,* 674–701.

Morey, L. C., & Ochoa, E. S. (1989). An investigation of adherence to diagnostic criteria: Clinical diagnosis of the DSM–III personality disorders. *Journal of Personality Disorders, 3,* 180–192.

Obiakor, F. E., Merhing, T. A., & Schwenn, J. O. (1997). *Disruption, disaster, and death: Helping students deal with crises.* Reston, VA: The Council for Exceptional Children. (ERIC Document Reproduction Service No. ED 403 709)

Pfeiffer, A. M., Whelan, J. P., & Martin, J. L. (2000). Decision-making in psychotherapy: Effects of hypothesis source and accountability. *Journal of Counseling Psychology, 47,* 429–436.

Robertson, J., & Fitzgerals, L. F. (1990). The (mis) treatment of men: Effects of client gender role and life-style on diagnosis and attribution of pathology. *Journal of Counseling Psychology, 37,* 3–9.

Rosenhan, D. L. (1973). On being sane in insane places. *Science, 179,* 240–248.

Saleebey, D. (1996). The strengths perspective in social work practice: Extensions and cautions. *Social Work, 41*(3), 296–305.

Satcher, D. (2001). *Mental health: Culture, race, and ethnicity. A supplement to mental health: A report of the Surgeon General.* Retrieved May 23, 2004, from http://www.surgeongeneral.gov/library/mentalhealth/cre/release.asp

Sharp, W. S., Walter, J. M., & Marsh, W. L. (1999). ADHD in girls: Clinical comparability of a research sample. *Journal of the American Academy of Child and Adolescent Psychiatry, 38*, 40–47.

Sprague, J. R., & Walker, H. M. (2000). Early identification and intervention for youth with antisocial and violent behavior. *Exceptional Children, 66*(3), 367–379.

Stewart, K. B., & Richards, A. B. (2000). Recognizing and managing your patient's alcohol abuse. *Nursing, 30*, 56–60.

Walker, H. M., & Severson, H. H. (1990). *Systematic screening for behavior disorders.* Longmont, CO: Sopris West.

Werner, E., & Smith, R. S. (1992). *Overcoming the odds: High-risk children from birth to adulthood.* Ithaca, NY: Cornell University Press.

Whaley, A. L. (2001). Cultural mistrust: An important psychological construct for diagnosis and treatment of African Americans. *Psychology: Research and Practice, 32*(6), 555–562

Wilke, D. (1994). Women and alcoholism: How a male-as-norm bias affects research, assessment, and treatment. *Health and Social Work, 19*, 29–35.

Chapter 6

Bisman, C. (1994). *Social work practice: Cases and principles.* Belmont, CA: Brooks/ Cole.

Brent, D. A. (1998, February). Psychotherapy: Definitions, mechanisms of action, and relationship to etiological models. *Journal of Abnormal Child Psychology, 26*(1), 17–25. Retrieved October 15, 2003, from http://www.findarticles.com/ cf_0/m0902/n1_v26/20565425/print.jhtml

Burns, D. D., & Nolen-Hoeksema, S. (1992). Therapeutic empathy and recovery from depression in cognitive-behavioral therapy: A structural equation model. *Journal of Consulting and Clinical Psychology, 60*, 441–449.

Cooley, E. J., & Lajoy, R. (1980). Therapeutic relationship and improvement as perceived by clients and therapists. *Journal of Clinical Psychology, 36*, 562–570.

Connors, G. J., Carroll, K. M., DiClemente, C. C., Longabaugh, R., & Donovan, D. M. (1997). The therapeutic alliance and its relationship to alcoholism treatment participation and outcome. *Journal of Consulting and Clinical Psychology, 65*, 588–598.

Entwistle, V. A., Sheldon, T. A., Sowden, A., & Watt, I. S. (1998). Evidence-informed patient choice. Practical issues of involving patients in decisions about health care technologies. *International Journal of Technology Assessment in Health Care, 14*, 212–225.

Evidence-Based Medicine Working Group. (1992). Evidence-based medicine: A new approach to teaching the practice of medicine. *Journal of the American Medical Association, 268,* 2420–2425.

Gambrill, E. (1999). Evidence-based practice: An alternative to authority-based practice. *Journal of Contemporary Human Services, 80,* 341–350.

Gambrill, E. (2000, October). *Evidence-based practice. A handout to the dean and directors of schools of social work.* Huntington Beach, CA.

Gehart-Brooks, D. R., & Lyle, R. R. (1999). Client and therapist perspectives of change in collaborative language systems: An interpretive ethnography. *Journal of Systemic Therapies, 18,* 78–97.

Gehart, D. R., & Lyle, R. D. (2001). Client experience of gender in therapeutic relationships: An interpretive ethnography. *Family Process, 40,* 443–458.

Glicken, M. D. (2004a). *Using the strengths perspective in social work practice: A positive approach for the helping professions.* Boston: Allyn & Bacon/Longman.

Glicken, M. D. (2004b). *Violent young children.* Boston: Allyn & Bacon/Longman.

Henry, W. P., Schacht, T. E., & Strupp, H. H. (1986). Structural analysis of social behavior: Application to a study of interpersonal process in differential psychotherapeutic outcome. *Journal of Consulting and Clinical Psychology, 54,* 27–31.

Horvath, A. O., & Greenberg, L. S. (Eds.). (1994). *The working alliance: Theory, research, and practice.* New York: Wiley.

Horvath, A. O., & Symonds, B. D. (1991). Relation between working alliance and outcome in psychotherapy: A meta-analysis. *Journal of Consulting and Clinical Psychology, 38,* 139–149.

Jones, E. E., & Zoppel, C. L. (1982). Impact of client and therapist gender on psychotherapy process and outcome. *Journal of Consulting and Clinical Psychology, 50,* 259–272.

Keith-Lucas, A. (1972). *Giving and taking help.* Chapel Hill: University of North Carolina Press.

Kopta, M. S., Lueger, R. J., Saunders, S. M., & Howard, K. I. (1999). Individual psychotherapy outcome and process research: Challenges leading to greater turmoil or a positive transition? *Annual Review of Psychology, 50,* 441–469. Retrieved April 13, 2001, from http://www.findarticles.com/cf_0/ m0961/1999_Annual/ 54442307/print.jhtml

Krupnick, J. L., Sotsky, S. M., Simmens, S., Moyer, J., Elkin, I., Watkins, J., & Pilkonis, A. (1996). The role of the therapeutic alliance in psychotherapy and pharmacotherapy outcome: findings in the National Institute of Mental Health Treatment of Depression Collaborative Research Program. *Journal of Consulting and Clinical Psychology, 64,* 532–539.

Lanzillo, A. B. (1999, October 31). A new psychotherapy for traditional men. *Journal of Men's Studies, 8*(1), 119.

Luborsky, L., McLellan, A. T., Woody, G. E., O'Brien, C. P., & Auerbach, A. (1985). Therapist success and its determinants. *Archives of General Psychiatry, 42,* 602–611.

Murphy, G. E., Simons, A. D, Wetzel, R. D., & Lustman, P. J. (1984). Cognitive therapy and pharmacotherapy: Singly and together in the treatment of depression. *Archives of General Psychiatry, 41,* 33–41.

Orlinsky, D. E., Grawe, K., & Parks, B. K. (1994). Process and outcome in psychotherapy—noch einmal. In A. E. Bergin & S. L. Garfield (Eds.), *Handbook of psychotherapy and behavior change* (4th ed., pp. 270–378). New York: Wiley.

Saleebey, D. (1996). The strengths perspective in social work practice: Extensions and cautions. *Social Work, 41,* 296–305.

Saleebey, D. (2000). Power to the people: Strength and hope. *Advancements in Social Work, 1,* 127–136.

Scher, M. (1979). On counseling men. *Personnel and Guidance Journal,* 252–254.

Seligman, M. E. P. (1995). The effectiveness of psychotherapy: The *Consumers Report* study. *American Psychologist, 50,* 965–974.

Sells, S. P., Smith, T. E., Coe, M. J., Yoshioka, M., & Robbins, J. (1994). An ethnography of couple and therapist experiences in reflecting team practice. *Journal of Marital and Family Therapy, 20,* 247–266.

Shields, C. G., & McDaniel, S. H. (1992). Process differences between male and female therapists in a first family interview. *Journal of Marital and Family Therapy, 18,* 143–151.

Warren, C. S. (2001). [Review of the book *Negotiating the therapeutic alliance: A relational treatment guide*]. *Psychotherapy Research, 11*(3), 357–359.

Weiss, W. D., Sampson, H., & O'Connor. L. (1995, Spring). How psychotherapy works: The findings of the San Francisco Psychotherapy Research Group. *Bulletin of the Psychoanalytic Research Society, 4,* 48–69.

Werner-Wilson, R. J., Price, S. J., Zimmerman, T. S., & Murphy, M. J. (1997). Client gender as a process variable in marriage and family therapy: Are women clients interrupted more than men clients? *Journal of Family Psychotherapy, 11,* 373–377.

Werner-Wilson, R. J., Zimmerman, T. S., & Price, S. J. (1999). Are goals and topics influenced by gender modality in the initial marriage and family therapy session? *Journal of Marital and Family Therapy, 25,* 253–262.

Chapter 7

Bly, R. (1986, April–May). The initiation rites of men. *Utne Reader, 6*(2), 14–19.

Brooks, G. R. (1998). *A new psychotherapy for traditional men.* San Francisco: Jossey-Bass.

Brooks, G. R. (1999). A new psychotherapy for traditional men. *Journal of Men's Studies, 8,* 119–125.

Cochran, S. V., & Rabinowitz, F. E. (2003). Gender-sensitive recommendations for assessment and treatment of depression in men. *Professional Psychology: Research and Practice, 34,* 132–140.

DeMaris, A. (1989). Attrition in batterers counseling: The role of social and demographic factors. *Social Service Review, 63,* 355–383.

Gambrill, E. (1999). Evidence-based practice: An alternative to authority-based practice. *Journal of Contemporary Human Services, 80,* 341–350.

Glicken, M. D. (1995). *A guide to working with abusive men.* Unpublished manuscript.

Glicken, M. D. (2004). *The strengths perspective: A positive approach for the helping professions.* Boston: Allyn & Bacon/Longman.

Kelly, K. R., & Hall, A. S. (1992a). Toward a developmental model of counseling men. *Journal of Mental Health Counseling, 14,* 257–273.

Kelly, K. R., & Hall, A. S. (1992b). Mental health counseling for men: A special issue. *Journal of Mental Health Counseling, 14,* 255–256.

Kelly, K. R., & Hall, A. S. (1994). Counseling men. *Journal of Mental Health Counseling, 16,* 475–483

Lanzillo, A. B. (1999). [Review of the book *A new psychotherapy for traditional men*]. *Journal of Men's Studies, 8,* 119–131.

O'Neill, J. M. (1982). Gender-role conflict and strain in men's lives. In K. Solomon & N. B. Levy (Eds.), *Men in transition: Theory and therapy* (pp. 5–44). New York: Plenum.

Pollack, W. (1990). Men's development and psychotherapy. *Psychotherapy, 27,* 27–39.

Robertson, J., & Fitzgerald, L. (1990). The mistreatment of men: Effects of client gender role and life style on diagnosis and attrition on pathology. *Journal of Counseling Psychology, 37,* 3–9.

Robertson, J., & Fitzgerald, L. (1992). *Journal of Counseling Psychology, 39,* 240–246.

Robertson, J. M., Lin, C., Woodford, J., Danos, K. K., & Hurst, M. A. (2001). The (un)emotional male: Physiological, verbal, and written correlates of expressiveness. *Journal of Men's Studies, 9,* 393–415.

Saleebey, D. (1996). The strengths perspective in social work practice: Extensions and cautions. *Social Work, 41,* 296–305.

Saleebey, D. (2000). Power in the people; strength and hope. *Advances in Social Work, 1,* 127–136.

Scher, M. (1979, January). On counseling men. *Personnel and Guidance Journal, 12,* 252–254.

Scher, M. (1990). Effect of gender role incongruencies on men's experiences as clients in psychotherapy. *Psychotherapy, 27,* 322–326.

Chapter 8

Allen, J., & Laird, J. (1998). Tales of absent fathers: Applying the "story" metaphor in family therapy. *Family Process, 32*(4), 441–458.

Eisikovits, Z. C., & Edelson, J. L. (1989). Intervening with men who batter: A critical review of the literature. *Social Service Review, 63,* 441–463.

Franklin, A. J. (1992). Therapy with African American men. *Families in Society: The Journal of Contemporary Human Services, 26*(7), 350–355.

Glicken, M. D. (1995). *Abusive men: A research report.* Unpublished manuscript.

Kelly, K. R., & Hall, A. S. (1994). Counseling men. *Journal of Mental Health Counseling, 16,* 475–483.

Haley, J. (1986). *Uncommon therapy: The psychiatric techniques of Milton H. Erickson, MD.* New York: Norton.

Hendrix, D. H. (1986). Metaphors as nudges toward understanding in mental health counseling. *Journal of Mental Health Counseling, 14,* 234–242.

Heston, M. L., & Kottman, S. (1997). Movies as metaphors: A counseling intervention. *Journal of Humanistic Education & Development, 36,* 92–100.

MacLeod, J. M. (2000, Winter). The two of us. *Grinnel Review, 16,* 49–50.

Martin, J., Cummings, A. L., & Hallberg, E. T. (1992). Therapists' intentional use of metaphor: Memorability, clinical impact, and possible epistemic/motivational functions. *Journal of Counseling and Clinical Psychology, 60,* 143–145.

Myers, J. E. (1998). Bibliotherapy and DCT: Co-constructing the therapeutic metaphor. *Journal of Counseling & Development, 76,* 243–251.

Pardeck, J. T. (1995). Bibliotherapy: An innovative approach for helping children. *Early Childhood Development and Care, 110,* 83–88.

Penn, P. (2001). Chronic illness: Trauma, language, and writing: Breaking the Silence. *Family Process, 40,* 33–52.

Rosen, J. (2003). My kafka problem. *American Scholar, 72,* 85–91.

Salloum, A., Avery, L., & McClain, R. P. (2001). Group psychotherapy for adolescent survivors of homicide victims: A pilot study. *Pediatrics, 107,* 1125–1132

Scapillato, D., & Manassis, K. (2002, June). Cognitive-behavioral/interpersonal group treatment for anxious adolescents. *Journal of the American Academy of Child and Adolescent Psychiatry, 41*(6), 739–741.

Zuniga, M. E. (1992). Using metaphors in therapy: Dichos and Latino clients. *Social Work, 37*(1), 55–60.

Chapter 9

Bly, R. (1986, April–May). Men of wisdom. *Utne Reader, 6*(3), 14–19.

Caserta, M. S., & Lund, D. A. (1993). Intrapersonal resources and the effectiveness of self-help groups for bereaved older adults. *Gerontologist, 33,* 619–629.

Christo, G., & Sutton, S. (1994). Anxiety and self-esteem as a function of abstinence time among recovering addicts attending narcotics anonymous. *British Journal of Clinical Psychology, 33,* 198–200.

Emrick, C. D., & Tonigan, J. S. (1993). Alcoholics Anonymous: What is currently known? In B. S. McCrady & W. R. Miller (Eds.), *Research on Alcoholics Anonymous: Opportunities and alternatives* (pp. 41–75). New Brunswick, NJ: Rutgers Center of Alcohol Studies.

Fetto, J. (2000). Lean on me. *American Demographics, 22,* 16.

Galanter, M. (1988). Zealous self-help groups as adjuncts to psychiatric treatment: A study of Recovery, Inc. *American Journal of Psychiatry, 145,* 1248–1253.

Gilden, J. L., Hendryx, A. S., Clar, S., Casia, P., & Singh, S. P. (1992). Diabetes support groups improve health care of older diabetic patients. *Journal of the American Geriatrics Society, 40,* 147–150.

Hinrichsen, G. A., & Revenson, T. A. (1985). Does self-help help? An empirical investigation of scoliosis peer support groups. *Journal of Social Issues, 5*(45), 946–947.

Hughes, J. M. (1977). Adolescent children of alcoholic parents and the relationship of Alateen to these children. *Journal of Consulting and Clinical Psychology 45,* 946–947.

Humphreys, K., Mavis, B. E., & Stoffelmayr, B. E. (1994). Are twelve step programs appropriate for disenfranchised groups? Evidence from a study of post- treatment mutual help involvement. *Prevention in Human Services, 11*(1), 165–179.

Humphreys, K., & Moos, R. H. (1996). Reduced substance-abuse-related health care costs among voluntary participants in Alcoholics Anonymous. *Psychiatric Services, 47,* 709–713.

Humphreys, K., & Rappaport, J. (1994). Researching self-help/mutual aid groups and organizations: Many roads, one journey. *Applied & Preventive Psychology, 3,* 217–231.

Kennedy, M. (1990, July). *Psychiatric hospitalizations of growers.* Paper presented at the Second Biennial Conference on Community Research and Action, East Lansing, MI.

Kessler, R. C., Frank, R. G., Edlund, M., Katz, S. J., Lin, E., & Leaf, P. (1997). Differences in the use of psychiatric outpatient services between the United States and Ontario. *New England Journal of Medicine, 336,* 551–557.

Kessler, R. C., Mickelson, K. D., & Zhao, S. (1997). Patterns and correlates of self-help group membership in the United States. *Social Policy, 27,* 27–46.

Kurtz, L. F. (1990). The self-help movement: Review of the past decade of research. *Social Work with Groups, 13,* 101–115.

Levy, L. H. (1984). Issues in research and evaluation. In A. Gartner & F. Riessman (Eds.), *The self-help revolution* (pp. 155–172). New York: Human Sciences Press.

Lewis, E. A., & Suarez, Z. E. (1995). Natural helping networks. *Encyclopedia of social work* (19th ed., pp. 1765–1772). Silver Spring, MD: National Association of Social Workers.

Lieberman, M. A., & Borman, L. D. (1991). The impact of self-help groups on widows' mental health. *National Reporter, 4,* 2–6.

Lieberman, M. A., & Videka-Sherman, L. (1986). The impact of self-help groups on the mental health of widows and widowers. *American Journal of Orthopsychiatry, 56,* 435–449.

Marmar, C. R., & Horowitz, M. J. (1988). A controlled trial of brief psychotherapy and mutual-help group treatment of conjugal bereavement. *American Journal of Psychiatry, 145*(2), 203–209.

McCallion, P., & Toseland, R. W. (1995). Supportive group interventions with caregivers of frail older adults. *Social Work with Groups, 18,* 11–25.

McKay, J. R., & Alterman, A. I. (1994). Treatment goals, continuity of care, and outcome in a day hospital substance abuse rehabilitation program. *American Journal of Psychiatry, 151,* 254–259.

Memmott, J. L. (1993). Models of helping and coping: A field experiment with natural and professional helpers. *Social Work Research & Abstracts, 29,* 11–22.

Nash, K. B., & Kramer, K. D. (1993). Self-help for sickle cell disease in African American communities. *Journal of Applied Behavioral Science, 29,* 202–215.

Patterson, S. L., Holzhuter, J. L., Struble, V. E., & Quadagno, J. S. (1972). *Final report, utilization of human resources for mental health.* (Grant No. MH 16618). Unpublished report.

Patterson, S. L., & Marsiglia, F. F. (2000). Mi casa es su casa: Beginning exploration of Mexican Americans' natural helping. *Families in Society, 81,* 22–31.

Pisani, V. D., & Fawcett, J. (1993). The relative contributions of medication adherence and AA meeting attendance to abstinent outcome for chronic alcoholics. *Journal of Studies on Alcohol, 54,* 115–119.

Riessman, F. (2000). Self-help comes of age. *Social Policy, 30,* 47–49.

Reissman, F., & Carroll, D. (1995). *Redefining self-help: Policy and practice.* San Francisco: Jossey-Bass.

Seligman, M. E. P. (1995). The effectiveness of psychotherapy: The Consumer Reports study. *American Psychologist, 50,* 965–974.

Simmons, D. (1992). Diabetes self help facilitated by local diabetes research: The Coventry Asian Diabetes Support Group. *Diabetic Medicine, 9,* 866–869.

Tattersall, M. L., & Hallstrom, C. (1992). Self-help and benzodiazepine withdrawal. *Journal of Affective Disorders, 24,* 193–198.

Videcka-Sherman, L., & Lieberman, M. A. (1985). The effects of self-help and psychotherapy intervention on child loss: The limits of recovery. *American Journal of Orthopsychiatry, 55,* 70–82.

Waller, M. A., & Patterson, S. (2002). Natural helping and resilience in a Dine (Navajo) community. *Society, 81,* 73–84.

Walsh, D. C., Hingson, R. W., & Merrigan, D. M. (1991). A randomized trial of treatment options for alcohol-abusing workers. *The New England Journal of Medicine, 325*(11), 775–782.

Wituk, S., Shepherd, M. D., Slavich, S., Warren, M. L., & Meissen, G. (2000). A topography of self-help groups: An empirical analysis. *Social Work, 45,* 157–165.

Wuthnow, R. (1994). *Sharing the journey: Support groups and America's new quest for community.* New York: Free Press.

Chapter 10

Alexander, R., Jr. (2000). *Counseling, treatment, and intervention methods with juvenile and adult offenders.* Pacific Grove, CA: Brooks/Cole.

Andrews, D., Zinger, I., Hoge, R., Bonta, J., Gendreau, P., & Cullen, F. (1990). Does correctional treatment work? A clinically-relevant and psychologically-informed meta-analysis. *Criminology, 28,* 369–404.

Baer, J. (1976). *How to be an assertive (not aggressive) woman in life, in love, and on the job: A total guide to self-assertiveness.* New York: New American Library.

Berliner, L. (1998). Juvenile sex offenders: Should they be treated differently? *Journal of Interpersonal Violence, 13,* 645–646.

Blumstein, A. (1995). Violence by young people: Why the deadly nexus? *National Institute of Justice Journal, 2*(9), 229–241.

Briscoe, J. (1997). Breaking the cycle of violence: A rational approach to at-risk youth. *Federal Probation, 61,* 3–13.

Butts, J. A., & Snyder, H. N. (1997). *The youngest delinquents: Offenders under age 15.* Washington, DC: U.S. Department of Justice Office of Juvenile Justice and Delinquency Prevention. (OJJDP No. 95-JN-FX-0008)

Caputo, A. A., Frick, P., & Brodsky, S. L. (1999). Family violence and juvenile sex offending: The potential mediating role of psychopathic traits and negative attitudes toward women. *Criminal Justice & Behavior, 26,* 338–356.

Currie, E. (1993). *Reckoning: Drugs, the cities, and the American future.* Washington, DC: U.S. Department of Justice, Office of Juvenile Justice Delinquency Prevention.

Ellickson, P. L., & McGuigan, K. A. (2000). Early predictors of adolescent violence. *American Journal of Public Health, 90,* 566–572

Elliott, D. S. (1994). Serious violent offenders: Onset, developmental course, and termination: The American society of criminology, 1993 Presidential Address. *Criminology, 32,* 1–21.

Elliott, D. S., Hamburg, B., & Williams, K. R. (1998). *Violence in American schools: A new perspective.* Boulder, CO: Center for the Study and Prevention of Violence.

Fagan, J. (1996, July). *Recent perspectives on youth violence.* Paper presented at the Northwest Conference on Youth Violence, Seattle, WA.

Glicken, M. D. (2004). *Violent young children.* Boston: Allyn & Bacon/Longman.

Glicken, M. D., & Sechrest, D. H. (2003). *The role of the helping professions in treating and preventing violence.* Boston: Allyn & Bacon/Longman.

Goldstein, A. P., & Glick, B. (1996). Aggression replacement training: Methods and outcomes. In C. R. Hollin & K. Howells (Eds.), *Clinical approaches to working with young offenders* (pp. 151–179). Chichester, England: Wiley.

Gramckow, H. P., & Tompkins, E. (1999). *Enhancing prosecutors' ability to combat and prevent juvenile crime in their jurisdictions.* Washington, DC: U.S. Department of Justice, Office of Justice Programs, Office of Juvenile Justice and Delinquency Prevention.

Groth, N. A., Longo, R. E., & McFadin, J. B. (1982). Undetected recidivism among rapists and child molesters. *Crime and Delinquency, 128,* 450–458.

Guetzloe, E. (1999, Fall). Violence in children and adolescents—A threat to public health and safety: A paradigm of prevention. *Preventing School Failure, 44,* 21–24

Hamburg, M. A. (1998). Youth violence is a public health concern. In D. S. Elliott, B. Hamburg, & K. R. Williams (Eds.), *Violence in American Schools: A New Perspective* (pp. 31–54). New York: Cambridge University Press.

Hawkins, J. D., & Catalano, R. F. (1992). *Communities that care.* San Francisco: Jossey-Bass.

Hawkins J. D., Catalano, R. F., Morrison, D. M., O'Donnell, J., Abbott, R. D., & Day, L. E. (1992). The Seattle Social Development Project: Effects of the first four years on protective factors and problem behaviors. In J. McCord & R. Tremblay (Eds.), *The Prevention of Antisocial Behavior in Children* (pp. 133–164). New York: Guilford.

Herrenkohl, T. I., Huang, B., Kosterman, R., & Hawkins, J. (2001). A comparison of social development processes leading to violent behavior in late adolescence for childhood initiators and adolescent initiators of violence. *Journal of Research in Crime & Delinquency, 38,* 45–63.

Huey, W. C., & Rank, R. C. (1984). Effects of counselor and peer-led groups' assertive training on Black adolescent aggression. *Journal of Counseling Psychology, 31,* 95–98.

Izzo, R., & Ross, R. (1990). Meta-analysis of rehabilitation programs for juvenile delinquents, a brief report. *Criminal Justice and Behavior, 17*, 134–142.

Johnson, D. L. (1990). The Houston Parent–Child Development Center Project: Disseminating a viable program for enhancing at-risk families. *Prevention in the Human Services, 7*, 89–108.

Kaplan, S. J., Pelcovitz, D., & Labruna, V. (1999). Child and adolescent abuse and neglect research: A review of the past 10 years. Part I: Physical and emotional abuse and neglect. *Journal of the American Academy of Child and Adolescent Psychiatry, 38*, 1214–1222.

Lane, P. S., & McWhirter, J. J. (1992). A peer mediation model: Conflict resolution for elementary and middle school children. *Elementary School Guidance & Counseling, 27*, 15–21.

Lukefahr, J. L. (2001). Treatment of child abuse [Review of the book *Treatment of child abuse: Common ground for mental health medical and legal protections*]. *Journal of the American Academy of Child and Adolescent Psychiatry, 40*, 383.

Mathias, C. E. (1992). Touching the lives of children: Consultative interventions that work. *Elementary School Guidance & Counseling, 26*, 190–201.

Mayer, G. R. (1995). Preventing antisocial behavior in the schools. *Journal of Applied Behavior Analysis, 28*, 467–478.

McCord, J. (1999). Family relationships, juvenile delinquency, and adult criminality. In F. R. Scarpitti & A. L. Nielson (Eds.), *Crime and criminals: Contemporary and classic readings* (pp. 167–176). Los Angeles: Roxbury.

Morales, A. (1982). The Mexican American gang member: Evaluation and treatment. In R. Becerra, M. Karno, & J. Escolar (Eds.), *Mental health and Hispanic Americans: Clinical perspective* (pp. 43–67). New York: Grune & Stratton.

Murray, B. A., & Myers, M. A. (1998). Conduct disorders and the special-education trap. *The Education Digest, 63*(8), 48–53.

Myles, B. S., & Simpson, R. L. (1998). Aggression cycle and prevention/intervention strategies. *Intervention in School and Clinic, 33*, 259–264.

Oates, R. K., & Bross, D. C. (1995). What have we learned about treating child physical abuse? A literature review of the last decade. *Journal of Child Abuse & Neglect, 19*, 463–473.

Olds, D. L., Henderson, C. R., Tatelbaum, R., & Chamberlin, R. (1988). Improving the life-course development of socially disadvantaged mothers: A randomized trial of nurse home visitation. *American Journal of Public Health, 78*, 1436–1444.

Osofsky, H. J., & Osofsky, J. D. (2001). Violent and aggressive behaviors in youth: A mental health and prevention perspective. *Psychiatry, 64*, 285–295.

Patterson, G., & Narrett, C. (1990), The development of a reliable and valid treatment program for aggressive young children. *International Journal of Mental Health, 19,* 19–26.

Rae-Grant, N., McConville, B. J., & Fleck, S. (1999). Violent behavior in children and youth: Preventive intervention from a psychiatric perspective. *Journal of the American Academy of Child and Adolescent Psychiatry, 38,* 235–241.

Reece, R. M. (Ed.). (2000). *Treatment of child abuse: Common ground for mental health, medical, and legal practitioners.* Baltimore: John Hopkins University Press.

Scahill, M. C. (2000, November). *Female delinquency cases, 1997 series: Fact sheet.* Retrieved May 27, 2004, from www.ojjdp.ncjrs.org

Schrumpt, F., Crawford, D., & Usadel, H. C. (1991). *Peer mediation: Conflict resolution in schools.* Champaign, IL: Research Press.

Sechrest, D. (2001). *Juvenile crime: A predictive study.* Unpublished manuscript.

Skiba, R. J., Peterson, R. L., & Williams, T. (1997). Office referrals and suspensions: Disciplinary intervention in middle schools. *Education and Treatment of Children, 20,* 295–315.

Sprague, J. R., & Walker, H. M. (2000). Early identification and intervention for youth with antisocial and violent behavior. *Exceptional Children, 66,* 367–379.

Steiner, H., & Stone, L. A. (1999). Introduction: Violence and related psychopathology. *Journal of the American Academy of Child and Adolescent Psychiatry, 38,* 232–234.

Studer, J. (1996). Understanding and preventing aggressive responses in youth. *Elementary School Guidance & Counseling, 30,* 194–203.

Tate, D., Reppucci, N., & Mulvey, E. (1995). Violent juvenile delinquents, treatment effectiveness and implications for future action. *American Psychologist, 50,* 777–781.

Thornberry, T. P., Huizinga, D., & Loeber, R. (1995). The prevention of serious delinquency and violence: Implications from the program of research on the causes and correlates of delinquency. In J. C. Howell, B. Krisberg, J. D. Hawkins, & J. J. Wilson (Eds.), *A sourcebook: Serious, violent, and chronic juvenile offenders* (pp. 213–237). Thousand Oaks, CA: Sage.

Veneziano, C., Veneziano, L., & LeGrand, S. (2000). The relationship between adolescent sex offender behaviors and victim characteristics with prior victimization. *Journal of Interpersonal Violence, 15,* 363–374.

Walker, H. M., Colvin, G., & Ramsey, E. (1995). *Antisocial behavior in school: Strategies and best practices.* Pacific Grove, CA: Brooks/Cole.

Walker, H. M., & Severson, H. H. (1990). *Systematic screening for behavior disorders.* Longmont, CO: Sopris West.

Widom, C. S. (1999). The cycle of violence. In F. R. Scarpitti & A. L. Nielson (Eds.), *Crime and criminals: Contemporary and classic readings* (pp. 332–334). Los Angeles: Roxbury.

Wolfgang, M. E. (1972). *Delinquency in a birth cohort.* Chicago: University of Chicago Press.

Wolfgang, M. E. (1987). *From boy to man, from delinquency to crime.* Chicago: University of Chicago Press.

Zigler, E., Tussig, C., & Black, K. (1992). Early childhood intervention: A promising preventative for juvenile delinquency. *American Psychologist, 47,* 997–1006.

Zolondek, S. C, Abel, G., Northey, W. F., & Jordan, A. D. (2000). The self-reported behaviors of juvenile sexual offenders. *Journal of Interpersonal Violence, 16*(1), 73–85.

Chapter 11

Adams, D. (1988). Counseling men who batter: A Profeminist analysis of five treatment models. In K. Yllo & M. Bograd (Eds.), *Feminist perspectives on wife abuse* (pp. 176–199). Newbury Park, CA: Sage.

Babcock, J. C., & Steiner, R. (1999, March). The relationship between treatment incarceration, and recidivism of battering: A program evaluation of Seattle's coordinated community response to domestic violence. *Journal of Family Psychology, 13*(1), 46–59.

Bagley, C. (1990). Development of a measure of unwanted sexual contact in childhood, for use in community mental health surveys. *Psychological Reports, 66,* 401–402.

Berlin, F. S. (1982). Sex offenders: A biomedical perspective. In J. Greer & I. Stuart (Eds.), *The sexual aggressor: Current perspectives on Treatment* (pp. 83–126). New York: Van Nostrand Reinhold.

Bernard, J. L., & Bernard, M. L. (1984). The abusive male seeking treatment: Jekyll and Hyde. *Family Relations, 33,* 543–547.

Davis, R. C., Smith, B. E., & Nickles, L. B. (1998, July). The deterrent effect of prosecuting domestic violence misdemeanors. *Crime & Deliquency, 44*(3), 434–442.

Dewhurst, A. M., Moore, R. J., & Alfano, D. P. (1992). Aggression against women by men: Sexual and spousal assault. *Journal of Offender Rehabilitation, 18,* 41–65.

Dodge, K. A., & Richard, B. A. (1986). Peer perceptions, aggression and peer relations. In L. Pryor & R. Day (Eds.), *The development of social cognition* (pp. 35–58). New York: Springer-Verlag.

Eisikovits, Z. C., & Edelson, J. L. (1989). Intervening with men who batter: A critical review of the literature. *Social Service Review, 63,* 384–414.

Fagan, J. A., Steward, D. K., & Hansen, K. V. (1983). Violent men or violent husbands: Background factors and situational correlates. In R. J. Finkelhor, G. T.

Gelles, M. A. Hotaling, & M. A. Straus (Eds.), *The dark side of families* (pp. 49–67. Beverly Hills, CA: Save.

Frinter, M., & Rubinson, L. (1993). Acquaintance rape: The influence of alcohol, fraternity membership and sports teams. *Journal of Sex Education and Therapy, 19,* 272–284.

Giles-Sims, P. (1983). *Wife battering: A systems theory.* New York: Guilford.

Glicken, M. D. (2005). *Improving the effectiveness of the helping professions: An evidence based approach to practice.* Thousand Oaks, CA: Sage.

Glicken, M. D. (2004). *Violent young children.* Boston: Allyn & Bacon/Longman.

Glicken, M. D., & Sechrest, D. (2003). *The role of the helping professions in treating the victims and perpetrators of violence.* Boston: Allyn & Bacon/Longman.

Gondolf, E. W. (1997). Patterns of reassault in batterer programs. *Violence and Victims, 12,* 373–387.

Greenfeld, L. A. (1997, February). *Sex offenses and offenders: An analysis of rape and sexual assault.* Washington, DC: U.S. Department of Justice (Publication No. NCJ–163392).

Groth, N. A. (1978). Patterns of sexual assault against children and adolescents. In A. Burgess et al. (Eds.), *Sexual assault of children and adolescents* (pp. 3–24). Lexington, MA: Heath.

Grusznski, R. J., & Carillo, T. E. (1988). Who completes batterer's treatment groups? An empirical investigation. *Journal of Family Violence, 3,* 141–150.

Hale, G., Duckworth, L., Zimostrad, N., & Scott, D. (1988). Abusive partners: MMPI profiles of male batterers. *Journal of Mental Health Counseling, 10,* 214–224.

Hamberger, K., & Hastings, J. (1993). Court-mandated treatment of men who assault their partner: Issues, controversies, and outcomes. In N. Z. Hilton (Ed.), *Legal responses to wife assault* (pp. 188–229). Newbury Perk, CA: Sage.

Hotaling, G. T. & Sugarman, D. B. (1984). An identification of risk factors. In G. L. Bowen, M. A. Straus, A. J. Seklak, G. T. Hotaling, & D. B. Sugarman (Eds.), *Domestic violence surveillance system feasibility study. Phase I report: Identification of outcome and risk factors* (pp. 3-1–3-66). Rockville, MD: Westat, Inc.

Jacobson, N. (1998, September 28). Treatment programs for batterers must be tested. *Women's Health Weekly, 26,* 10–12.

Johnson, P., Hudson, S. M., & Marshall, R. W. (1992). The effects of masturbatory reconditioning with nonfamilial child molesters. *Behavior Research and Therapy, 30,* 559–561.

Jouard, S., & Landsman, M. (1969). Cognition and the "didactic effect." Men's self-disclosing behavior. *Merrill-Palmer Quarterly, 6,* 176–184.

Kalmuss, D. (1984). The intergenerational transmission of marital aggression. *Journal of Marriage and the Family, 46,* 11–19.

Koss, M. P., & Dinero, T. E. (1988). A discriminate analysis of risk factors among a national sample of college women. *Journal of Consulting and Clinical Psychology, 57,* 133–147.

Lerman, L. (1984). A model state act: Remedies for domestic abuse. *Harvard Journal on Legislation, 21,* 453–459.

Looman, J., Abracen, J., & Nicholaichuk, T. P. (2000). Recidivism among treated sexual offenders and matched controls. *Journal of Interpersonal Violence, 15*(3), 279–290.

Los Angeles Police Department Data. (1997, January). *The Family Bulletin, 23*(1), 9–17.

Loza, W., & Loza-Fanous, A. (1999). The fallacy of reducing rape and violent recidivism by treating anger. *International Journal of Offender Therapy and Comparative Criminology, 43*(4), 492–502.

Malamuth, N. M. (1989). Predictors of naturalistic social aggression. In M. A. Prigg-Good & J. E. Stets (Eds.), *Violence in dating relationships: Emerging social issues* (pp, 219–240). New York: Praeger.

Mayer, A. (1988). *Sex offenders: Approaches to understanding and management.* Holmes Beach, FL: Learning Perspectives.

Murphy, W. D., Coleman, E. M., & Haynes, M. R. (1986, Winter). Factors related to coercive sexual behavior in a non-clinical sample of males. *Violence-and-Victims, 1*(4), 255–278.

National Institute on Alcohol Abuse and Alcoholism. (2001, October 1). *Alcohol-related problems among college students: Epidemiology and prevention.* RFA-AA-02-001. Washington, DC: Author.

Neuman, E. (1995, Winter). The trouble with domestic violence. *Media Critic, 2*(1), 67–73.

Peterson, R. (1980). Social class, social learning and wife abuse. *Social Service Review, 54,* 390–406.

Rosen, R. C., & Fracher, J. C. (1983). Tension-reducing training in the treatment of compulsive sex offenders. In J. G. Greer & I. Stuart (Eds.), *The sexual aggressors* (pp. 144–159). New York: Van Nostrand Reinhold.

Rosenfeld, B. D. (1992). Court-ordered treatment of spouse abuse. *Clinical Psychology Review, 12,* 205–226.

Roy, M. (Ed.). (1982). *The abusive partner: An analysis of domestic battering.* New York: Van Nostrand Reinhold.

Scher, E., & Stevens, M. (1985). Men and violence. *Journal of Counseling and Development, 65*(7), 47–95.

Schuerger, J. M., & Reigle, N. (1988). Personality and biographic data that characterize men who abuse their wives. *Journal of Clinical Psychology, 44,* 75–84.

Sherman, L., & Bark, R. A. (1984). The specific deterrent effect of arrest for domestic assault. *American Sociological Review, 49,* 261–272.

Straus, M. A., & Gelles, R. J. (1990). *Physical violence in American families: Risk factors and adaptations to violence in families.* New Brunswick, NJ: Transaction Publishers.

Straus, M. A., & Walsh, M. R. (1997). *Women, men and gender.* New Haven, CT: Yale University Press.

Tjaden, P., & Thoenner, N. (1998). *Prevalence, incidence, and consequences of violence against women: Findings from the National Violence Against Women Survey.* Atlanta, GA: Centers for Disease Control and Prevention and National Institute of Justice.

University of Nebraska. (1996). *Dating violence and acquaintance assault.* Nebraska Cooperative Extension NF 95-244. Retrieved from http://www.lanr.uni.edu/pubs/family/nf244.htm

Waldo, M. (1987). Also victims: Understanding and treating men arrested for spousal abuse. *Journal of Counseling and Development, 65,* 68–87.

Widom, C. S. (1989). Does violence beget violence? A critical review of the literature. *Psychology Bulletin, 106,* 3–28.

Wiederholt, I. C. (1992). The psychodynamics of sex offenses and implications for treatment. *The Haworth Press, 18,* 19–24.

Wolf-Smith, J. H., & LaRossa, J. R. (1992). After he hits her. *Family Relations, 41,* 16–19.

Yang, J. (1992, November 1). The aroused, the conqueror, the angry, the abused. *Psychology Today, 17*(11), 46.

Chapter 12

Bernstein, R. (1994, January 13). Guilty if charged. *Los Angeles Times,* pp. 11–14.

Bureau of Justice Statistics. (1998, July). *Workplace safety.* U.S. Department of Justice. NCJ 168634.

Burgess, D., & Borgida, E. (1997). Sexual harassment: An experimental test of sex-role spillover theory. *Personality and Social Psychology Bulletin, 21,* 63–75.

Cochran, C. C., Frazier, P. A., & Olson, A. M. (1997). Predictors of responses to unwanted sexual attention. *Psychology of Women Quarterly, 21,* 207–226.

Fitzgerald, L., & Ormerod, M. (1991). Perceptions of sexual harassment: The influence of gender and academic context. *Psychology of Women Quarterly, 15,* 281–294.

Glicken, M. (1988, January 24). Resolving office conflict. *National Business Employment Weekly, 28*(3), 12–14.

Glicken, M. (1996, February 1). Dealing with workplace stress. *National Business Employment Weekly, 36*(5), 22–23.

Glicken, M. D., & Ino, S. (1997). *Workplace violence: A description of the levels of potential for violence.* Unpublished manuscript.

Glicken, M. D., & Sechrest, D. K. (2003). *The role of the helping professions in treating the victims and perpetrators of violence.* Boston: Allyn & Bacon/Longman.

Grauerholz, E. (1989). Sexual harassment of women professors by students: Exploring the dynamics of power, authority, and gender in a university setting. *Sex Roles, 21,* 789–801.

Gutek, A. G. (1995). How subjective is sexual harassment? An examination of rater effects. *Basic and Applied Social Psychology, 17,* 447–467.

Jossi, F. (1999, February 1). Defusing workplace violence. *Business and Health, 12*(2). Retrieved April 7, 2003, from http://www.findarticles.com/cf_0/m2294/2000_Feb/63787377/print.jhtml

Katz, N. V. (2003). Sexual harassment statistics. Retrieved October 1, 2004 from http://www.womenissues.about.com/library/blsexharassmentstats.htm

Kim, H., & Fiske, S. T. (1999, June). *Are the motives of men who sexually harass women misunderstood?: An investigation linking ambivalent sexism and sexual harassment.* Poster session presented at the 11th annual conference of the American Psychological Society, Denver, CO.

Leo, J. (1994, April 18). De-escalating the gender war. *U.S. News and World Report, 166*(15), 24.

MacKinnon, C. A. (1979). *The sexual harassment of working women: A case of sex discrimination.* New Haven, CT: Yale University Press.

Matchen, J., & DeSouza, E. (2000, February 9). The sexual harassment of faculty members by students. *Sex Roles: A Journal of Research, 28*(2). Retrieved May 7, 2004, from http://www.findarticles.com/cf_0/m2294/2000_Feb/63787377/print.jhtml

McKinney, K. (1990). Sexual harassment of university faculty by colleagues and students. *Sex Roles, 23,* 421–438.

Robinson, J. L. (1996). *Ten facts every employer and employee should know about workplace violence: It may save your life.* Smart Business Supersite. Retrieved August 4, 2002, from http://wwwsmartbiz.com

Tangri, S. S., Burt, M. R., & Johnson, L. B. (1982). Sexual harassment at work: Three explanatory models. *Journal of Social Issues, 38*(11), 33–54.

Waldo, C. R., Berdahl, J. L., & Fitzgerald, L. F. (1998). Are men sexually harassed? If so by whom? *Law and Human Behavior, 22,* 59–79.

Chapter 13

Aboramph, O. M. (1989). Black male–female relationships. Some observations. *Journal of Black Studies, 19,* 320–342.

372

Adebimpe, V. R. (1981). Overview: White norms and psychiatric diagnosis of black patients. *American Journal of Psychiatry, 138,* 279–285.

Bell, A. P. (1978). Black sexuality: Fact and fancy. In R. Staples (Ed.), *The Black family: Essays and studies* (pp. 78–80). Belmont, CA: Wadsworth.

Christian, J. (1990, February 12). An epidemic of Black violence. *The Los Angeles Times,* p. A3.

DiIulio, J. J., Jr. (1996a). Fill churches, not jails: Youth crime and super predators: Statement before the United States Senate Subcommittee on Youth Violence, February 28, 1996. Retrieved June 13, 2004, from http://www.brook.edu/pa/hot/diiulio.htm

DiIulio, J. J., Jr. (1996b, July 13). Stop crime where it starts. *The New York Times.* Retrieved July 13, 2004, from http://www.brook.edu/pa/hot/arttoppics/diiulio.htm

FBI Uniform Crime Report for 2001. (2002). U.S. Department of Justice Web site. Retrieved April 13, 2004, from http://www.fbi.gov/ucr/o1cius.htm

Flaherty, J. A., & Meagher, R. (1980). Measuring racial bias in inpatient treatment. *American Journal of Psychiatry, 137,* 679–682.

Franklin, A. J. (1992). Therapy with African American men. *Families in Society: The Journal of Contemporary Human Services, 26*(6), 350–355.

Garretson, D. J. (1993). Psychological misdiagnosis of African Americans. *Journal of Multicultural Counseling and Development, 21,* 119–126.

Hamill, P. (1996, November 1). Mike Tyson in prison. *Esquire, 56*(11), 100–108.

Harris, I. (1990). Media myths and the reality of men's work. In M. Kimmel & M. Messner (Eds.), *Men's Lives* (pp. 225–231). New York: Macmillan.

Lawson, E. J., & Sharpe, T. L. (2000, July). Black men and divorce: Implications for culturally competent practice. *Minority Health Today, X.* Retrieved April 17, 2003, from http://www.findarticles.com/cf_0/m0HKU/5_1/66918338/ print.jhtml

Laszloffy, T. A., & Hardy, C. B. (2000). Uncommon strategies for a common problem: Addressing racism in family therapy. *Family Process, 39,* 35–50.

Marin, P. (1991, July 8). The prejudice against men. *Nation, 253*(2), 46–51.

Pena, J. M., Bland, I. J., Shervinton, D., Rice, J. C., & Foulks, E. F. (2000, February 1). Racial identity and its assessment in a sample of African-American men in treatment for cocaine dependence. *American Journal of Drug and Alcohol Abuse.* Retrieved March 17, 2004, from http://www.findarticles.com/cf_0/PI/search.jhtml?magR=all+magazines&key=psychotherapy+%2B+race

Poussaint, A. F. (1993, February). Enough already. *Ebony, 48,* 86–89.

Satcher, D. (1999, January 7). *Mental health, A report of the surgeon general.* Retrieved February 21, 2002, from http://www.mentalhealth.org/features/surgeongeneralreport/chapter8/sec1.asp#ensure

Satcher, D. (2001). *Mental health: Culture, race, and ethnicity a supplement to mental health: A Report of the Surgeon General.* Retrieved February 22, 2002, from http://www.surgeongeneral.gov/library/mentalhealth/cre/release.asp

Slater, E. (2003, June 23). Democratic candidates skewer Bush in appeal to Black voters. *Los Angeles Times*, p. A13.

Solomon, A. (1992). Clinical diagnosis among diverse populations: A multicultural perspective. *Families in Society, 73*, 371–377.

Staples, R. (1986). Stereotypes of Black male sexuality: The facts behind the myths. In M. Kimmel & M. Messner (Eds.), *Men's lives* (pp. 432–438). New York: Macmillan.

Whaley, A. L. (2001). Cultural mistrust: An important psychological construct for diagnosis and treatment of African Americans. *Psychology: Research and Practice,. 32*, 555–562.

Williams, O. J. (1992, December). Ethnically sensitive practice to enhance treatment participation of African American men who batter. *Families in Society: The Journal of Contemporary Human Sciences, 26*(12), 588–595.

Chapter 14

Altarriba, J., & Bauer, L. M. (1998). Counseling the Hispanic client: Cuban Americans, Mexican Americans, and Puerto Ricans. *Journal of Counseling and Development, 76*, 389–396.

Baca Zinn, M. (1980). Gender and ethnic identity among Chicanos. *Frontiers, 2*, 18–24.

Chafetz, J. S. (1974). *Masculine/feminine or human.* Itasca, IL: F. E. Peacock Publishers.

Congress, E. (1990). Crisis intervention with Hispanic clients in an urban mental health clinic. In A. Roberts (Ed.), *Crisis intervention handbook* (pp. 221–236). Belmont, CA: Wadsworth.

Glicken, M. D., & Garza, M. A. (1996, October). *Crisis intervention with newly immigrated Latino clients.* Paper presented at the California Conference for Latino Social Workers, Sacramento, CA.

Gonzalez, M. J. (2000, October). *Provision of mental health services to Hispanic clients.* Retrieved February 3, 2004, from http://www.naswnyc.org/d16.html

Hernandez, R. (1990, September 9). Please stand up if you are a real Hispanic. *Los Angeles Times*, p. 57.

Howe, C. (1994). Improving the achievement of Hispanic students. *Educational Leadership, 51*(8), 42.

Latino USA. (2002, May 31). *Julio can't read.* Retrieved August 2, 2004, from http://www.latinousa.org/program/lusapgm477.html

Mirande, A. (1979). A reinterpretation of male dominance in the Chicano family. *Family Coordinator, 28*, 473–497.

Monsivais, C. (1996, August 25). The immigrant's view of education. *Los Angeles Times*, p. M2.

Neff, J. A., Prihoda, T. J., & Hoppe, S. K. (1991). "Machismo," self-esteem, education, and high maximum drinking among Anglo, Black and Mexican-American male drinkers. *Journal of Studies on Alcohol, 52*, 458–463.

Pena, M. (1991). Class, gender, and machismo: The "treacherous woman" folklore of Mexican male workers. *Gender and Society, 5*(1), 30–46.

Randolph, W. M., Stroup-Benham, C., & Black, S. A. (1998). Alcohol use among Cuban-Americans, Mexican-Americans, and Puerto Ricans. *Alcohol Health and Research World, 22*, 265–269.

Roger, L., & Malgady, R. (1987). What do culturally sensitive mental services mean? The case of Hispanics. *American Psychologist, 42*, 565–570.

Shai, D., & Rosenwaithe, I. (1988). Violent deaths among Mexican, Puerto Rican, and Cuban born migrants in the United States. *Social Science Medicine, 26*(2), 269–276.

University of Arizona. (2000, January 4). Crime statistics paint a gloomy future for Latino communities. *The Arizona Report*. Retrieved July 28, 2002, from W3fp.Arizona.edu/masrc/pubs/av1n1f.htm

Velasquez, R. J., Arellano, L. M., & McNeill, B. W. (2004). The handbook of chicana/o psychology and mental health. Mahwah, NJ: Lawrence Erlbaum Associates.

Zuniga, M. E. (1992). Using metaphors in therapy: Dichos and Latino clients. *Social Work, 37*(1), 55–60.

Chapter 15

Ewing, C. P. (1990). Crisis intervention as brief psychotherapy. In R. A. Wells & V. J. Giannetti (Eds.), *Handbook of brief psychotherapies* (pp. 277–294). New York: Plenum.

Furuto, S. M., Biswas, R., Chung, D., Murase, K., & Ross-Sheriff, F. (Eds.). (1992). *Social work practice with Asian Americans*. Newbury Park, CA: Sage.

Gaw, A. C. (1993). Psychiatric care of Chinese Americans. In A. Gaw (Ed.), *Culture, ethnicity, and mental illness* (pp. 245–280). Washington DC: American Psychiatric Association Press.

Glicken, M. D. (2004). Using the strengths perspective in social work practice. Boston, MA: Allyn and Bacon/Longman.

Golan, N. (1978). *Treatment in crisis situations*. New York: Free Press.

Gong-Guy, E. (1987). *California Southeast Asian Mental Health Needs Assessment*. Oakland, CA: Asian Community Mental Health Association.

Ho, M. K. (1987). *Family therapy with ethnic minorities*. Newberry Park, CA.: Sage.

Ino, S. (1985a). *Close relationships: Their subjective construction and contribution to the sense of self*. Ann Arbor, MI: University Microfilms International.

Ino, S. (1985b, August). *The concept of an Asian American collective self.* Paper presented at the Pacific/Asian American Research Methods Workshop (P/AAMHRC), Ann Arbor, MI.

Ino, S. (1987, August). *The sense of collective self in Asian American psychology.* Paper presented at the Asian American Psychological Association's National Convention, New York.

Ino, S. (1991, August). *The sense of collective self in Asian American psychology.* Paper presented at the American Psychological Association's 99th Annual Convention, San Francisco.

Ino, S. M., & Glicken, M. D. (1999). Treating Asian American clients in crisis: A collectivist approach. *Smith College Studies in Social Work, 69,* 525–540.

Ino, S. M., & Glicken, M. D. (2002). Understanding and treating the ethnically Asian client: A collectivist approach. *Journal of Health and Social Policy, 14,* 37–48.

Lee, E. (1996). Asian American families: An overview. In M. Mcgoldrick, J. Giordana, & J. Pearce (Eds.), *Ethnicity and family therapy* (2nd ed., pp. 58–87). New York: Guilford.

Leong, F. T. L. (1986). Counseling and psychotherapy with Asian-Americans: Review of the literature. *Journal of Counseling Psychology, 33,* 196–206.

Roberts, A. R. (1990). *Crisis intervention handbook: Assessment, treatment, and research.* Belmont, CA: Wadsworth.

Root, M. (1993). Guidelines for facilitating therapy with Asian American clients. In D. Atkinson, G. Morten, & D. W. Sue (Eds.), *Counseling American minorities: A cross-cultural perspective* (pp. 349–356). Madison, WI: Brown and Benchmark Publishers.

Sue, S., & Morishima, J. K. (1982). *The mental health of Asian Americans: Contemporary issues in identifying and treating mental problems.* San Francisco: Jossey-Bass.

Uba, L. (1994). *Asian Americans: Personality patterns, identity, and mental health.* New York: Guilford.

Chapter 16

American Psychiatric Association. (1994). *Diagnostic and statistical manual of mental disorders* (4th ed.). Washington, DC: Author.

Atkinson, R. (1995). Treatment programs for aging alcoholics. In T. Beresford & E. Gomberg (Eds.), *Alcohol and aging* (pp. 186–210). New York: Oxford University Press.

Babor, T. F., & Higgins-Biddle, J. C. (2000). Alcohol screening and brief intervention: Dissemination strategies for medical practice and public health. *Addiction, 95,* 677–687.

Backer, K. L., & Walton-Moss, B. (2001). Detecting and addressing alcohol abuse in women. *Nurse Practitioner, 26,* 13–22.

Bakeland, F. E., & Lundwall, L. (1975). Dropping out of treatment: A critical review. *Psychological Bulletin, 82,* 738–783.

Bien, T. J., Miller, W. R., & Tonigan, J. S. (1993). Brief interventions for alcohol problems: A review. *Addictions, 88,* 315–335.

Biernacki, P. (1986). *Pathways from heroin addiction: Recover without treatment.* Philadelphia: Temple University Press.

Bisson, J., Nadeau, L., & Demers, A. (1999). The validity of the CAGE scale to screen heavy drinking and drinking problems in a general population. *Addiction, 94,* 715–723.

Burge, S. K., Amodei, N., Elkin, B., Catala, S., Andrew, S. R., Lane, P. A., et al. (1997). An evaluation of two primary care interventions for alcohol abuse among Mexican-American patients. *Addiction, 92,* 1705–1716.

Burtscheidt, W., Wolwer, W., & Schwartz, R. (2002, September). Alcoholism, rehabilitation and comorbidity. *Acta Psychiatrica Scandinavica, 106*(3), 227–233.

Chang, G., Wilkins-Haug, L., Berman, S., & Goetz, M. A. (1999). Brief intervention for alcohol use in pregnancy: A randomized trial. *Addiction, 94,* 1499–1508.

Dahlgren, L., & Willander, A. (1989). Are special treatment facilities for female alcoholics needed? *Alcoholism, Clinical and Experimental Research, 13,* 499–504.

Epperly, T., & Moore, K. E. (2000, July 1). Health issues in men: Part II. Common psychosocial disorders. *American Family Physician.* Retrieved January 25, 2005, from http://www.findarticles.com/cf_0/m3225/1_62/65864000/print.jhtml

Fleming, M. F., Barry, K. L., Manwell, L. B., Johnson, K., & London, R. (1997). Brief physician advice for problem alcohol drinkers: A randomized controlled trial in community-based primary care practices. *Journal of the American Medical Association, 277,* 1039–1045.

Fleming, M., & Manwell, L. B. (1998). Brief intervention in primary care settings: A primary treatment method for at-risk, problem, and dependent drinkers. *Alcohol Research and Health, 23,* 128–137.

Gentilello, L. M., Donovan, D. M., Dunn, C. W., & Rivara, F. P. (1995). Alcohol interventions in trauma centers: Current practice and future directions. *Journal of the American Medical Association, 274,* 1043–1048.

Glicken, M. D. (2005). *Improving the effectiveness of the helping professions: An evidence-based approach to practice.* Thousand Oaks, CA: Sage.

Granfield, R., & Cloud, W. (1996). The elephant that no one sees: Natural recovery among middle-class addicts. *Journal of Drug Issues, 26,* 45–61.

Grant, B. F., & Dawson, D. A. (1997). Age at onset of alcohol use and its association with DSM–IV alcohol abuse and dependence: Results from the national longitudinal alcohol epidemiologic survey. *Journal of Substance Abuse, 9,* 103–110.

Gupta, S. (2003, May 12). Why men die young. *Time, 161*(19), 84.

Herman, M. (2000). Psychotherapy with substance abusers: Integration of psychodynamic and cognitive-behavioral approaches. *American Journal of Psychotherapy, 54,* 574–579.

Higgins-Biddle, J. C., Babor, T. F., Mullahy, J., Daniels, J., & Mcree, B. (1997). Alcohol screening and brief interventions: Where research meets practice. *Connecticut Medicine, 61,* 565–575.

Hingson, R., Scotch, N., Day, N., & Culbert, A. (1980). Recognizing and seeking help for drinking problems. *Journal of Studies on Alcohol, 41,* 1102–1117.

Hingson, R. W., Heeren, T., & Zakocs, R. C. (2002). Magnitude of alcohol-related mortality and morbidity among U.S. college students ages 18–24. *Journal of Studies on Alcohol, 63,* 136–144.

Humphreys, K. (1998). Can addiction-related self-help/mutual aid groups lower demand for professional substance abuse treatment? *Social Policy, 29,* 13–17.

Johnston, L. D., O'Malley, P. M., & Bachman, J. G. (2001). *Monitoring the Future: National Survey Results on Drug Use, 1975–2000. Volume I: Secondary School Students* (NIH Publication No. 01–4924). Bethesda, MD: National Institute on Drug Abuse.

Kann, L. (2001). Commentary. *Journal of Drug Issues, 31,* 725–727.

Kirchner, J. E., Booth, B. M., Owen, R. R., Lancaster, A. E., & Smith, G. R. (2000). Predictors of patient entry into alcohol treatment after initial diagnosis. *Journal of Behavioral Health Services & Research, 27,* 339–347.

Kuperman, S., Schlosser, S. S., Kramer, J. R., Bucholz, K., Hesselbrock, V., Reich, T., et al. (2001, April). Risk domains associated with adolescent alcohol dependence diagnosis. *Addiction, 96*(4), 629–637.

Leigh, G., Osborne, A. C., & Cleland, P. (1984). Factors associated with dropout from an outpatient alcoholism treatment service. *Journal of Studies of Alcoholism, 45,* 359–362.

Lennox, R. D., & Mansfield, A. J. (2001). A latent variable model of evidence-based quality improvement for substance abuse treatment. *Journal of Behavioral Health Services & Research, 28,* 164–177.

Liberto, J. G., & Oslin, D. W. (1995). Early versus late onset of alcoholism in the elderly. *International Journal of Addiction, 30,* 1799–1818.

Lu, M., & McGuire, T. G. (2002). The productivity of outpatient treatment for substance abuse. *Journal of Human Resources, 37,* 309–335.

Menninger, J. A. (2002, Spring). Source assessment and treatment of alcoholism and substance-related disorders in the elderly. *Bulletin of the Menninger Clinic, 66,* 166–184.

Miller, K. E. (2001). Can two questions screen for alcohol and substance abuse? *American Family Physician, 64,* 1247.

Miller, W. R., & Rollnick, S. (1991). *Motivational interviewing: Preparing people to change addictive behavior.* New York: Guilford.

Miller, W. R., & Sanchez, V. C. (1994). Motivating young adults for treatment and lifestyle change. In G. S. Howard & P. E. Nathan (Eds.), *Alcohol use and misuse by young adults* (pp. 55–81). Notre Dame, IN: University of Notre Dame Press.

Monti, P. M., Colby, S. M., Barnett, N. P., et al. (1999). Brief intervention for harm reduction with alcohol-positive older adolescents in a hospital emergency department. *Journal of Consulting and Clinical Psychology, 67,* 989–994.

Moxley, D. P., & Olivia, G. (2001). Strengths-based recovery practice in chemical dependency: A transperson perspective. *Families in Society, 82,* 251–262.

National Institute of Alcohol Abuse and Alcoholism. (2000). *Alcohol Alert.* NIAAA, Vol. 49.

National Institute on Drug Abuse. (1999). *Principles of drug addiction treatment: A research-based guide.* Rockville, MD: National Institute on Drug Abuse. DHHS publication (ADM)99-4180.

Peele, S. (1989). *The diseasing of America: Addiction treatment out of control.* Lexington, MA: Lexington Books.

Pennington, H., Butler, R., & Eagger, S. (2000). The assessment of patients with alcohol disorders by an old age psychiatric service. *Aging & Mental Health, 4,* 182–185.

Rees, D. W. (1986). Changing patient health beliefs to improve compliance with alcoholism treatment: A controlled trial. *Journal of Studies of Alcoholism, 47,* 436–439.

Roizen, R., Cahalan, D., Lambert, E., Wiebel, W., & Shanks, P. (1978). Spontaneous remission among untreated problem drinkers. In. D. Kandel (Ed.), *Longitudinal research on drug use* (pp. 46–83). Washington, DC: Hemisphere Publishing.

Reuben, D. B., Yoshikawa, T. T., & Besdine, R. W. (Eds.). (1996). *Geriatrics review syllabus; a core curriculum in geriatric medicine* (3rd ed.). New York: American Geriatric Society.

Seligman, M. E. P. (1995). The effectiveness of psychotherapy: The Consumers Reports study. *American Psychologist, 50,* 965–974.

Snow, M. (1973). Maturing out of narcotic addiction in New York City. *International Journal of the Addictions, 8,* 932–938.

Sobell, L., Sobell, M., Toneatto, T., & Leo, G. (1993). What triggers the resolution of alcohol problems without treatment? *Alcoholism: Clinical and Experimental Research, 17,* 217–224.

Stall, R., & Biernacki, P. (1989). Spontaneous remission from the problematic use of substances. *International Journal of the Addictions, 21,* 1–23.

Stewart, K. B., & Richards, A. B. (2000). Recognizing and managing your patient's alcohol abuse. *Nursing, 30,* 56–60.

Trice, H., & Roman, P. (1970). Delabeling, relabeling, and Alcoholics Anonymous. *Social Problems, 17,* 538–546.

U.S. Department of Health and Human Services. (2000a). *Healthy people 2010 (2nd ed.). With understanding and improving health and objectives for improving health, 2 Vols.* Washington, DC: U.S. Government Printing Office.

U.S. Department of Health and Human Services. (2000b). *National household survey on drug abuse.* Retrieved October 13, 2002, from http://www.samhsa.gov/ oas/dependence/chapter2.htm

Waldorf, D., Reinarman, C., & Murphy, S. (1991). *Cocaine changes: The experience of using and quitting.* Philadelphia: Temple University Press.

Walitzer, K. S., Dermen, K. H., & Connors, G. J. (1999). Strategies for preparing clients for treatment: A review. *Behavior Modification, 12,* 129–151.

Winick, C. (1962). Maturing out of narcotic addiction. *Bulletin on Narcotics, 6,* 1.

Chapter 17

American Psychiatric Association. (1994). *Diagnostic and statistical manual of mental disorders* (4th ed.). New York: Author.

Angier, C. (2002). *The double bond of Primo Levi.* New York: Farrar, Strauss & Giroux.

Baron, L., Eisman, H., Scuello, M., Veyzer, A., & Lieberman, M. (1996). Stress resilience, locus of control, and religion in children of Holocaust victims. *Journal of Psychology, 130,* 513–525.

Beck, J. G., & Stanley, M. A. (1997). Anxiety disorders in the elderly: The emerging role of behavior therapy. *Behavior Therapy, 28*(6), 83–100.

Beekman, A. T., Bremmer, M. A., Deeg, D. J. H., van Balkou, A. J., Smit, J. H., Debeurs, E., et al. (1998). Anxiety disorders in later life: A report from the Longitudinal Aging Study, Amsterdam. *International Journal of Geriatric Psychiatry, 12,* 717–726.

Casey, D. A. (1994). Depression in the elderly. *Southern Medical Journal, 87,* 559–564.

Cochran, S. V., & Rabinowitz, F. E. (2003). Gender-sensitive recommendations for assessment and treatment of depression in men. *Professional Psychology: Research and Practice, 34,* 132–140.

Gallagher-Thompson, D., Hanley-Peterson, P., & Thompson, L. W. (1990). Maintenance of gains versus relapse following brief psychotherapy for depression. *Journal of Consulting and Clinical Psychology, 58,* 371–374.

Glicken, M. D. (2004). *The strengths perspective in social work practice: A positive approach for the helping professions.* Boston: Allyn & Bacon/Longman.

Glicken, M. D. (2005). *Improving the effectiveness of the helping professions: An evidence-based approach to practice.* Thousand Oaks, CA: Sage.

Huffman, G. B. (1999). Preventing recurrence of depression in the elderly. *American Family Physician, 59,* 2589–2591.

Kennedy, G. J., & Tannenbaum, S. (2000). Psychotherapy with older adults. *American Journal of Psychotherapy, 54,* 386–407.

Kogan, J. N., Edelstein, B. A., & McKee, D. R. (2000). Assessment of anxiety in older adults: Current status. *Journal of Anxiety Disorders, 14*(2), 109–132

Lang, A. J., & Stein, M. B. (2001). Anxiety disorders. *Geriatrics, 56,* 24–30.

Lenze, E. J., Dew, M. A., Mazumdar, S., Begley, A. E., Cornes, C., Miller, M. D., et al. (2002). Combined pharmacotherapy and psychotherapy as maintenance treatment for late-life depression: Effects on social adjustment. *American Journal of Psychiatry, 159,* 466–468.

Levi, P. (1995a). *If not now, when?* New York: Viking Penguin.

Levi, P. (1995b). *The periodic table.* Stockholm: Raymond Rosenthal.

Mills, T. L., & Henretta, J. C. (2001). Racial, ethnic, and socio-demographic differences in the level of psychosocial distress among older America. s. *Research on Aging, 23,* 131–152.

Newman, L. (1979). Emotional disturbances in children of Holocaust survivors. *Social Casework: The Journal of Contemporary Social Work, 5,* 43–50.

O'Connor, R. (2001). Active treatment of depression. *American Journal of Psychotherapy, 55,* 507–530.

Rush, A. J., & Giles, D. E. (1982). *Cognitive therapy: Theory and research in short term psychotherapies for depression.* New York: Guilford.

Saleeby, D. (1992). *The strengths perspective in social work practice.* White Plains, NY: Longman.

Smith, S. S., Sherrill, K. A., & Celenda, C. C. (1995, April 4). Anxious elders deserve careful diagnosing and the most appropriate interventions. *Brown University Long-Term Care Letter, 7,* 5–7.

Stanley, M. A., & Novy, D. M. (2000). Cognitive-behavior therapy for generalized anxiety in late life: An evaluative overview. *Journal of Anxiety Disorders, 14,* 191–207.

Tech, N. (2003). *Resilience and courage: Women, men, and the holocaust.* New Haven, CT: Yale University Press.

Tyler, K. A., & Hoyt, D. R. (2000). The effects of an acute stressor on depressive symptoms among older adults. *Research on Aging, 22,* 143–164.

Vaillant, G. E., & Mukamal, K. (2001). Successful aging. *American Journal of Psychiatry, 158,* 839–847.

Waern, M., Runeson, B. S., Allebeck, P., & Beskau, J. (2002). Mental disorder in elderly suicides: A case-control study. *American Journal of Psychiatry, 159*(3), 450–455.

Wallis, M. A. (2000). Looking at depression through bifocal lenses. *Nursing, 30,* 58–62.

Weick, A., Rapp, C., Sullivan, W. P., & Kisthardt, W. (1989). A strengths perspective for social work practice. *Social Work, 34,* 350–354.

Chapter 18

Ash, P., Kellermann, A., Fuqua-Whitley, D., & Johnson, D. (1996). Gun acquisition and use by juvenile offenders. *Journal of the American Medical Association, 275,* 1754–1758.

Barlow, D. H. (1996). Health care policy, psychotherapy research, and the future of psychotherapy. *American Psychologist, 51,* 1007–1016.

Bereska, T. M. (2003). The changing boys' world in the 20th century: Reality and "fiction." *Journal of Men's Studies, 11,* 157–192.

Borduin, C. M. (1999). Multisystemic treatment of criminality and violence in adolescents. *Journal of the American Academy of Child and Adolescent Psychiatry, 38,* 242–249.

Caplan, M., Weissberg, R. P., Grober, J. S., Sivo, P. J., Grady, K., & Jacoby, C. (1992). Social competence promotion with inner-city and suburban young adolescents: Effects on social adjustment and alcohol use. *Journal of Consulting and Clinical Psychology, 60,* 56–63

Farrell, W. (2002). *9/11s' survival dilemma.* Retrieved April 13, 2004 from http://www.warrenfarrell.com

Forbes, D. (2003). Turn the wheel: Integral school counseling for male adolescents. *Journal of Counseling & Development, 81,* 142–150.

Glicken, M. D. (2004). *Using the strengths perspective: A positive approach for the helping professions.* Boston: Allyn & Bacon.

Goffman, E. (1979). *Gender advertisements.* Cambridge, MA: Harvard University Press.

Greenwood, P. W., Model, K. E., Rydell, C. P., & Chiesa, J. (1996). *Diverting children from a life of crime: Measuring costs and benefits.* Santa Monica, CA: Rand Corporation.

Hansen, W. B., & Graham, J. W. (1991). Preventing alcohol, marijuana, and cigarette use among adolescents: Peer pressure resistance training versus establishing conservative norms. *Preventative Medicine, 20,* 414–430.

Hawkins, J. D., Catalano, R. F., Morrison, D. M., O'Donnell, J., Abbott, R. D., & Day, L. E. (1992). The Seattle Social Development Project: Effects of the first four years on protective factors and problem behaviors. In J. M. McCord & R. Tremblay (Eds.), *The prevention of antisocial behavior in children* (pp. 103–136). New York: Guilford.

Huey, W. C., & Rank, R. C. (1984). Effects of counselor and peer-led groups' assertive training on Black adolescent aggression. *Journal of Counseling Psychology, 31,* 95–98.

Johnson, D. L. (1990). The Houston parent–child development center project: Disseminating a viable program for enhancing at-risk families. *Prevention in Human Services, 7*(6), 89–108.

Kimmel, M. S. (1994). Masculinity as homophobia: Fear, shame, and silence in the construction of gender identity. In H. Brod & M. Kaufman (Eds.), *Theorizing masculinities* (pp. 119–141). Thousand Oaks, CA: Sage.

Mathias, C. E. (1992). Touching the lives of children: Consultative interventions that work. *Elementary School Guidance and Counseling, 26,* 190–201.

Migliaccio, T. A. (2001). Marginalizing the battered male. *Journal of Men's Studies, 9,* 205–225.

Morrow, L., & Dickerson, J. (1994, February 14). Men are they really that bad? *Time, 143,* 52–60.

Olds, D. L., Henderson, C. R., Tatelbaum, R., & Chamberlin, R. (1988). Improving the life-course development of socially disadvantaged mothers: A randomized trial of nurse home visitation. *American Journal of Public Health, 78,* 1436–1444.

O'Neill, T. (2000). Sex differences in education. *Report/Newsmagazine (Alberta Edition), 27,* 54–56.

Parloff, M. B. (1979). Can psychotherapy research guide the policymaker? A little knowledge may be a dangerous thing. *American Psychologist, 34,* 296–306.

Parloff, M. B., & Elkin, I. (1992). The NIMH Treatment of Depression Collaborative Research Program. In D. K. Freedheim (Ed.), *History of psychotherapy: A century of change* (pp. 442–450). Washington, DC: American Psychological Association.

Peebles, J. (2000). The future of psychotherapy outcome research: Science or political rhetoric? *Journal of Psychology, 134,* 659–670.

Rae-Grant, N., McConville, B. J., & Fleck, S. (1999, March). Violent behavior in children and youth: Preventive intervention from a psychiatric perspective. *Journal of the American Academy of Child and Adolescent Psychiatry, 38*(3), 235–241.

Studer, J. (1996, February). Understanding and preventing aggressive responses in youth. *Elementary School Guidance and Counseling, 30,* 194–203.

Wampold, B. E., Mondin, G. W., Moody, M., et al. (1997). A meta-analysis of outcome studies comparing bona fide psychotherapies: Empirically. *Psychological Bulletin, 122,* 203–215.

Weikart, D. P., Schweinhart, L. J., & Larner, M. B. (1986). A report on the High/Scope Preschool Curriculum Comparison Study: Consequences of three preschool curriculum models through age 15. *Early Child Research, 1,* 15–45.

Zigler, E., Taussig, C., & Black, K. (1992). Early childhood intervention: A promising preventative for juvenile delinquency. *American Psychologist, 47*(7), 997–1006.

Chapter 19

Bergin, A. E. (1971). The evaluation of therapeutic outcomes. In A. E. Bergin & S. Garfield (Eds.), *Handbook of psychotherapy and behavior change* (pp. 217–270). New York: Wiley.

Bidsrup, S. (2000). *Homophobia: The fear behind the hatred.* Retrieved August 27, 2004, from http://www.bidstrup.com/phobia.htm

Flaherty, R. J. (2001, September 15). Medical myths: Today's perspectives. *Patient Care, 6*(9). Retrieved February 17, 2003, from http://www.findarticles.com/cf_0/m3233/17_35/78547389/print.jhtml

Heckert, T. M., Droste, H. E., Adams, P. J., Griffin, C. M., Roberts, L. L., Mueller, M. A., & Wallis, H. A. (2002, August). Gender differences in anticipated salary: Role of salary estimates for others, job characteristics, career paths, and job inputs. *Sex Roles: A Journal of Research, 42,* 341–345.

Issacs, D. (1999). Seven alternatives to evidence based medicine. *British Medical Journal, 39,* 1619–1625.

Kopta, M. S., Lueger, R. J., Saunders, S. M., & Howard, K. I. (1999). Individual psychotherapy outcome and process research: Challenges leading to greater turmoil or a positive transition? *Annual Review of Psychology, 50,* 441–469. Retrieved May 19, 2002, from http://www.findarticles.com/cf_0/m0961/ 1999_Annual/ 54442307/print.jhtml

Migliaccio, T. A. (2001). Marginalizing the battered male. *Journal of Men's Studies, 9,* 205–222

O'Donnell, M. (1997). *A skeptic's medical dictionary.* London: BMJ Books.

Poussaint, A. F. (1993). Enough already. *Ebony, 48,* 86–89.

Author Index

A

Aaron, F., 40, *351*
Abel, G., 163, *367*
Abernethy, M., 54, 55, *353*
Abbott, R. D., 172, 321, *364, 381*
Aboramph, O. M., 231, *371*
Abracen, J., 196, *369*
Adams, D., 181, *367*
Adams, P. J., 331, *383*
Adebimpe, V. R., 232, *371*
Alexander, R., Jr., 173, 174, *363*
Alfano, D. P., 179, 184, *367*
Alkon, A., 52 *353*
Allebeck, P., 305, *380*
Allen, J., 7, 131, 132, *347, 360*
Altarriba, J., 254, 255, *373*
Alterman, A. I., 153, *362*
Amodei, N., 282, *376*
Anderson, R., 44, *351*
Andrew, S. R., 282, *376*
Andrews, D., 172, *363*
Angier, C., 304, 306, *379*
Arellano, L. M., 253, *374*
Ash, P., 320, *381*
Atkinson, R., 283, 284, *375*
Auerbach, A., 82, *358*
Avery, L., 140, *360*

B

Babcock, J. C., 187, *367*
Babor, T. F., 284, *375, 377*
Baca Zinn, M., 246, 247, *373*
Bachman, J. G., 276, *377*

Backer, K. L., 278, *376*
Baer, J., 166, *363*
Bagley, C., 179, *367*
Bakeland, F. E., 286, *376*
Balcom, D. A., 9, 10, *347*
Bard, K. A., 29, *349*
Bark, R. A., 186, *369*
Barlow, D. H., 318, *381*
Barnett, M. P., 285, *378*
Baron, L., 306, *379*
Barry, K. L., 283, *376*
Bauer, L. M., 254, 255, *373*
Begley, A. E., 302, *380*
Beck, J. G., 298, *379*
Beekman, A. T., 297, *379*
Bell, A. P., 237, *371*
Berdahl, J. L., 205, *371*
Bereska, T. M., 17, 315, 323, *349, 381*
Bergin, A. E., 342, *383*
Berlin, F. S., 195, *367*
Berliner, L., 164, *363*
Berman, S., 282, *376*
Bernard, J. L., 184, *367*
Bernard, M. L., 184, *367*
Bernstein, R., 207, 208, *370*
Besdine, R. W., 34, *353, 276, 378*
Beskau, J., 305, *380*
Bidsrup, S., 343, *383*
Bien, T. J., 282, 283, *376*
Biernacki, P., 289, 290, *376, 378*
Bisman, C., 81, 87, *356*
Bisson, J., 76, 277, 278, *354, 375*
Biswas, R., 263, *374*
Black, K., 172, 321, *367, 383*
Black, S. A., 246, *374*

Bland, I. J., 234, 372
Blashfield, R. K., 69, 354
Blumstein, A., 162, 363
Bly, R., 106, 125, 149, 361
Bonta, J., 363
Booth, B. M., 287, 377
Borduin, C. M., 320, 381
Borgida, E., 204, 370
Borman, L. D., 152, 362
Brannon, R. C., 16, 18, 349
Bremmer, M. A., 297, 379
Brent, D. A., 80, 82, 83, 356
Briscoe, J., 161, 363
Brittan-Powell, C., 26, 351
Brodsky, S. L., 164, 363
Brooks, G. R., 30, 104, 116, 349, 359
Bross, D. C., 170, 365
Bucholz, K., 280, 377
Buehler, J., 40, 351
Burns, D. D., 82, 356
Burge, S. K., 282, 376
Burgess, D., 204, 370
Burt, M. R., 204, 371
Burtscheidt, W., 289, 376
Butler, R., 279, 378
Butts, J. A., 162, 363

C

Cahalan, D., 289,
Caplan, M., 320, 381
Caputo, A. A., 164, 363
Carrillo, T. E., 188, 368
Carroll, D., 148, 362
Carroll, K. M., 82, 356
Cary, S., 52, 53, 353
Caserta, M. S., 146, 154, 361
Casey, D. A., 300, 301, 379
Casia, P., 146, 361
Catala, S., 282, 376
Catalano, R. F., 165, 172, 321, 364, 381
Celenda, C. C., 297, 298, 299, 380
Chafetz, J. S., 248, 373
Chamberlin, R., 171, 320, 365, 382
Chang, G., 282, 376
Chiesa, J., 320, 381
Chin, J., 34, 38, 39, 352
Christian, J., 229, 371
Christo, G., 153, 360
Chung, D., 263, 374
Clar, S., 146, 361

Cleland, P., 286, 377
Cloud, J., 68, 354
Cloud, W., 289, 290, 291, 376
Cochran, C. C., 370
Cochran, S. V., 44, 101, 204, 301, 302, 351,
    359, 379
Coe, M. J., 83, 358
Colby, S. M., 285, 378
Coleman, E. M., 180, 369
Colvin, G., 166, 366
Congress, E., 251, 373
Conlin, M., 6, 12, 13, 347
Connors, G. J., 82, 285, 286, 356, 379
Cooley, E. J., 82, 83, 356
Cornes, C., 302, 380
Cournoyer, R. J., 26, 349
Courtenay, W., 5, 37, 40, 41, 42, 347, 351
Cowley, G., 20, 349
Crawford, D., 167, 366
Culbert, A., 289, 377
Cullen, F., 363
Cummings, A. L., 133, 360
Currie, E., 161, 363

D

Dahlgren, L., 289, 376
Daniels, J., 284, 377
Danos, K. K., 105, 359
D'Antonio, M., 12, 13, 347
Darrow, C. N., 25, 26, 349
Davis, R. C., 186, 187, 367
Davis, R. T., 69, 354
Dawson, D. A., 280, 376
Day, L. E., 321, 364, 381
Day, N., 289, 377
Debeurs, E., 279, 379
Deeg, D. J. H., 297, 379
DeGrandpre, R., 69, 354
DeMaris, A., 103, 359
Demers, A., 76, 277, 278, 354, 376
Dermen, K. H., 285, 286, 379
DeSouza, E., 204, 371
Dew, M. A., 302, 380
Dewhurst, A. M., 179, 184, 367
Dickerson, J., 315, 382
DiClemente, C. C., 82, 356
DiIulio, J. J., Jr., 8, 229, 347, 371
Dinero, T. E., 192, 369
Dodge, K. A., 181, 367
Donovan, D. M., 82, 285, 356, 376

Droste, H. E., 331, *383*
Duckworth, L., 179, *368*
Dunn, C. W., 285, *376*
Dunn, J., 14, *347*
Dutton, 185, *367*
Dwyer, K. P., 73, *354*

E

Eagger, S., 279, *378*
Edelson, J. L., 140, 186, 189, *360, 367*
Edelstein, B. A., 298, *380*
Edlund, M., 147, *361*
Egan, J., 26, *350*
Eisenberg, N., 27, *349*
Eisikovits, Z. C., 140, 186, 189, *360, 367*
Eisman, H., 306, *379*
Elkin, B., 282, *376*
Elkin, I., 82, 318, *357, 382*
Ellickson, P. L., 171, *364*
Elliott, D. S., 162, 169, *364*
Ellum, F., 13, *347*
Elofsson, S., 39, *352*
Emrick, C. D., 152, 153, *361*
Entwistle, V. A., 80, *356*
Epperley, T. D., 34, 276, *351, 376*
Everingham, J., 9, *348*
Ewing, C. P., 265, *374*

F

Fabes, R. A., 27, *349*
Fagan, J., 165, 186, *364, 367*
Farrell, W., 27, 52, 53, 317, *349, 353, 381*
Fawcett, J., 153, *362*
Fetto, J., 147, *361*
Ficarrotto, T., 34, 38, 39, *352*
Figlio, R. M., 6, *349*
Fiske, S. T., 204, *371*
Fitzgerald, D., 341, *383*
Fitzgerald, L. F., 23, 69, 99, 100, 102, 103, 104, 205, *350, 355, 359, 370, 371*
Fivush, R., *349*
Flaherty, J. A., 232, *371*
Flaherty, R. J., 341, *383*
Fleck, S., 168, 171, 172, 320, 321, *366, 382*
Fleming, M. F., 283, 285, *376*
Forbes, D., 315, 318, *381*
Foulks, E. F., 234, *372*
Fracher, J. C., 195, *369*
Frank, R. G., 147, *361*

Franklin, A. J., 71, 140, 235, *355, 360, 372*
Frazier, P. A., 204, *370*
Freudenberger, H., 9, *347*
Frick, P., 164, *363*
Frinter, M., 192, *368*
Frodi, A. M., 53, 58, *354*
Frodi, M., 53, 58, *354*
Fuller, S. G., 42, *352*
Fuqua-Whitley, D., 320, *381*
Furstenberg, F. F., Jr., 9, *348*
Furuto, S. M., 263, *374*

G

Galanter, M., 155, *361*
Gallagher-Thompson, L. W., 302, *379*
Gambrill, E., 72, 89, 102, *355, 357, 359*
Garretson, D. J., 232, *372*
Garza, M. A., *373*
Gaw, A. C., 263, *374*
Gehart, D. R., 84, *357*
Gehart-Brooks, D. R., 83, *357*
Gelles, R. J., 179, 185, *370*
Gendreau, P., *363*
Gentilello, L. M., 285, *376*
Gilden, J. L., 146, *361*
Giles, D. E., 310, *380*
Giles-Sims, P., 181, *368*
Gilligan, C., 24, *349*
Glick, B., 167, 173, *364*
Glicken, M. D., 72, 74, 75, 81, 84, 86, 124,
    141, 161, 166, 170, 174, 178, 197,
    215, 219, 221, 255, 259, 260, 272,
    291, 296, 304, 308, *355, 357, 359,*
    360, 364, 368, 370, 373, 374, 375,
    376, 379, 380
Goetz, M. A., 282, *376*
Goffman, E., 319, *381*
Golan, N., 263, *374*
Goldstein, A. P., 167, 173, 174, *364*
Gondolf, E. W., 187, *368*
Gong-Guy, E., 263, *374*
Gonzalez, M. J., 249, *373*
Grady, K., 320, *381*
Graham, J. W., 320, *381*
Gramckow, H. P., 161, *364*
Granfield, R., 289, 290, 291, *376*
Grant, B. F., 280, *376*
Grant-Bowman, C., 58, *353*
Grauerholz, E., 204, *371*
Grawe, K., 80, *358*

Greenberg, L. S., 82, 357
Greenfeld, L. A., 192, 368
Greenwood, P. W., 320, 381
Griffin, C. M., 331, 383
Grimm, R., 40, 351
Grober, J. S., 320, 381
Groth, N. A., 164, 195 364, 368
Grusznski, R. J., 188,368
Guetzloe, E., 172, 173, 364
Gupta, S., 33, 34, 276, 351, 377
Gutek, A. G., 205, 371

H

Hale, G., 179, 368
Haley, J., 133, 360
Hall, A. S., 56, 113, 115, 132, 353, 354, 359,
        360
Hallberg, E. T., 133, 360
Hallstrom, C., 154, 363
Hamberger, K., 187, 368
Hamburg, B., 364
Hamburg, M. A., 163, 169, 364
Hammill, P., 229, 230, 372
Hanley-Peterson, P., 302, 379
Hansen, K. V., 186, 367
Hansen, W. B., 320, 381
Hardy, C. B., 232, 234, 372
Harris, I., 229, 372
Harrison, J., 34, 38, 39, 352
Hastings, J., 187, 368
Haverkamp, B., 70 355
Hawkins, J. D., 162, 165, 172, 321, 364, 381
Hayes, C. D., 29, 351
Haynes, M. R., 180, 369
Heckard, I. D., 59, 353
Heckert, T. M., 331, 383
Heeren, T., 276, 377
Heifner, C., 44, 352
Henderson, C. R., 171, 320, 365, 382
Hendrix, D. H., 133, 360
Hendryx, A. S., 146, 361
Henretta, J. C., 301, 380
Henry, W. P., 83, 357
Herman, M., 282, 287, 288, 377
Hernandez, R., 245, 373
Herrenkoh, T. I., 162, 364
Herzog, E., 9, 348
Hesselbrock, V., 280, 377
Heston, M. L., 133, 360
Higgins-Biddle, J. C., 284, 375, 377

Hingson, R. W., 153, 276, 289, 363, 377
Hinrichsen, G. A., 154, 361
Ho, M. K., 261, 374
Hoge, R., 172, 363
Holzhuter, J. L., 149, 362
Hopkins, W. D., 29, 349
Hoppe, S. K., 247, 374
Horowitz, M. J., 155, 362
Horvath, A. O., 82, 357
Hotaling, G. T., 180, 183, 368
Howard, K. I., 79, 82, 342, 357, 383
Howe, C., 246, 373
Hoyt, D. R., 301, 380
Huang, B., 364
Hudson, S. M., 196, 368
Huey, W. C., 167, 322, 364, 382
Huffman, G. B., 302, 380
Hughes, J., 40, 351
Hughes, J. M., 153, 361
Huizinga, D., 162, 366
Humphreys, K., 146, 152, 153, 291, 294,
        361, 377
Hurst, M. A., 105, 359
Huyck, M. H., 44, 352
Hwang, C. -P., 53, 58, 162, 354

I

Ino, S., 215, 266, 267, 271, 370, 374
Isaacs, D., 341, 383
Izzo, R., 172, 365

J

Jacobs, D., 40, 351
Jacobson, N., 178, 182, 183, 368
Jacoby, C., 320, 381
Johnson, D. L., 171, 172, 320, 321, 365,
        381, 382
Johnson, K., 283, 376
Johnson, L. B., 204, 371
Johnson, P., 196, 368
Johnston, L. D., 276, 377
Jones, E. E., 83, 357
Jordan, A. D., 163, 367
Jossi, F., 215, 371
Jouard, S., 184, 368

K

Kalmuss, D., 180, 368

Kann, L., 275, *377*
Kaplan, S. J., 170, *365*
Karbon, M., 27, *329*
Karlberg, L., 39, *352*
Katz, N. V., 203, *371*
Katz, S. J., 147, *361*
Kaufman, G., 53, 58, *353*
Keightley, M. L., 27, *350*
Keith-Lucas, A., 80, 81, *357*
Keller, A. K., 27, *349*
Kellerman, A., 320, *381*
Kelly, K. R., 56, 113, 115, 132, *353, 354,
     359, 360*
Kempton, C., 28, *350*
Kennedy, G. J., 303, 304, *380*
Kennedy, M., 155, *361*
Kessler, R. C., 146, 147, 152, *361*
Kim, H., 204, *371*
Kimmel, M. S., 319, *382*
Kirchner, J. E., 287, *377*
Kisthardt, W., 308, *381*
Klein, E. B., 25, 26, *349*
Kochanek, K., 44, *351*
Kogan, J. N., 298, *380*
Kohlberg, L., 24, *349*
Kolko, D. J., 80, 82, 83, *356*
Kopta, M. S., 79, 82, 342, *357, 383*
Korgan, M. J., 38, *352*
Koss, M. P., 192, *369*
Kosterman, R., 162, *364*
Kottman, S., 133, *360*
Kraemer, S., 28, 29, 37, 38, *349, 352*
Kramer, J. R., 280, *377*
Kramer, K. D., 154, *362*
Krakau, I., 39, *352*
Kruger, A., 45, 46, *352*
Krugman, S., 9, *348*
Krupnick, J. L., 82, *357*
Kuperman, S., 280, *377*
Kurtz, L. F., 146, 155, *362*

L

Labruna, V., 170, *365*
Laird, J., 131, 132, *360*
Lajoy, R., 82, 83, *356*
Lamb, M. E., 53, 58, *354*
Lambert, E., 289, *378*
Lancaster, A. E., 287, *377*
Landsman, M., 184, *368*
Lane, P. A., 282, *376*
Lane, P. S., 167, *365*

Lang, A. J., 297, 299, *380*
Lanzillo, A. B., 86, 104, *358, 359*
LaRossa, J. R., 184, *370*
Larner, M. B., 321, *382*
Laszloffy, T. A., 232, 234, *372*
Lawson, E. J., 231, 232, 238, *372*
Leaf, P., 147, *361*
Lee, E., 261, *375*
LeGrand, S., 165, *366*
Lehrman, K., 58, *354*
Leigh, G., 286, *377*
Lennox, R. D., 289, *377*
Lenze, E. J., 302, *380*
Leo, G., 289, *378*
Leo, J., 57, 201, *354, 371*
Leong, F. T. L., 264, *375*
Lerman, L., 185, *369*
Levant, R. F., 9, 12, *348*
Levi, P., 304, *380*
Levinson, D. J., 25, 26, 45, *349, 352*
Levinson, M. H., 25, 26, *349*
Levy, L. H., 152, *362*
Lewis, E. A., 149, *362*
Liberto, J. G., 283, *377*
Lieberman, M. A., 152, 155, 306, *362, 363,
     379*
Lin, C., 105, *359*
Lin, E., 147, *361*
Lloyd, B. F., 26, *349*
Locke, B. D., 26, *349*
Loeber, R., 162, *366*
London, R., 283, *376*
Longabaugh, R., 82, *356*
Longo, R. E., 164, *364*
Looman, J., 196, *369*
Loza, W., 196, 197, *369*
Loza-Fanous, A., 196, 197, *369*
Lu, M., 285, *377*
Luborsky, L., 82, *358*
Lucca, J. S., 14, *348*
Lueger, R. J., 79, 82, 342, *357, 383*
Lukefahr, J. L., 170, *365*
Lund, D. A., 146, 155, *361*
Lundwall, L., 286, *376*
Lustman, P. J., 82, 83, *358*
Lyle, R. R., 83, 84, *357*
Lynam, D., 73, *355*

M

MacDoniels, J., 44, *352*
MacKinnon, C. A., 204, *371*

MacLeod, J. M., 137, 360
Mahalik, J. R., 26, 349
Malamuth, N. M., 192, 369
Malgady, R., 249, 374
Manassis, K., 140, 360
Mansfield, A. J., 289, 377
Manwell, L. B., 283, 285, 376
Marin, P., 10, 11, 230, 348, 372
Markowitz, F. E., 71, 355
Marmar, C. R., 155, 362
Marsh, W. L., 69, 356
Marshall, R. W., 196, 368
Marsiglia, F. F., 149, 362
Martin, J. L., 70, 133, 355, 360
Matchen, J., 204, 371
Mathias, C. E., 167, 322, 365, 382
Mavis, B. E., 153, 361
Mayer, A., 195, 369
Mayer, G. R., 163, 365
Mazumdar, S., 302, 380
McCallion, P., 146, 362
McClain, R. P., 140, 360
McConville, B. J., 168, 171, 172, 320, 321,
        366, 382
McCord, J., 170, 365
Mcree, B., 284, 377
McDaniel, S. H., 84, 358
McElroy, R. A., 69, 354
McFadin, J. B., 164, 364
McGuigan, K. A., 171, 364
McGuire, T. G., 285, 377
McKay, J. R., 153, 362
McKee, B., 25, 26, 349
McKee, D. R., 297, 380
McKinney, K., 204, 371
McLaughlin, J. E., 69, 70, 355
McLellan, A. T., 82, 358
McNeill, B. W., 253, 374
McWhirter, J. J., 167, 365
Mead, M., 26, 349
Meagher, R., 232, 371
Meissen, G., 146, 148, 363
Memmott, J. L., 149, 362
Menninger, J. A., 284, 377
Merhing, T. A., 74, 355
Merrigan, D. M., 153, 363
Mickelson, K. D., 146, 152, 361
Migliaccio, T. A., 319, 346, 382, 383
Miller, M. D., 302, 380
Miller, K. E., 277, 378
Miller, W. R., 282, 283, 376, 378

Mills, T. L., 301, 380
Mirande, A., 247, 373
Misener, T. R., 42, 352
Mittelmark, M., 40, 351
Model, K. E., 320, 381
Moffitt, T. E., 73, 355
Mondin, G. W., 319, 382
Monsivais, C., 246, 252, 373
Monti, P. M., 285, 378
Moody, M., 319, 382
Moore, K. E., 34, 276, 351, 376
Moore, R. J., 179, 184, 367
Moore, T., 40, 352
Moos, R. H., 146, 152, 361
Moralis, A., 169, 365
Morey, L. C., 69, 355
Morishima, J. K., 263, 375
Morrison, D. M., 172, 321, 364, 381
Morrison, P., 58, 354
Morrow, L., 55, 56, 58, 315, 354, 382
Moxley, D. P., 294, 378
Moyer, J., 82, 357
Mueller, M. A., 331, 383
Mukamal, K., 301, 380
Mullahy, J., 284, 377
Mulvey, E., 172, 366
Murase, K., 263, 374
Murphy, G. E., 82, 83, 358
Murphy, M. J., 84, 358
Murphy, S., 44, 351, 290, 379
Murphy, W. D., 180, 369
Murray, B. A., 165, 365
Murray, L., 28, 350
Myers, J. E., 136, 360
Myers, M. A., 165, 365
Myles, B. S., 169, 365

N

Nadeau, L., 76, 277, 278, 354, 376
Narrett, C., 169, 366
Nash, K. B., 154, 362
Nathanson, P., 55, 354
Neff, J. A., 247, 374
Neuman, E., 179, 369
Newman, L., 306, 380
Nicholaichuk, T. P., 196, 369
Nickels, L. B., 186, 187, 367
Nolen-Hoeksema, S., 82, 356
Nord, C. W., 9, 348
Northey, W. F., 163, 367
Novy, D. M., 298, 380

O

Oates, R. K., 170, *365*
Obiakor, F. E., 74, *355*
O'Brien, C. P., 82, *358*
Ochoa, E. S., 69, *355*
O'Connor, L., 81, *358*
O'Connor, R., 303, 310, *380*
O'Donnell, J., 172, 321, *364, 381*
O'Donnell, M., 341, *383*
Olds, D. L., 171, 320, *365, 382*
Olivia, G., 294, *378*
Olson, A. M., 204, *370*
O'Malley, P. M., 276, *377*
O'Neil, J. M., 23, 26, 100, *350, 359*
O'Neill, T., 6, 7, 315, *348, 382*
Orlinsky, D. E., 80, *358*
Ormerod, M., 204, *370*
Osborne, A. C., 286, *377*
Osher, D., 73, *354*
Oslin, D. W., 283, *377*
Osofsky, H. J., 6, 162, *348, 365*
Osofsky, J. D., 6, 162, *348, 365*
Owen, R. R., 287, *377*

P

Pardeck, J. T., 136, *360*
Parker, J. D., 27, *350*
Parks, B. K., 80, *358*
Parloff, M. B., 318, *382*
Patterson, G., 169, *366*
Patterson, S. L., 149, *362, 363*
Peebles, J., 318, *382*
Peele, S., 276, 290, *378*
Pelcovitz, D., 170, *365*
Pena, J. M., 234, *372*
Pena, M., 247, 248, *374*
Penn, P., 134, *360*
Pennington, H., 279, *378*
Peterson, J. L., 9, *348*
Peterson, R. L., 166, 180, *366, 396*
Pfeiffer, A. M., 70, *355*
Pilkonis, A., 82, *357*
Pisani, V. D., 153, *362*
Pitman, F. S., 23, *350*
Pleck, J. H., 25, 26, 30, *350*
Pollack, W., 32, 122, *350, 359*
Poussaint, A. F., 237, 238, 340, 342, *372, 383*
Price, S. J., 84, *358*
Prihoda, T. J., 247, *374*

Q

Quadagno, J. S., 149, *362*

R

Rabinowitz, F. E., 44, 101, 301, 302, *351, 359, 379*
Rae-Grant, N., 168, 171, 172, 320, 321, *366, 382*
Ramsey, E., 166, *366*
Randolph, W. M., 246, *374*
Rank, R. C., 167, 322, *364, 382*
Rapp, C., 308, *381*
Rappaport, J., 152, *361*
Reece, R. M., 170, *366*
Rees, D. W., *378*
Reich, T., 280, *377*
Reigle, N., 183, *369*
Reinarman, C., 290, *379*
Repucci, N., 172, *366*
Reuben, D. B., 34, *353*, 276, *378*
Revenson, 154, *361*
Rice, J., 234, *372*
Richard, B. A., 181, *367*
Richards, A. B., 76, 277, 278, 281, *356, 379*
Riessman, F., 146, 147, 148, 154, *362*
Rivara, F. P., 285, *376*
Roach, R., 5, *348*
Robbins, J., 83, *358*
Roberts, A. R., 263, *375*
Roberts, L. L., 331, *383*
Robertson, J., 23, 69, 99, 100, 102, 103, 104, 105, *350, 355, 359*
Robinson, J. L., 213, *371*
Roger, L., 249, *374*
Roizen, R., 289, *378*
Rollnick, S., 283, *378*
Roman, P., 290, *378*
Root, M., 262, *375*
Rosen, J., 135, *360*
Rosen, R. C., 195, *369*
Rosenfeld, B. D., 187, *369*
Rosenhan, D. L., *70*, 355
Rosenwaithe, I., 247, *374*
Ross, R., 172, *365*
Ross-Sheriff, F., 263, *374*
Roy, M., 180, *369*
Rout, U., 28, *350*
Rubinson, L., 192, *368*
Runeson, B. S., 305, *380*
Rush, A. J., 310, *380*

Rydell, C. P., 320, *381*

S

Sackett, G. P., 29, *350*
Saleeby, D., 68, 79, 81, 113, 308, *355, 358,*
    359, 380
Salloum, A., 140, *360*
Sampson, H., 81, *358*
Sanchez, V. C., 283, *378*
Sargent, J., 32, *350*
Satcher, D., 75, 233, *355, 372*
Saunders, C. S., 34, *353*
Saunders, S. M., 79, 82, 342, *357, 383*
Scahill, M. C., 161, *366*
Scapillato, D., 140, *360*
Schacht, T. E., 83, *357*
Schenk, R., 9, *348*
Scher, E., 182, *369*
Scher, M., 16, 23, 24, 31, 85, 101, 121, *350,*
    358, 359
Schlosser, S. S., 280, *377*
Schrumpt, F., 167, *366*
Schuerger, J. M., 183, *369*
Schwartz, R., 289, *376*
Schweinhart, L. J., 321, *382*
Schwenn, J. O., 74, *355*
Scotch, N., 289, *377*
Scott, D., 179, *368*
Scuello, M., 306, *379*
Sechrest, D., 168, 170, 178, 221, *366, 368,*
    370
Seligman, D., 43, *353*
Seligman, M. E. P., 79, 152, 282, *358, 362,*
    378
Selling, T., 6, *349*
Sells, S. P., 83, *358*
Severson, H. H., 73, 163, *356, 366*
Shai, D., 247, *374*
Shanks, P., 289, *378*
Sharp, W. S., 69, *356*
Sharpe, T. L., 231, 232, 238, *372*
Shek, D. T. L., 45, *353*
Sheldon, T. A., 80, *356*
Shepherd, M. D., 146, 148, *363*
Sherman, L., 186, *369*
Sherrill, K. A., 297, 298, 299, *380*
Shervinton, D., 234, *372*
Shields, C. G., 84, *358*
Simmens, S., 82, *357*
Simmons, D., 154, *362*

Simons, A. D., 82, 83, *358*
Simpson, R. L., 169, *365*
Singh, S. P., 146, *361*
Sivo, P. J., 320, *381*
Skiba, R. J., 166, *366*
Slater, E., 5, 229, *348, 373*
Slavich, S., 146, 148, *363*
Smit, J. H., 279, *379*
Smith, B. E., 186, 187, *367*
Smith, C. T., 27, *350*
Smith, G. R., 287, *377*
Smith, R. S., 75, *356*
Smith, S. S., 297, 298, 299, *380*
Smith, T. E., 83, *358*
Snow, M., 290, *378*
Snyder, H. N., 162, *363*
Sobell, L., 289, *378*
Sobell, M., 289, *378*
Solomon, A., 232, *373*
Sotsky, S. M., 82, *357*
Sowden, A., 80, *356*
Speilberg, W. E., 31, *350*
Sprague, J. R., 73, 163, 165, 166, 168, *356,*
    366
Stall, R., 289, 290, *378*
Stanley, M. A., 298, *379, 380*
Staples, R., 230, *373*
Stein, M. B., 297, 299, *380*
Steiner, H., 170, 171, *366*
Steiner, R., 187, *367*
Steinmetz, S. K., 14, *348*
Stevens, M., 182, *369*
Steward, D. K., 186, *367*
Stewart, K. B., 76, 277, 278, 281, *356, 379*
Stillman, D., *354*
Stoffelmayr, B. E., 153, *361*
Stone, L. A., 170, 171, *366*
Straus, M. A., 179, 185, *370*
Stroup-Benham, C., 246, *374*
Struble, V. E., 149, *362*
Strupp, H. H., 83, *357*
Studer, J., 166, 321, *366, 382*
Suarez, Z. E., 149, *362*
Sudia, C., 9, *348*
Sue, S., 263, *375*
Sugarman, D. B., 180, 183, *368*
Sullivan, W. P., 308, *381*
Sutton, S., 153, *360*
Svoboda, S., 6, 22, 24, *348, 351*
Switzer, G., 27, *349*
Symonds, B. D., 82, *357*

T

Tangri, S. S., 204, *371*
Tannenbaum, S., 303, 304, *380*
Tate, D., 172, *366*
Tatelbaum, R., 171, 320, *365, 382*
Tattersall, M. L., 154, *363*
Taussig, C., 321, *383*
Taylor, G., 27, *350*
Tech, N., 306, *380*
Theodore, H., 26, *349*
Thoenner, N., 179, *370*
Thompson, L. W., 302, *379*
Thornberry, T. P., 162, *366*
Tjaden, P., 179, *370*
Tompkins, E., 161, *364*
Toneatto, T., 289, *378*
Tonigan, J. S., 152, 153, 282, 283, *361, 376*
Toseland, R. W., 146, *362*
Trice, A. B., 290, *379*
Troyer, D., 27, *349*
Tussig, C., 172, *367*
Tyler, K. A., 301, *380*

U

Uba, L., 263, *375*
Unden, A.-L., 39, *352*
Usadel, H. C., 167, *366*

V

Vaillant, G. E., 301, *380*
van Balkou, A. J., 279, *379*
Van Wormer, K., 19, *350*
Velasquez, R. J., 253, *374*
Veneziano, C., 165, *366*
Veneziano, L., 156, *366*
Veyzer, A., 306, *379*
Videka-Sherman, L., 152, 155, *362, 363*

W

Wade, J. C., 26, *351*
Waern, M., 305, *380*
Waldo, C. R., 205, *371*
Waldo, M., 180, 181, 184, *370*
Waldorf, D., 290, *378*
Walitzer, K. S., 285, 286, *379*
Walker, H. M., 73, 163, 165, 166, 168, *356, 366*

Waller, M. A., 149, *363*
Wallis, H. A., 331, *383*
Wallis, M. A., 300, *381*
Walsh, D. C., 153, *363*
Walsh, M. R., 179, *370*
Walter, J. M., 69, *356*
Walton-Moss, B., 278, *376*
Wampold, B. E., 319, *382*
Warner, W., 75, *356*
Warren, C. S., 79, *358*
Warren, M. L., 146, 148, *363*
Watkins, J., 82, *357*
Watt, I. S., 80, *356*
Weibel, W., 289, *378*
Weick, A., 308, *381*
Weikart, D. P., 321, *382*
Weiss, W. D., 81, *358*
Weissberg, R. P., 320, *381*
Werner, E., 74, *356*
Werner-Wilson, R. J., 84, *358*
West, M., 27, *349*
Wetzel, R. D., 82, 83, *358*
Wetzstein, C., 52, *354*
Whaley, A. L., 68, 233, *356, 373*
Whelan, J. P., 70, *355*
Widom, C. S., 170, 185, *367, 370*
Wiederholt, I. C., 180, *370*
Wilke, D., 69, *356*
Wilkins-Haug, L., 282, *376*
Willander, A., 289, *376*
Williams, K. R., 169, *364*
Williams, O. J., 236, *372*
Williams, T., 166, *366*
Wilson, J. Q., 24, 29, *351*
Winick, C., 290, *379*
Wituk, S., 146, 148, *363*
Wolfgang, M. E., 6, 161, *349, 367*
Wolf-Smith, J. H., 184, *370*
Wolwer ,W., 289, *376*
Woodford, J., 105, *359*
Woody, G. E., 82, *358*
Woolgar, M., 28,
Worell, J., 24, *351*
Wuthnow, R., 147, *363*

Y

Yacovene, D., 18, *351*
Yang, J., 193, 194, *370*
Yoshikawa, T. T., 34, *353,* 276, *378*
Yoshioka, M., 83, *358*

Young, C., 53, *354*
Young, K., 55, *354*

Z

Zakocs, R. C., 276, *377*
Zaslow, M. J., 29, *351*
Zhao, S., 146, 152, *361*

Zigler, E., 172, 321, *367, 383*
Zill, N., 9, *348*
Zimmerman, T. S., 84, *358*
Zimostrad, N., 179, *368*
Zinger, I., 172, *363*
Zolondek, S. C., 163, *367*
Zoppel, C. L., 83, *357*
Zuniga, M. E., 133, 134, 252, *360, 374*

Subject Index

A

Abandonment, 9–10, 107–108, 324, 331, 333
Abuse (*see* Alcohol abuse *and* Child abuse
    and Sexual abuse *and* Spousal
    abuse)
African American
    community, 5
    men, 230–236
    women, 6
    youth, 163
Aggression, 12, 17, 39, 73–74, 166,
    168–169, 175, 180–182, 320–322
    sexual, 50, 58, 192–194
    among Spanish speaking groups, 248
Aggression Replacement Training (ART),
    173
Alcohol abuse, (*see also* Drinking), 34, 142,
    152–154, 156–158, 275–295
    in females, 279–280
    long-term treatments of, 286–287
    natural recovery, 289–291
    related medical problems, 281–282
    short-term treatment of, 282–286
    treatment strategies, 287–289
Alcohol Alert, 275
Alcoholics Anonymous, 152–153, 284
Anger, 19, 53, 74, 190, 216–217, 221, 225,
    235, 253, 307–309
    at women, 193–196
Anger management, 166, 172–173, 185,
    195–196, 321
Anxiety, 36, 39, 43, 50, 105, 117, 119, 153,
    287

    in Asian men, 260
    in Latino men, 250
    in older males, 297–298
        treating, 298–300
    performance, 47
Asian men
    as collective self, 260, 266–267
    understanding the elements of,
        261–263
    and treatment, 263–264
        reasons for seeking, 267–268
    unique treatment situations, 264–267
Assertive behavior, 13, 55, 180
Assertiveness training, 166–167, 195,
    321–322
Attention-deficit disorder (ADD), 12
Attention Deficit Hyperactivity Disorder
    (ADHD), 69

B

Behavioral difficulties, 38–39
Behavior(s)
    abusive, 110–111
    antisocial, 75
    at risk, 42, 320
    men's patterns of, 140
    that negatively affect health, 40–41
    positive aspects of, 316–317
    violent, 73–74
Bereavement, 27, 130, 155, 270, 296,
    303–304
Bibliotherapy, 136–140
Black family structure, 231

Black men
    and (their) fathers, 239–244
    and homicide, 229
    imprisoned, 5, 229
    level of education, 229–230
    and employment, 230–231
    treatment issues and, 232–238
Boys
    abandoned, 9
    coping with aggression, 321–322
    destructive effects on, 316
    male difficulties placed on, 12
    natural assertiveness of, 13
    school performance of, 7
    in young adult fiction, 316
Brain (see Male brain physiology)
Bridges of Madison County, 137

C

CAGE questionnaire, 76, 277–278
Cancer, 35–37
Child abuse, xii, 73, 166, 170–171, 247
Child-support, 8–10
Coaching (see Personal coaching)
Cobras, 182–185
Compensatory masculinity, 17, 39–40, 49
Competitiveness, 16, 20
Conflict
    mediation, 167
    resolution, 188, 221, 320–321
Crime, 179
    Black mens involvement in, 229
    juvenile, 161–162
    Latino mens involvement in, 245–246
    overstressing, 14

D

Death
    camps, 306
    causes of (men), 33
    premature, 40, 56
    rates (of men), 5, 33–35
    by violence, 15, 38
Depression, 44
    alcohol-related, 156–158
    in older males, 296–297, 300–301
        treating, 301–311
Developmental model for work with men,
    113

Diagnosing male clients (see also
    Misdiagnosis)
    concerns about, 67–70
    reducing errors in, 70–71
Diagnostic and Statistical Manual of Mental
        Disorders (DSM), 67–68
    criticism of, 67–68
Dichos, 139, 252–253
Divorce, 8–9, 31, 130–131
    among Blacks, 231–232, 238
    declining, 54
Domestic violence, 3, 7, 13, 43, 56–58, 163,
        178–179, 186–188, 247
Drinking, 49–50, 156, 276–277
DWI, 3, 35, 156, 223, 276
Dysfunctional
    behavior, 12
    family, 165, 271–272

E

Educational underperformance, 315–316
Emotional
    danger, 260–261
    expression, 17
    indicators of at risk behavior, 42
    needs, 80
    problems, 155–156, 344–345
    of older patients, 303
Emotions
    internalizing, 33
Evidence-based practice (EBP), 72
Explosive disorders, 183

F

Facilitation, 220
Family
    Asian, 261–267
    Black, 231, 326
    deterioration in, 8–9, 305
    expulsion, 270–271
    identity, 260–261
    illnesses, 50
    Latino, 247–248
    origin, 70, 89
    pathology, 117
    treatment, 84
    violence, 150, 170, 179–180, 331, 345
Family-oriented culture, 139

Fathering roles, 30
Father(s)
    abandonment by, 17
    absent, 8–10, 106–110, 322
    Black men and their, 239–244
    competent, 58
    issues with, 141–143
    loss of, 333
    roles of, 53–55
Feminine mystique, 25
Feminist
    attitude, 53
    literature, 55–56
    movement, 331
FRAMES, 283

G

Gangs, 17
Gay men, 339–340, 343–344
    Latino, 138–139
Gender
    issues, 4, 323
    misdiagnosis, 69
    stereotyping, 346
Gender role strain, 30–32
Gossip, 264–265
Grief, 10, 109, 155, 238, 270, 282, 302, 304, 308
Group therapy (*see* Men's groups)

H

Health problems (*see* Male health problems)
Higher education
    of men, 6–7
    of women, 6
Hispanic men, 245
Homelessness, 10–12
Homicide, 33, 49
    among Blacks, 163, 229
    of spouses, 14
    by coworkers, 212–214, 217
    of young males in the U.S., 6, 162
Homophobia, 62, 316, 343–344
Honeymoon period, 181
Humor, 134–136

I

Ideal mate, 111–112

Impotence, 47–48
Incarceration, 168, 173, 187–188, 244
Interventions, 168–171, 189, 215, 234, 239, 253, 261, 264–265, 271
    with alcohol abusers, 282–287, 291–295, 320
    early, 172–173
    in the workplace, 218

J

Juvenile
    arrests, 12
    crime, 6, 161–170
    violence, 22

L

Labeling men, 71–72, 117–118
Latino men, 245
    attitudes toward psychotherapy, 249–250
    cultural issues, 254–258
    areas of difficulty, 245–246
    and feelings, 253–254
    and treatment, 248–250
    treatment suggestions with, 251–252
Levi, Primo, 304–306
Life expectancy, 38
Loss, 101, 238, 267, 270, 296–297, 304
    of father, 333
    fear of, 98
    of trust, 180

M

Machismo, 246–247
Male
    bashing, 52–57, 330–331, 340–341
        responding to, 61–63, 316–317
        themes, 60–61
    brain physiology, 12
    code of conduct, 16
    development, 18–23
        genetic factors in, 27–30
    difficulties
        evidence of, 5–7
    educational underperformance, 315–316
    health problems, 34–37, 49–50

avoidable reasons for, 38–43
insensitivity, 60
sexual inadequacy, 61
socialization, 23–27, 99, 113–116
    positive aspects of, 316–317
    understanding the aspects of,
        102–103
stereotypes, 57–60, 116–117
    of gay men, 139
stupidity, 60
therapy
    developmental state of, 4
Masculinity (*see also* Compensatory
    masculinity)
    cultural perceptions of, 18
    discourse surrounding, 316
    traditional notions of, 49, 103–104
    validation of, 25, 30
Medical problems, 154, 279, 301
    alcohol related, 287
    as symptoms of anxiety, 298
Men (*see also* Asian men *and* Black men
    and Latino men)
    dysfunctional, 110
    as natural helpers, 150–152
    portrayal of in commercials, 53–55
    traditional, 30
Men's groups, 140–143
Mid-life crisis, 44–47
Misandry, 55
Misdiagnosis, 68–71, 75–78
    negative consequences of, 72–73
Mothers
    abuse by, 210
    moods of, 28
    resolving issues related to, 106–107
    single, 333, 337

N

Narcissistic Personality Disorder (NPS), 69
Narcotics Anonymous, 153
Nurturance, 30, 141

O

Ombudsmen, 219

P

Patient-therapist relationship, 79

Peer review, 220
Personal coaching, 127–131
Pit Bulls, 182–185
Poetry, 137–138
Political correctness, 4, 15, 67
Posttraumatic stress disorder (PTSD), 189,
    331, 334
Primary issues of therapy with men,
    106–112
Problem-solving, 102, 104, 119, 166–168,
    172, 188, 284, 320–321
Pseudo-transference, 69
Psychotherapy
    anti-male attitudes in, 57
    defined, 80
    effectiveness of, 79, 152, 342
    Latino men's attitude toward, 249–250
    mens' avoidance of, 38
    poor outcome, 83
    traditional notions of, 99–100, 194

R

Racism, 68–69, 71, 229, 231–237, 266
Rape, 7, 13–14, 138, 194, 197–200
    alcohol and drugs in, 192
    in feminist literature, 55–56
Rapists, 194
Research, 317–318
Resilience, 75
Resistence to therapy, 99–100
Respect, 3, 83, 99, 116, 125, 216, 233, 238,
    251
Risk-taking, 33, 41, 281, 339
Ritalin, 12–13
Role playing, 143–145

S

Self-awareness, 99–100, 185
Self-destructive behavior, 3, 41, 110, 124,
    271, 338, 341
Self-help groups, 141, 156–158
    defining, 146–149
    effectiveness of, 152
    indigenous leaders of, 149–150
Self-restraint, 262
Self-righting capabilities, 74
Sexual
    abuse, 58, 74, 170, 191–200

aggression, 50, 58
assault, 192–193
harassment, 3–4, 15, 42, 56, 59
inadequacy, 60–61
offenses, 164–165
perpetrators, 193–197
problems, 47–48
violence, 163–164
Sexuality, 25–26, 195, 343
Sexually transmitted diseases (STDs), 5, 37, 41
Social programs, 320–322
Sports, 16
Spousal abuse, 179–180
dynamics of, 180–182
predicting potential for, 182–185
treating, 185–191
Spreading Misandry: The Teaching of Contempt for Men in Popular Culture
Stalking, 183, 192–193, 211
Stereotypes (see also Male stereotypes)
cultural, 69
gender, 302, 343
Latino, 246
racial, 237
Storytelling, 131–133
Strength(s)
focusing on, 124–125
Stress, 32, 118, 129–131, 213–214
gender, 105
internalized, 49
Stress-related diseases, 34
Substance abuse, 49, 77, 152–154, 183–184, 275
diagnostic markers of, 277–282
Suicide, 35, 44, 304–306
Symptoms
of anxiety, 296–298, 311
checklist of, 69
of mental illness, 255
paranoid, 233
of withdrawal, 283

T

Therapeutic relationships, 80–81
attentiveness in, 88
empathy in, 82
evidence-based practice, 88–89
and gender, 83–86
humility in, 90
importance of (with male clients), 82–83
independent client solutions, 89–90
opinions in, 90
rapport in, 87–88
Therapeutic metaphors, 133–134
Therapists
effective, 81
female, 76, 83–86, 117
gender-sensitive, 101
mistreatment by, 100
shopping around for, 79–80
Therapy
culture of, 104
description of (for men), 118
guidelines for work with men, 113–126
men's view of, 102–106
men's primary issues in (see Primary issues of therapy with men)
as problem-solving, 118–119
Transference, 91–92, 94–98
Treatment
of alcoholism (long-term), 286–287
of alcoholism (short-term), 282–286
of anxiety in older men, 298–300
of Asian men, 263–264
attrition, 4
collaboration in, 113–114
for conduct disorder, 174–177
depression in older males, 301–311
effectiveness, 80–81
men's unwillingness to seek, 100–102
new approaches to, 318–319
of sexual perpetrators, 194–197
for violence, 172–174
Treatment of Child Abuse, 170
Trust, 121–123
Type A behavior, 39–40

U

Unemployment, 10–12, 41, 79, 165, 229, 235

V

Value system, 110

Viagra, 48
Victimization, 163
Violence (see also Domestic violence and
    Sexual violence)
    in boys, 13, 73, 161–165
    and compensatory masculinity, 17
    data, 13–15
    early onset, 73, 163
        predictors of, 165–166

    treating, 166–171
    physical, 7
    prevention, 171–174
    in the workplace, 3

W

Wolpe, Paul R., 13
Woman Can't Hear What Men Don't, 53